BRADY

Medical Assistant Test Review Programmed Learner

Bonnie Fremgen, PhD
Kathleen Wallington, CMA
Mary King-Lesniewski, CMA

BRADY
Prentice Hall
Upper Saddle River, New Jersey 07458

Library of Congress Cataloging-in-Publication Data

Fremgen, Bonnie F.
   Medical assistant test review programmed learner / Bonnie Fremgen,
Kathleen Wallington, Mary King-Lesniewski.
      p.   cm
   Includes bibliographical references.
   ISBN 0-8359-5137-5 (alk. paper)
   1. Medical assistants—Examinations, questions, etc.   2. Medical
assistants—Programmed instruction.   I. Wallington, Kathleen.
II. King-Lesniewski, Mary, 1963-   III. Title.
   [DNLM: 1. Physician Assistants programmed instruction.
2. Physician Assistants examination questions.   W 18.2F869m 1999]
R728.8.F726   1999
610.73'7'076—dc21

DNLM/DLC
for Library of Congress   98-38632
                                                               CIP

PUBLISHER: Susan Katz
ACQUISITIONS EDITOR: Barbara Krawiec
MANAGING PRODUCTION EDITOR: Patrick Walsh
PRODUCTION EDITOR: Navta Associates
DIRECTOR OF MANUFACTURING & PRODUCTION:
   Bruce Johnson
SENIOR PRODUCTION MANAGER: Ilene Sanford
MARKETING MANAGER: Tiffany Price
MARKETING COORDINATOR: Cindy Frederick
EDITORIAL ASSISTANT: Stephanie Camangian
COVER DESIGN: Paul Gourhan
INTERIOR DESIGN: Barbara J. Barg
PRINTING AND BINDING: Banta Harrisonburg

© 1999 by Prentice-Hall, Inc.
A Simon & Schuster Company
Upper Saddle River, New Jersey 07458

Printed in the United States of America
10 9 8 7 6 5 4 3 2 1

ISBN 0-8359-5137-5

PRENTICE HALL INTERNATIONAL (UK) LIMITED, *London*
PRENTICE HALL OF AUSTRALIA PTY. LIMITED, *Sydney*
PRENTICE HALL CANADA INC., *Toronto*
PRENTICE HALL HISPANOAMERICANA, S.A., *Mexico*
PRENTICE HALL OF INDIA PRIVATE LIMITED, *New Delhi*
PRENTICE HALL OF JAPAN, INC., *Tokyo*
SIMON & SCHUSTER ASIA PTE. LTD., *Singapore*
EDITORA PRENTICE HALL DO BRASIL, LTDA., *Rio de Janeiro*

Dedication

The authors gratefully dedicate this book to their families.

CONTENTS

PREFACE

The purpose of this book, *Medical Assistant Test Review Programmed Learner,* is fourfold:

1. To assist the medical assistant student to prepare for either the Certified Medical Assistant (CMA) examination, offered by the American Association of Medical Assistants (AAMA), or the Registered Medical Assistant (RMA) examination, sponsored by the American Medical Technologists (AMT).
2. To facilitate learning with a programmed instruction method that moves the student through material covered in certified medical assistant programs.
3. To offer study hints and tips to assist the student in performing well on a timed examination.
4. To offer a wide range of examination questions that provide the student with experience in taking a timed examination (both pre-test and post-test examination questions are provided).

The material covered in this textbook mirrors the course material taught throughout the United States in certified medical assistant programs. Therefore, no matter which state you reside in, this textbook can be used to review for the CMA or RMA exam.

However, this book is not intended to replace work experience or a comprehensive medical assistant textbook. The student should use this test preparation book diligently as an additional source of study and review material.

The CMA/RMA Exam

The Certified Medical Assistant (CMA) examination is offered twice a year, on the last Friday in January and the last Friday in June. There are numerous test locations throughout the United States. The examination is based on the process for developing a curriculum (DACUM), which was developed by the American Association of Medical Assistants in 1979. DACUM was based on the skills performed daily by medical assistants. In 1997, the DACUM list was revised to reflect major changes in medicine and the health care delivery system. The revision is called the Role Delineation Study. Information on taking the CMA certification/recertification examination can be obtained by calling 1-800-228-2262 or writing:

AAMA Certifying Board
20 North Wacker Drive
Chicago, IL 60606-2903

The Registered Medical Assistant (RMA) examination is offered by the American Medical Technologists (AMT) three times a year: the second Saturday of March, June, and November. There are numerous test locations throughout the United States. The RMA examination is based on the material covered in the *Registered Medical Assistant Competency Areas Outline.* A candidate handbook for the RMA examination can be obtained by calling 1-800-275-1268 or writing:

Registered Medical Assistants of the American Medical Technologists
710 Higgins Road
Park Ridge, IL 60068-5765

How to Use This Programmed Instruction Book

Programmed instruction is a time-proven method for learning. It is based on the premise that topics already mastered will assist the student in learning new material. In most test questions, all the answers will provide valuable information that answers either that particular question or future questions.

The answer for each question is provided directly at the end of the question. The student should cover all the answers with a folded sheet of paper as he or she reads through the question. Then the answer should be read, as well as all the explanations for the other four answers.

For example: The word root ileum means

- **(A)** hipbone
- **(B)** thigh bone
- **(C)** large intestine
- **(D)** small intestine
- **(E)** groin area

(D) is correct. The word root ileum means a portion of the small intestine.
(A) The word root for hipbone is ilium.
(B) The word root/combining form for thigh bone is femor/o.
(C) The word root/combining form for large intestine or colon is col/o.
(E) The word root/combining form for groin or inguinal area is inguin/o.

If, after answering this question, the student is still confused about the difference between ileum and ilium, then a check mark should be placed next to these terms for further review. In addition, the terms for thigh bone, large intestine, and groin area have been reviewed in this question. Some of the terms will appear again in later questions to reinforce learning.

If the student has difficulty understanding the material in any one of the five answer options, then that material should be examined with further study. *Essentials of Medical Assisting* by Bonnie Fremgen can be used as a reference for further study. The student should also use any other reference material that he or she has, such as lecture notes and textbooks.

Ideally, at the end of each chapter, the student should review and understand every incorrect answer before going on to the next chapter. In this manner, material will be mastered in manageable segments rather than by trying to go back later over incorrect answers.

The book is divided into chapters that relate to the subject matter taught in certified medical assistant programs. In addition, a pre-test of 150 multiple-choice questions is included at the beginning of the book. There are 50 general, 50 administrative, and 50 clinical questions on this pre-test. The student can use this as a simulation of an actual exam by taking the exam in a 2-hour time frame.

A 300-question comprehensive examination is included at the end of this review book. This post-test should be timed by the student to simulate the actual 4-hour examination. This is also broken into three components: 100 general questions, 100 administrative questions, and 100 clinical questions.

References

Fremgen, Bonnie. *Essentials of Medical Assisting.* Upper Saddle River, NJ: Brady/Prentice Hall, 1998.

Fremgen, Bonnie. *Medical Terminology.* Upper Saddle River, NJ: Brady/Prentice Hall, 1997.

Taber's Cyclopedic Medical Dictionary. 18th edition. Philadelphia: F.A. Davis Company, 1997.

Acknowledgments

The following reviewers provided valuable feedback during the writing process. We thank all these professionals for their contribution and attention to detail.

Lynn Augenstern, MA, CMA
Program Director, Medical Assisting
Ridley-Lowell Business and Technical Institute
Binghamton, New York

Sherry Boutin
Hartford Hospital
Morse School of Business
Hartford, Connecticut

Michelle A. Green, MPS, RRA, CMA
Alfred State College
Alfred, New York

Leila Kissick, CMA, RN, BSN
Former Instructor, Medical Assisting Program
Northwest Kansas Technical School
Goodland, Kansas

Cris McTighe, CMA, RMA
Medical Assisting Program Director
San Leandro, California

Marilyn Pooler, RN, CMA-C, MEd
Professor of Medical Assisting
Springfield Technical Community College
Springfield, Massachusetts

Lori Reddington, BA, CMA, CPT
Chair, Medical Assisting Program
Southern Ohio College
Cincinnati, Ohio

Kathleen Tozzi, CLPN/RMA
Director of Education
Cleveland Dental-Medical Assistant, Inc.
Mentor, OH

INTRODUCTION

Test-Taking Strategies

Since this examination is the culmination of many hours of hard work and study in a certified medical assistant program, the student should do everything possible to pass on the first attempt. The following study methods and tips may help.

Study Methods

Every student will develop a slightly different study method. The actual time of day spent in study, the location for study, and the presence of other people during study time may not be important. What is important is that the student MUST establish the discipline of continual study and preparation for this examination.

The most frequently heard complaint from students relates to the inability to find time to study. A plan of study, ideally established at least 3 months before the examination, should be placed in writing by the student. For example, the student may only have 2 hours a day between the hours of 8:00 PM and 10:00 PM every night. But these hours must be adhered to, without taking time out for television or social gatherings. During the final 4 weeks before the examination, the hours should be increased.

Key Advice: Set out a study schedule and do not vary—try to add an extra hour or two of study as the exam date nears.

Never go anywhere without a bag of notes, review book, and/or textbook for study whenever you find a few minutes while waiting for transportation, for children, or in dental and doctor waiting rooms.

Try to eliminate all distractions. While this is difficult to do in a busy household or a busy library, it is possible. Set up another study space if TV, noise, and children interrupt study. Many students find it a good investment to hire a baby-sitter while he or she goes to a quiet library to study.

Study past quizzes and tests from your medical assistant program. Some students take the time to rewrite all their notes; this is not always considered to be a good use of time. It is better to use the notes along with the textbook, and add any other important facts that were not included in the notes. The lecture notes are a good place to start the study process. The student should move quickly through the notes and quizzes and on to a formal examination review book.

If time allows, write your own multiple-choice questions and also use these to study. Break test preparation into small bites. Never try to learn an entire chapter of material at one time.

Note Taking

Twenty-five to 30 percent of your time should be spent learning the material, and the remaining 70 to 75 percent of the time drilling on the facts. Reading material over and over has not been found to be a particularly effective means of learning and retaining material. Therefore, note taking becomes an important skill.

During the study period, it is wise to take notes on any material that is new or needs reinforcement. Do not expect to remember everything the first time you read it. Important numbers—such as the ranges of normal for vital signs, normal hematology values, and microscope settings—should be summarized in brief notes. Many students find that index cards are useful when taking study notes. These cards come in a wide range of colors and sizes. Different colors can be used for separate topics: yellow for vital signs and measurements; red or pink for hematology ranges; blue for medical terms; and white for administrative functions. Flash cards that contain a medical term on one side and the answer on the other side are extremely useful.

Some students dictate their notes into a recording device and then play back these important facts while they drive or take public transportation.

You may develop "tricks" to aid in memorizing long lists, such as the sequence On Old Olympus's Towering Top A Fin And German Viewed Some Hops to aid in remembering the 12 cranial nerves:

1. On—Olfactory
2. Old—Optic
3. Olympus's—Oculomotor
4. Towering—Trochlear
5. Top—Trigeminal
6. A—Abducens
7. Fin—Facial
8. And—Acoustic
9. German—Glossopharyngeal
10. Viewed —Vagus
11. Some—Spinal Accessory
12. Hops—Hypoglossal

Using the alphabet (ABC) has helped us to remember A—Airway, B—Breathing, C—Circulation.

When studying, be sure to tackle all the difficult areas first; then study the areas you are comfortable with. An effective method of taking notes when reading a textbook is to use the same headings the author did. The author believed the heading topics were important enough to highlight them by placing them as headings.

Highlighter pens are not always effective when used to highlight almost every word. Use them sparingly to bring attention to critical points or figures.

When using a textbook to study, jot the key words in the margin next to the material you are studying. To do a quick final review, just review the key words.

Set a timer when studying. Know that when 20 minutes are up, you should have completed reviewing a certain section. This will force you to concentrate on what you are reading and reviewing.

Don't wait until the night before to study material for the first time. Keep a list of key words or concepts; review them just before going to sleep the night before the exam.

Practice timing yourself by using the final comprehensive exam at the end of this book.

The Day Before the Examination

Have clear directions on how to find the location and room. If you have never been to the exam location before, it is wise to visit it beforehand, if possible.

Assemble all the material you MUST have to enter the examination:

1. Registration card
2. Picture ID
3. Three number 2 pencils (a pair and a spare) with good erasers

You are not allowed to bring any calculators or food into the examination room. Be sure to get a good night's sleep. The student should NOT spend all night cramming for this long examination. Careless mistakes are made when the test-taker is suffering from a lack of sleep.

The Actual Exam

You should arrive at the room site at least 15 to 20 minutes early. No personal items, such as books and papers, can be taken into the room with you. It is wise to visit the rest room before entering the examination room. However, you will be allowed to use the rest room, if necessary, during the examination. You must hand your test to the proctor if you have to leave the room.

The proctor will give some preliminary instructions, and tell you when you can open the exam and begin. The proctor will also announce a 30-minute and 10-minute warning before the end of the exam. You will not be allowed to take longer than the allotted 4 hours. If you finish before the 4 hours are up, you can hand your paper to the proctor and leave.

A frequent omission on the answer sheet is the student's name. In addition to placing your name and Social Security number in the bubble spaces, you must also print your name in the correct space.

Be sure to check that all the bubble spaces are filled in on your answer sheet before turning it in. Follow these steps:

1. Pace yourself. Place your wristwatch on the desk and pace yourself throughout the exam. In order to complete all 300 questions within a 4-hour (240-minute) time frame, you will have to take less than 1 minute per question.

2. Read the questions and directions very carefully. Don't jump at what appears to be the right answer without reading ALL the answers first.

3. Work as rapidly as possible, with accuracy. Always double-check to make sure that you are placing your answer in the correct bubble on the answer sheet. It is wise to check for this at least at every fifth question.

4. If a question stumps you completely, skip it and come back to it later. Place a line next to it on the answer sheet. Avoid skipping too many items.

5. If you do not know the answer to a question after skipping over it once, then guess at the answer. You have something to gain by guessing since the test is based on the number of correct answers only. If you leave a question blank, you have no chance of receiving any credit for that question. In addition, the blank bubble space may confuse you and get you off-course in answering the other questions.

6. Select the one BEST answer.

7. Do not rely on flaws in the test construction. For example, don't predetermine that the longest or shortest answer is always correct. Do not look for trends in the answers, such as so many C responses in a row. Answers occur in a random pattern.

8. Read the question as it is stated, not as you would like it to be stated.

9. Note key words in the question, such as "always," "never," "rarely," "most important," and "first."

10. Do not stare blankly at the question if you have no idea about the correct answer. Precious time is lost puzzling over the difficult questions. Always focus on what you are doing. Either move on to the next question or take an educated guess at the answer.

11. Many test-takers believe that your first response to a multiple-choice question is the best. However, if you really believe you have made a mistake, then thoroughly erase the first answer and change it.

12. Be careful not to turn over two pages of the exam at once. Double-check that you are placing the answer next to the correct number on the answer sheet.

13. Remember that the right answer is ALWAYS one of the five options. Don't try to second-guess the test and worry about an option that wasn't given.

14. Concentrate intensely. If you find your mind wandering, then stop briefly and regroup. Do not worry about what anyone else in the exam room is doing.

15. Eliminate the incorrect answers first. This will narrow the answers down to one or two options.

16. You may wish to use your finger as a pointer on difficult questions to make sure you haven't missed a word.

17. Everybody takes tests at their own speed. Don't pace yourself based on what others are doing.

18. Read quickly through the entire examination before answering the first question. Many times, a later question will help you answer an earlier one.

19. Do not look for tricks in examination questions. Examinations are meant to be a determination of your knowledge of the subject.

20. One of the most common errors is to misread the exam question. Try to read the question twice before answering it.

21. Always review the entire test before handing it in. Double-check that the correct bubbles are filled in next to the right number.

Good luck!

Pre-Test Simulation

(150-question, 2-hour pre-test)

GENERAL

(Covers medical terminology; anatomy and physiology; medical science and type of medical practice; medical law and ethics; quality assurance and government regulations; and human relations and psychology.)

Directions: Select the ONE best answer for each of the following multiple-choice questions.

1. The word root is

   (A) an acronym for a word
   (B) an abbreviation for a word
   ✓**(C)** the foundation for a word
   (D) able to stand alone as a medical term
   (E) a synonym

2. Medical ethics is

   (A) courtesy physicians extend to one another
   (B) an authorization to practice one's profession
   (C) a form of contract that must be honored by law
   ✓**(D)** moral conduct based on principles regulating the behavior of health care professionals
   (E) the regulations and standards set up by federal, state, and local governments to direct the medical treatment of patients

3. The major categories of tissue are

   (A) striated, smooth, and cardiac
   (B) voluntary and involuntary
   ✓**(C)** muscle, epithelial, connective, and nerve
   (D) bones, tendons, and fatty
   (E) sagittal, frontal, and transverse

4. A person who represents or acts on behalf of another person is called a/an

   (A) expert witness   **(D)** minor
   (B) appellant   ✓**(E)** agent
   (C) defendant

5. The filtration of waste products takes place in the

   (A) ureters   **(D)** bladder
   ✓**(B)** nephrons   **(E)** meatus
   (C) urethra

6. The 19th-century surgeon who introduced the antiseptic system in surgery was

✓**(A)** Lister
(B) Pasteur
(C) Semmelweiss
(D) Koch
(E) Roentgen

7. The word root ileum means

(A) hipbone
(B) thigh bone
(C) large intestine
✓**(D)** small intestine
(E) groin area

8. The doctrine that applies to the law of negligence, which means "The thing speaks for itself," is

(A) *respondeat superior*
✓**(B)** *res ipsa loquitur*
(C) standard of care
(D) informed consent
(E) statute of limitations

9. To protect the physician from legal claims when a patient is angry, the medical assistant should

(A) tell the patient to keep his or her voice down
(B) interrupt the patient and ask him or her to return to the office when calm
(C) do what the patient is asking
✓**(D)** document the incident on the medical record and complete an incident report
(E) all of the above

10. A lengthwise body plane running from side to side is the

(A) frontal plane
(B) coronal plane
(C) horizontal plane
✓**(D)** sagittal plane
(E) transverse plane

11. A New York City physician who founded a school for training persons to work in the medical office is

(A) Läennec
(B) Hahnemann
✓**(C)** Mandl
(D) Domagk
(E) Curie

12. Performing surgery on a patient without the proper informed consent of the patient is an example of

(A) intentional tort
(B) battery
(C) assault
✓**(D)** A and B
(E) A and C

13. The prefix meaning bad is

(A) medi-
✓**(B)** mal-
(C) meso-
(D) medi-
(E) macro-

14. What law requires a full disclosure concerning the payment of any fee that will be collected in more than four installments and is also referred to as Regulation Z of the Consumer Protection Act?

✓**(A)** Truth in Lending Act of 1969
  (B) Fair Credit Reporting Act of 1971
  (C) Fair Debt Collection Practice Act of 1978
  (D) Equal Credit Opportunity Act of 1975
  (E) none of the above

15. A person under the age of 18 who is free of parental care and is financially responsible is an example of a/an

  (A) mature minor
  (B) minor
✓**(C)** emancipated minor
  (D) guardian *ad litum*
  (E) appellant

16. The suffix -rrhage means

  (A) to stitch or suture
  (B) discharge
✓**(C)** excessive, abnormal flow
  (D) to rupture
  (E) drooping

17. The Latin phrase that means the physician as employer is responsible for the action of the employee is

  (A) *res ipsa loquitur*
✓**(B)** *respondeat superior*
  (C) subpoena *duces tecum*
  (D) proximate cause
  (E) guardian *ad litum*

18. The state regulations that direct the practice of medicine in that state are known as the

  (A) Hippocratic oath
  (B) Code of Hammurabi
✓**(C)** Medical Practice Act
  (D) United States Medical Licensing Examination
  (E) National Board Medical Examination

19. To move toward the median or midline of the body is called

✓**(A)** adduction
  (B) abduction
  (C) lateral
  (D) inversion
  (E) eversion

20. The person best known for the study of death and dying is

  (A) Dr. Benjamin Spock
✓**(B)** Dr. Elisabeth Kübler-Ross
  (C) Dr. Jonas Salk
  (D) Abraham Maslow
  (E) Dr. Sigmund Freud

21. A word ending in -a will change to the plural by

  (A) changing -a to -ata
  (B) changing -a to -um
  (C) adding an -es
✓**(D)** keeping the -a and adding -e
  (E) none of the above

22. Defamation of character, which occurs when a defaming statement is spoken, is called

    (A) a deposition
    (B) libel
    ✓**(C)** slander

    (D) consent
    (E) abandonment

23. The rule for word building is

    (A) start at the beginning of the word and translate each component
    (B) memorize the definition of each medical term
    ✓**(C)** read the term from the end of the word (or the suffix) back to the beginning (prefix) and then pick up the word root
    (D) there are no hard-and-fast rules when building medical terms
    (E) none of the above

24. When a patient's medical record has been subpoenaed, the patient should be notified by

    (A) telephone, as soon as possible
    (B) registered mail
    (C) next-day mail

    ✓**(D)** certified mail
    (E) in person

25. The suffix -stalsis means

    (A) twitch
    (B) to visualize
    (C) the study of

    (D) surgical removal
    ✓**(E)** constriction

26. A mental disorder that is characterized by delusions and hallucinations is

    (A) dissociative disorder
    (B) cognitive disorder
    (C) anxiety disorder

    ✓**(D)** schizophrenia
    (E) personality disorder

27. Which of the following organs and structures is/are NOT found in the endocrine system?

    (A) pineal
    (B) ovaries
    (C) thymus

    (D) testes
    ✓**(E)** spleen

28. Ankyl/o is the word root/combining form meaning

    (A) cartilage
    (B) joint
    (C) digit

    ✓**(D)** stiff joint
    (E) rib

29. The time period during which a patient has the right to file a suit against a physician is known as the

    ✓**(A)** statute of limitations
    (B) rule of discovery
    (C) *res ipsa loquitur*

    (D) *respondeat superior*
    (E) precedent

30. A jejunoileostomy is the

   (A) surgical creation of a gastric fistula or opening through the abdominal wall
   (B) surgical removal of part or the whole of the stomach
   (C) surgical removal of the colon
   ✓**(D)** surgical creation of an opening between the jejunum and the ileum
   (E) surgical removal of a lobe of the lung

31. A program in which hospitals and medical practices evaluate the services they provide by comparing their services with accepted standards is known as a

   (A) peer review organization   **(D)** CPR
   ✓**(B)** quality assurance program   **(E)** all of the above
   (C) standard of care

32. Tars/o is the word root/combining form for

   ✓**(A)** foot   **(D)** chest
   (B) tendon   **(E)** tibia
   (C) stretch

33. Examples of psychoses are

   (A) hysteria and hypochondriasis
   (B) anxiety, obsessions, and compulsions
   (C) delusions, depression, and a manic-depressive state
   (D) hallucinations and schizophrenia
   ✓**(E)** C and D

34. One who specializes in disorders of the gastrointestinal tract is a/an

   (A) urologist   ✓**(D)** proctologist
   (B) gynecologist   **(E)** endocrinologist
   (C) neurologist

35. Another name for an otorhinolaryngologist is a/an

   (A) throat specialist   **(D)** oncologist
   ✓**(B)** ENT   **(E)** orthopedist
   (C) ophthalmologist

36. Hard or horny is the word root/combining form

   (A) host/o   ✓**(D)** kerat/o
   (B) hidr/o   **(E)** cutane/o
   (C) lip/o

37. The number of individual cases of a disease within a defined population is known as the

   (A) mortality rate   **(D)** primary care
   ✓**(B)** morbidity rate   **(E)** terminally ill
   (C) DRG

38. The cheekbones are

    (A) mandibular bones   ✓(D) zygomatic bones
    (B) maxillary bones   (E) lacrimal bones
    (C) palatine bones

39. The federal agency that has the power to enforce regulations concerning the health and safety of employees is the

    (A) FDA
    (B) Department of Health and Human Safety
   ✓(C) OSHA
    (D) CLIA
    (E) none of the above

40. The dermis layer of the skin contains

    (A) keratin   ✓(D) blood vessels
    (B) melanin   (E) basal layer
    (C) stratified squamous epithelium

41. CLIA 88 divides laboratories into how many categories?

    (A) 2   (D) 5
   ✓(B) 3   (E) 6
    (C) 4

42. The word root/combining form meaning sugar is

    (A) gonad/o   (D) crin/o
    (B) gluc/o   ✓(E) B and C
    (C) glyc/o

43. The Fair Debt Collection Practices Act is a federal law that

    (A) mandates the collection of blood
    (B) regulates the wearing of PPE
    (C) controls the administration of controlled substances
   ✓(D) protects debtors from harassment
    (E) none of the above

44. Small laboratories that are located in physicians' offices and conduct routine diagnostic tests are referred to as

   ✓(A) POLs   (D) MRIs
    (B) CLTs   (E) CTs
    (C) EMTs

45. The pyloric sphincter controls the passage of food into what location?

    (A) jejunum of the small intestine
   ✓(B) duodenum of the small intestine
    (C) cecum of the large intestine
    (D) sigmoid colon
    (E) appendix

46. Cholangi/o refers to the

    (A) cecum
    (B) colon
    (C) gallbladder

    ✓**(D)** bile duct
    (E) lip

47. Severe mental disorders that interfere with a perception of reality are called

    (A) hysteria
    (B) anxiety
    (C) neuroses

    ✓**(D)** psychoses
    (E) hypochondria

48. How many bones are in the lumbar vertebra?

    (A) 1
    (B) 3
    ✓**(C)** 5

    (D) 7
    (E) 12

49. The suffix -tocia means

    (A) pregnancy
    ✓**(B)** labor or childbirth
    (C) turning of

    (D) to bear
    (E) beginning

50. A deficiency in vitamin D can cause what bone disorder?

    (A) gout
    (B) scurvy
    ✓**(C)** rickets

    (D) scoliosis
    (E) lordosis

ADMINISTRATIVE

(Covers oral and written communication; appointment scheduling; computers in medicine; fees, billing, collections, and credit; health information technology; insurance and coding; and office management.)

Directions: Select the ONE best answer for each of the following multiple-choice questions.

1. When an account has been referred for collection, the medical assistant should

    (A) send a reminder letter
    ✓**(B)** not attempt to collect
    (C) discuss payment with the patient
    (D) call the patient's employer
    (E) cancel the balance

2. Assignment of lifetime benefits is available with

    ✓**(A)** Medicare
    (B) Medicaid
    (C) workers' compensation

    (D) CHAMPUS
    (E) CHAMPVA

3. Which is NOT a basic component of a computer system?

✓**(A)** modem

(B) monitor

(C) keyboard

(D) CPU

(E) printer

4. A written authorization by the patient giving the insurance company the right to pay the physician directly for billed services is called a/an

(A) co-payment

✓**(B)** assignment of benefits

(C) preauthorization

(D) deductible

(E) premium

5. A record of services for billing and insurance processing is a/an

✓**(A)** superbill - *ENCOUNTER*

(B) ledger

(C) double-entry bookkeeping

(D) receipt

(E) aging account

6. The speed measurement of printers is in

(A) gigabytes

(B) kilobytes

✓**(C)** characters per second

(D) megahertz

(E) RAM

7. The CD-ROM disc is capable of storing more information than

(A) 10 floppy disks

(B) 50 floppy disks

(C) 100 floppy disks

(D) 500 floppy disks

✓**(E)** 1,000 floppy disks

8. Placing your own feelings onto another person is an example of which of the following defensive behaviors?

(A) rationalization

✓**(B)** projection

(C) compensation

(D) displaced anger

(E) disassociation

9. ICD-9 codes used in the medical office

(A) may be coded directly from Volume III

✓**(B)** may require a fifth digit

(C) never require a fifth digit

(D) always require a V code to support the diagnosis

(E) always require an E code to support the diagnosis

10. The newest transcription technology, which allows the physician to speak into a microphone connected to a computer program that then translates the dictation into a typed report, is known as

(A) TDD

✓**(B)** VRT

(C) TActile CONverter

(D) all of the above

(E) none of the above

11. Directing the conversation back to the patient by repeating the words is called mirroring or

  (A) restating
  ✓(B) reflecting
  (C) assessment
  (D) clarification
  (E) all of the above

12. Computer memory is measured in

  (A) DOS
  (B) CPUs
  ✓(C) kilobytes
  (D) RAM
  (E) megahertz

13. A condition in which a patient is protected by the court and all collection attempts must cease is

  (A) statute of limitations
  (B) claims against estates
  (C) accounts receivable insurance
  (D) assignment of benefits
  ✓(E) bankruptcy

14. VRT is an example of a/an

  (A) synonym
  ✓(B) acronym
  (C) antonym
  (D) phonetics
  (E) eponym

15. The Alpha-Z color-coded system of filing, using an alphabetical system, is based on

  (A) 4 colors
  (B) 10 colors
  (C) 12 colors
  ✓(D) 13 colors
  (E) 15 colors

16. In computer language, a network is another term for

  (A) format
  (B) input
  (C) output
  ✓(D) interface
  (E) menu

17. A peripheral device for communicating between the user and the computer hardware is

  (A) track ball
  (B) mouse
  (C) joystick
  (D) light wand
  ✓(E) all of the above

18. The process for determining when accounts are overdue is

  (A) accounts receivable insurance
  (B) a collection agency
  (C) the Fair Debt Collection Practices Act
  (D) statute of limitations
  ✓(E) aging of accounts

19. When handling an emergency telephone call from a patient, the FIRST thing a medical assistant should do is

  ✓**(A)** get the caller's name and telephone number
    (B) ascertain whether or not the call is an emergency
    (C) gather as much information as possible about the emergency in the shortest amount of time
    (D) ask to speak with someone other than the patient if the patient/caller is too hysterical to communicate the details of the situation
    (E) ask if an ambulance has been summoned

20. The "brain" or "heart" of the computer is the

    (A) ROM   **(D)** DOS
  ✓**(B)** CPU   **(E)** GIGO
    (C) RAM

21. "Blocking out" the appointment schedule book is called developing

    (A) a double-booking schedule   **(D)** a modified wave schedule
    (B) a wave schedule   **(E)** open office hours
  ✓**(C)** a matrix

22. The filing system that assigns a number to patients the first time they are seen or admitted to a hospital is known as

    (A) straight numerical filing   ✓**(D)** unit numbering
    (B) middle digit filing   **(E)** none of the above
    (C) serial numbering

23. How soon should a patient be greeted after arrival in the office?

    (A) immediately   **(D)** within 5 minutes
  ✓**(B)** within 1 minute   **(E)** within 10 minutes
    (C) within 3 minutes

24. A new employee's probationary period is usually

    (A) 30 days   **(D)** 6 months
    (B) 2 months   **(E)** none of the above
  ✓**(C)** 3 months

25. When a physician cancels a patient's debt, it is called

    (A) debt cancellation   **(D)** assignment of benefits
  ✓**(B)** write-off   **(E)** accounts receivable reversal
    (C) skip

26. When handling a request for a prescription refill, a medical assistant

    (A) may call in the request, but only for a noncontrolled substance
    (B) should ask the patient to come into the office to obtain a written prescription
  ✓**(C)** may never call in a refill without the physician's direct order
    (D) is certified to call in all prescription refills
    (E) should call in the prescription if directed to do so by a nurse

27. Employee records must be kept for all of the following EXCEPT

    (A) Social Security number   (D) number of claimed exemptions
  ✓(B) net salary   (E) deductions
    (C) gross salary

28. Elective surgery is a procedure that

    (A) is necessary for the patient to have but can be postponed until the patient has the time
    (B) is for a life-threatening condition
    (C) does not require a surgical consent
  ✓(D) is not for a life-threatening condition and is often left up to the discretion of the patient as to whether he or she wishes to have the procedure
    (E) C and D

29. A real or imaginary wrong regarded as the cause for a complaint is known as

    (A) citation   (D) fault
    (B) judgment   (E) illegal action
  ✓(C) grievance

30. The "birthday rule" is used when both parents have individual insurance plans and a dependent needs to be covered. According to this "rule," the insurance plan that would be designated the primary plan is that belonging to the parent

    (A) who obtained the insurance first
    (B) who is the youngest
    (C) who is the oldest
  ✓(D) whose birthday falls earliest in the year
    (E) none of the above

31. Adopting the feelings of someone else, as when a child is afraid of needles because the mother is afraid, is the defensive behavior of

    (A) projection   ✓(D) introjection
    (B) compensation   (E) sublimation
    (C) regression

32. The HCFA-1500 insurance claim form

    (A) must be filled out by the patient
    (B) must be filled out by the physician's billing staff
    (C) is accepted by every insurance company within the United States
    (D) is never used
  ✓(E) is commonly accepted by most carriers

33. It is unethical for a medical assistant to decide

    (A) a patient's chief complaint
    (B) how much time the patient's appointment requires
    (C) that a patient is lying about the need to be seen by a physician
    (D) if the patient can pay his or her bill
  ✓(E) C and D

34. The back of a check is endorsed or signed by the

    (A) payer   **(D)** signee
    ✓**(B)** payee   **(E)** all of the above
    (C) maker

35. In ICD-9 coding guidelines, E codes

    (A) stand alone
    (B) should never be used with V codes
    (C) are required for a diagnosis
    ✓**(D)** give external causes or factors for an illness or injury
    (E) are the same as CPT codes

36. What type of mail is used to send valuables, such as currency and jewelry?

    (A) special handling   **(D)** special delivery
    ✓**(B)** registered mail   **(E)** all of the above
    (C) priority mail

37. The process of turning verbal descriptions into numerical designations is called

    (A) rider   **(D)** modifying
    ✓**(B)** coding   **(E)** classifying
    (C) grouping

38. The process by which a patient gives a medical assistant demographic information over the telephone prior to an office visit is known as

    (A) precertification   ✓**(D)** preregistration
    (B) insurance verification   **(E)** none of the above
    (C) preadmission

39. The act that protects pension funds is

    ✓**(A)** ERISA   **(D)** Title VII
    (B) ADA   **(E)** ADEA
    (C) FLSA

40. The proofreader's mark that means "insert a space" is

    ✓**(A)** #   **(D)** [/]
    (B) /=   **(E)** sp
    (C) [

41. MICR refers to

    (A) the code number on the right upper corner of the printed check to identify the bank
    (B) an indication that there is not sufficient money in the account to honor payment of the check
    ✓**(C)** the characters and letters printed on the bottom of the check that are used as routing information to identify the bank and number of the individual account

(D) a blank endorsement
(E) a restrictive endorsement

42. A military medical insurance plan that is part of the government is

✓**(A)** CHAMPUS
(B) Medicare
(C) Medicaid
(D) HMO
(E) Blue Cross/Blue Shield

43. The type of scheduling that may produce the longest patient waiting time is

✓**(A)** wave
(B) specified time
(C) modified wave
(D) grouping
(E) double booking

44. Only the employer is required to make payments to

(A) FICA
(B) OASDI
(C) Medicare
✓**(D)** FUTA
(E) none of the above

45. What type of mail should be used to send contracts, mortgages, deeds, and checks?

(A) priority mail
(B) first class
✓**(C)** certified mail
(D) second class
(E) third class

46. Words that sound alike but have different meanings and spelling are

✓**(A)** homophones
(B) synonyms
(C) antonyms
(D) eponyms
(E) none of the above

47. Liabilities include

(A) land, buildings, and furniture
(B) machinery and equipment
✓**(C)** accounts payable
(D) accounts receivable
(E) A, B, and D

48. Which refers to the amount of eligible charges each patient must pay each calendar year before the plan pays benefits?

(A) claim
(B) coinsurance
✓**(C)** deductible
(D) premium
(E) co-payment

49. When a patient is given six 15-minute time slots for a complete physical examination requiring $1\frac{1}{2}$ hours, this is called

(A) wave scheduling
✓**(B)** specified wave scheduling
(C) modified wave scheduling
(D) open office hours
(E) double booking

50. A standard #10 envelope measures

✓**(A)** 9½″ × 4⅛″

(B) 7½″ × 3⅞″

(C) 6½″ × 3⅝″

(D) 8½″ × 11″

(E) none of the above

CLINICAL

(Covers infection control; vital signs and measurements; assisting with physical examinations; assisting with medical specialties; assisting with minor surgery; assisting patients with special physical needs; urinalysis; microbiology; hematology; pharmacology and medication administration; patient education and nutrition; electrocardiology, radiology, and physical therapy; and emergency services.)

Directions: Select the ONE best answer for each of the following multiple-choice questions.

1. When using the problem-oriented medical recording method for medical recording, which of the following areas is the patient's history housed in?

(A) objective findings

✓**(B)** database

(C) problem list

(D) initial plan

(E) progress notes

2. A cerebrovascular accident (CVA) caused by a clot forming in the body and traveling to the brain is called a

(A) compression

(B) cerebral hemorrhage

✓**(C)** cerebral embolism

(D) cerebral thrombosis

(E) cardioversion

3. When reading a mercury thermometer, each short line represents

(A) a degree

(B) two degrees

(C) one-tenth of a degree

✓**(D)** two-tenths of a degree

(E) three-tenths of a degree

4. The presence of which of the following in urine may signal the onset of liver disease?

(A) nitrites

(B) ketones

(C) erythrocytes

(D) leukocytes

✓**(E)** bilirubin

5. A microorganism, serum, or toxic substance that is introduced by inoculation is called the

(A) aerobe

(B) anaerobe

(C) swab

✓**(D)** inoculum

(E) inoculate

6. When preparing a smear, holding the slide and passing it over a flame

   (A) inoculates the slide
   (B) sterilizes the specimen
   ✓(C) fixes the smear to the slide
   (D) kills the bacteria on the slide
   (E) allows the technician to see the microorganisms

7. A temperature of 101 degrees F is equal to how many degrees Celsius?

   ✓(A) 38.3°C
   (B) 24.1°C
   (C) 88.1°C
   (D) 39.0°C
   (E) 37.6°C

8. The largest cellular component of the blood consists of

   (A) leukocytes
   ✓(B) erythrocytes
   (C) platelets
   (D) lymphocytes
   (E) phagocytes

9. The proprietary name of a drug is also known as the

   (A) trade name
   (B) brand name
   ✓(C) generic name
   (D) A & B
   (E) A & C

10. What part of the brain controls body temperature?

   (A) medulla oblongata
   (B) midbrain
   (C) thalamus
   ✓(D) hypothalamus
   (E) cerebrum

11. Approximately 23 percent of all the energy released by nutrients is used by the body to carry on functions. The rest becomes

   ✓(A) heat
   (B) fat
   (C) sugar
   (D) muscle
   (E) bone

12. Which site can be used for subcutaneous injections?

   (A) deltoid
   (B) forearm
   (C) upper chest
   (D) buttocks
   ✓(E) abdomen

13. Which of the following temperatures is considered normal?

   (A) oral, 98.6°F/37°C
   (B) rectal, 99.6°F/37.6°C
   (C) axillary, 97.6°F/36.4°C
   (D) aural, 98.6°F/37°C
   ✓(E) all of the above

14. Which of the following is appropriate when hand washing?

(A) use hot water and hold hands upward
(B) use cold water and hold hands downward
✓(C) use tepid or lukewarm water and hold hands downward
(D) use warm water under high pressure and hold hands outward
(E) use warm water and hold hands upward

15. In what part of the SOAP charting system is the diagnosis found?

✓(A) assessment
(B) subjective
(C) objective
(D) plan
(E) problem list

16. When taking a rectal temperature on a pediatric patient, insert the thermometer into the anal canal approximately

(A) 2 to 2½ inches
(B) ¼ of an inch
✓(C) ½ to 1 inch
(D) 1 to 1½ inches
(E) no more than 3 inches

17. Immunizations scheduled for a child 4 to 5 months of age are

(A) HBV 1, DPT 1, Oral Polio 1
✓(B) DPT 2, Oral Polio 2, Hib 2
(C) DPT 1, Oral Polio 2, HBV 2, Hib 1
(D) DPT 1, Oral Polio 2, HBV 2
(E) DPT 2, Oral Polio 2, MMR

18. Universal precautions (Ups) under OSHA are

(A) guidelines
(B) suggestions
(C) recommendations
(D) bills
✓(E) laws

19. When transferring sterile solutions to a sterile field

(A) discard the liquid remaining in the bottle
(B) place the cap on a surface with outside edges of the cap facing up
✓(C) place the cap on a surface with the inside edges of the cap facing up
(D) place the cap on the Mayo stand
(E) pour the liquid by stabilizing the bottle on the edge of the basin

20. An example of a water-soluble vitamin is

(A) vitamin A
✓(B) vitamin B
(C) vitamin D
(D) vitamin E
(E) vitamin K

21. A child less than 1 year old may have a pulse rate that ranges between

(A) 50 and 65
(B) 60 and 80
(C) 70 and 90
(D) 80 and 120
✓(E) 120 and 160

22. What type of immunity would one have if given tetanus immune serum globulin (TIG)?

   (A) active acquired natural immunity (AANI)
   (B) active acquired artificial immunity (AAAI)
   (C) passive acquired natural immunity (PANI)
   (D) passive acquired artificial immunity (PAAI)
   √(E) none of the above

23. Which of the following would be considered a symptom?

   (A) hypertension
   √(B) dizziness
   (C) diabetes
   (D) arthritis
   (E) pregnancy

24. The "little spark" that begins or starts the heartbeat originates in the

   (A) Purkinje fibers
   (B) vagus nerve
   √(C) SA node
   (D) AV node
   (E) artificial pacemaker

25. What type of bacteria forms pairs, stains gram-negative, and is seen in gonorrhea and pneumonia?

   (A) streptococci
   (B) staphylococci
   √(C) diplococci
   (D) bacilli
   (E) spirilla

26. When taking a pulse, the medical assistant should count for at least

   (A) 10 seconds
   (B) 15 seconds
   (C) 20 seconds
   (D) 30 seconds
   √(E) 60 seconds

27. What method of examination is used to gauge the growth of the body or to determine size?

   √(A) mensuration
   (B) inspection
   (C) palpation
   (D) percussion
   (E) auscultation

28. Anaphylactic shock can result in

   (A) edema and rash
   (B) convulsions
   (C) unconsciousness and death
   √(D) A, B, and C
   (E) B and C only

29. A mixture of 1:10 bleach and water is a substance that can kill microorganisms but not spores and is not used on people. It can be classified as a/an

   (A) bactericide
   (B) germicide
   √(C) disinfectant
   (D) antiseptic
   (E) formaldehyde

30. A COPD patient may use what instrument to monitor his or her breathing at home?

(A) oximeter
(B) spirometer
✓(C) peak flowmeter
(D) pressurized oxygen meter
(E) none of the above

31. If administered sugar, a patient suffering from an insulin reaction

(A) will have no response to the sugar
✓(B) will respond immediately
(C) will get worse
(D) would be given insulin
(E) none of the above

32. A person who is suffering cardiac arrest should be administered chest compressions at a rate of

(A) 12 times a minute
(B) 15 times a minute
(C) 50 to 70 times a minute
✓(D) 80 to 100 times a minute
(E) this person should not receive chest compressions at all

33. During an EKG, a tense muscle or a muscular contraction may produce an artifact called a/an

(A) erratic stylus defect
✓(B) somatic tremor
(C) AC interference
(D) baseline shift
(E) none of the above

34. Which of the following ratios is accurate for the proportion of respiratory rate to pulse rate?

(A) 10:1
(B) 20:1
✓(C) 1:4
(D) 5:1
(E) 1:5

35. A substance that prevents the growth of microorganisms without necessarily killing them and is generally safe for use on people is a/an

(A) bactericide
(B) germicide
(C) disinfectant
✓(D) antiseptic
(E) formaldehyde

36. A hemostat with clawlike teeth at the tip to grasp and hold tissue is called a

(A) thumb forceps
✓(B) tissue forceps
(C) sterilizer or transfer forceps
(D) needle holder
(E) splinter forceps

37. The drug classification that controls or relieves coughing is

(A) antibiotic
(B) decongestant
(C) bronchodilator
✓(D) antitussive
(E) expectorant

38. During which of the Korotkoff phases might an auscultatory gap occur?

(A) I
✓(B) II
(C) III
(D) IV
(E) V

39. A discomforting uneasiness that is often a sign of infection is

(A) metastasis
(B) acuity
(C) benign
✓(D) malaise
(E) contagious

40. HIV is transmitted by

(A) indirect transmission
(B) contact with cough droplets
✓(C) direct contact
(D) droplets produced by sneezing
(E) none of the above

41. The physician has ordered 250 mg of penicillin to be administered. Penicillin on hand is 0.25 g /5 cc. How much should be given?

(A) 1 cc
(B) 2 cc
(C) 3 cc
(D) 4 cc
✓(E) 5 cc

42. Which is a primary hypertension of unknown cause?

(A) renal
✓(B) essential
(C) benign
(D) malignant
(E) secondary

43. What is the infectious fungal skin disease that can be detected through the use of a Wood's light?

✓(A) tinea
(B) herpes zoster
(C) impetigo
(D) scabies
(E) herpes simplex

44. Pathogens that grow in oxygen-rich environments are known as

(A) spores
(B) normal flora
✓(C) aerobes
(D) anaerobes
(E) nosocomial

45. A tuberculin skin test is a

(A) Mantoux test
(B) tine test
(C) culture for tuberculosis
✓(D) A and B
(E) none of the above

46. Which artery is most commonly used for taking a patient's BP?

(A) carotid
✓(B) brachial
(C) popliteal
(D) dorsalis pedis
(E) apical

47. Mr. Duffy weighs 220 lbs. How many kilograms does he weigh?

    (A)   48.40 kg.   ✓**(D)**   99.00 kg.
    (B)   26.40 kg.   **(E)**   136.08 kg.
    (C)   102 kg.

48. An example of a small-gauge suture used for the skin is

  ✓**(A)**   stainless steel 5-0   **(D)**   plain gut 3-0
    (B)   stainless steel 0   **(E)**   nylon 2-0
    (C)   chromic gut 2-0

49. A substage condenser on a microscope is a

    (A)   control for vertical and horizontal movement of the slide
    (B)   part of the microscope that holds the illuminator
    (C)   lens system used to increase light for a sharper image
  ✓**(D)**   small knob atop a larger knob that adjusts the stage up and down
    (E)   directional light source

50. Glucose will "spill" into the urine when the blood glucose level exceeds

    (A)   120 to 140 mg/100 mL   **(D)**   180 to 200 mg/100 mL
    (B)   140 to 160 mg/100 mL   **(E)**   200 mg/100 mL
  ✓**(C)**   160 to 180 mg/100 mL

PRE-TEST ANSWERS

GENERAL

1. C
2. D
3. C
4. E
5. B
6. A
7. D
8. B
9. D
10. D
11. C
12. D
13. B
14. A
15. C
16. C
17. B
18. C
19. A
20. B
21. D
22. C
23. C
24. D
25. E
26. D
27. E
28. D
29. A
30. D
31. B
32. A
33. E
34. D
35. B
36. D
37. B
38. D
39. C
40. D
41. B
42. E
43. D
44. A
45. B
46. D
47. D
48. C
49. B
50. C

ADMINISTRATIVE

1. B
2. A
3. A
4. B
5. A
6. C
7. E
8. B
9. B
10. B
11. B
12. C
13. E
14. B
15. D
16. D
17. E
18. E
19. A
20. B
21. C
22. D
23. B
24. C
25. B
26. C
27. B
28. D
29. C
30. D
31. D
32. E
33. E
34. B
35. D
36. B
37. B
38. D
39. A
40. A
41. C
42. A
43. A
44. D
45. C
46. A
47. C
48. C
49. B
50. A

CLINICAL

1. B
2. C
3. D
4. E
5. D
6. C
7. A
8. B
9. C
10. D
11. A
12. E
13. E
14. C
15. A
16. C
17. B
18. E
19. C
20. B
21. E
22. D
23. B
24. C
25. C
26. E
27. A
28. D
29. C
30. C
31. B
32. D
33. B
34. C
35. D
36. B
37. D
38. B
39. D
40. C
41. E
42. B
43. A
44. C
45. D
46. B
47. D
48. A
49. D
50. C

PART I

GENERAL MEDICAL KNOWLEDGE

CHAPTER 1

MEDICAL TERMINOLOGY

1. The four components of most medical terms consist of

    (A) word root, combining form "e," prefix, and/or suffix
    (B) word root, combining form/vowel "o," prefix, and/or suffix
    (C) word root, combining consonant, prefix, and/or suffix
    (D) word abbreviation, combining vowel "e," prefix, and/or suffix
    (E) word abbreviation, combining consonant, prefix, and/or suffix

    (B) Word root, combining form "o," prefix, and/or suffix is correct. The general rule for forming medical terms is that most terms will consist of a word root, such as cardi- meaning heart, the combining form or vowel "o," a prefix at the beginning of the word, and/or a suffix at the end of the word.

2. A word root is

    (A) an acronym for a word
    (B) an abbreviation for a word
    ✓**(C)** the foundation of a word
    (D) able to stand alone as a medical term
    (E) a synonym

    (C) A word root is the foundation of a word is correct.
    (A) An acronym, in which the first letter of each word forms a short word, is never used as a word root when forming a medical term.
    (B) A word root represents the fundamental meaning of the word and, as such, is more than an abbreviation.
    (D) A word root does not generally stand alone to form a new word. The word root would need a prefix and/or suffix to explain it more completely.
    (E) A synonym, or a word that has approximately the same meaning as another word, is not used as a word root.

3. The word root ileum means

    (A) hipbone
    (B) thigh bone
    (C) large intestine
    (D) small intestine
    (E) groin area

    (D) The small intestine is correct.
    (A) The word root for hipbone is ilium.
    (B) The word root/combining form for thigh bone is femor/o.
    (C) The word root/combining form for large intestine or colon is col/o.
    (E) The word root/combining form for groin or inguinal area is inguin/o.

4. The combining vowel or form is

(A) used to make it possible to pronounce long medical terms with ease
(B) a word root and usually the vowel "o"
(C) used between two word roots
(D) either a consonant or a vowel
(E) A, B, and C only

    (E) is correct. Long medical terms such as nephrolithectomy, meaning removal of kidney stones, are easier to pronounce with the combining vowel "o" between the word roots nephro (kidney) and lith (stone). A combining vowel is usually "o" and may be found between two word roots, such as in osteoarthritis.

5. A prefix

(A) forms a new medical term when added in front of a word root
(B) can give information about the location of an organ
(C) can give information about a number of parts, measurement, or time
(D) can give information pertaining to color
(E) all of the above

    (E) is correct. A prefix added to the front of a word root forms a new word, such as adding the prefix peri-, meaning around, in front of the word root cardi-, meaning heart, to form pericardial, meaning "pertaining to around the heart." A prefix can represent the location of an organ, such as later/o meaning side, infra- meaning under, and hyper- meaning over. A prefix can give information about a number of parts: bi- meaning two or quad- meaning four; measurement, such as semi- meaning partial; and time, such as brady- meaning slow and tachy- meaning fast. A prefix can also give information pertaining to color, such as alb- meaning white, cyano- meaning blue, and erythr- meaning red.

6. The prefix meaning bad is

(A) medi-   **(D)** my/o-
(B) mal-   **(E)** macro-
(C) meso-

    (B) is correct. The prefix mal- means bad. For instance, the word malodorous means having a bad odor.
    (A) Medi- means middle.
    (C) Meso- means middle.
    (D) My/o- means muscle.
    (E) Macro- means large.

7. The prefix pertaining to double is

(A) semi-   **(D)** diplo-
(B) hemi-   **(E)** mono-
(C) bi-

    (D) Diplo- is correct, such as in the word diplopia meaning double vision.
    (A) Semi- means partial, such as in the term semicircle meaning a half circle.

(B)	Hemi- means half, such as in the word hemiplegia meaning paralyzed on one side of the body.

(C)	Bi- means two, such as in the term bicuspid meaning having two cusps.

(E)	Mono- means one, such as in the term mononucleosis meaning having one nucleus.

8.	A suffix is a small word or term

(A)	attached to the beginning of a word to add additional meaning
(B)	found in every medical term
(C)	added at the beginning of the combining form of the word root
(D)	that can stand alone as a medical term
(E)	attached to the end of a word to add additional meaning, such as a condition, disease, or procedure

(E)	is correct. A suffix is always attached after the word root and combining form. It can add a new meaning: a condition, as with the suffix -ectopy meaning displacement; a disease, such as in -cele meaning hernia or swelling; or a procedure, such as -ectomy meaning the surgical removal of a part or disease.
(A)	A prefix is attached to the beginning of a word and a suffix is attached at the end.
(B)	A suffix is not found in every medical term.
(C)	A suffix is added at the end of the combining form of the word root.
(D)	A suffix cannot stand alone as a medical term. It further explains the term or word root.

9.	The suffix -rrhage means

(A)	to stitch or suture	(D)	rupture
(B)	discharge	(E)	drooping
(C)	excessive, abnormal flow

(C)	is correct. For instance, hemorrhage means an abnormal flow of blood.
(A)	-Rrhaphy means to stitch or suture.
(B)	-Rrhea means a discharge or flow.
(D)	-Rrhexis is a rupture.
(E)	-Ptosis means drooping, such as in blepharoptosis.

10.	It is acceptable to vary the

(A)	pronunciation of medical terms	(D)	A and C are both correct
(B)	spelling of medical terms	(E)	none of the above
(C)	meaning of medical terms

(A)	is correct. The pronunciation may vary, depending on where a person is born or educated.
(B)	Spelling may never vary.
(C)	The meaning of medical terms is based on the word root, prefix, and suffix used. This does not vary; however, there may be more than one meaning for some words.

11. The rules for setting up singular and plural forms of some words follow the rules of

  (A) whatever sounds correct
  (B) English
  (C) Latin and Greek
  (D) individual cases when changing from singular to plural
  (E) B, C, and D only

  (E) is correct. Some words, such as changing the singular virus to the plural viruses, follow English rules. Other words, such as changing the singular sarcoma to sarcomata, follow Latin and Greek rules.

12. A word ending in -a, such as vertebra, will change to the plural by

  (A) changing -a to -ata   **(D)** keeping the -a and adding an -e
  (B) changing -a to -um   **(E)** none of the above
  (C) adding an -es

  (D) is correct. The singular vertebra becomes vertebrae for the plural.
  (A) A word ending in -ma will drop the -ma and add -mata for the plural (sarcoma to sarcomata).
  (B) A word ending in -um will drop the -um and add -a for the plural form (ovum to ova).
  (C) A word ending in -is will drop the -is and add -es for the plural form (metastasis to metastases).

13. The plural form of biopsy is

  (A) formed by dropping the -y and adding -ies
  (B) the same as the singular form
  (C) not necessary since there is never more than one biopsy performed at a time
  (D) formed by dropping the -y and adding -es
  (E) none of the above

  (A) is correct. Biopsy becomes biopsies in the plural form.
  (B) Very few terms are the same in the singular and plural forms.
  (C) Several biopsies can be performed on various tissue samples during the same surgical procedure.
  (D) A word ending in -is will drop the -is and add -es for the plural form. For instance, metastasis becomes metastases in the plural form.

14. To change the word phalanx, or finger, to its plural form, you would

  (A) change the x to g and add -es
  (B) leave the x and add -es
  (C) drop the x and add um
  (D) leave the word alone since it is the same in the plural as it is in the singular form
  (E) none of the above

  (A) is correct. Phalanx becomes phalanges in the plural form.

15. The rule for word building is

    (A) start at the beginning of the word and translate each component
    (B) memorize the definition of each medical term
    (C) read the term from the end of word (or the suffix) back to the beginning (prefix) and then pick up the word root
    (D) there are no hard-and-fast rules when building medical terms
    (E) none of the above

        (C) is correct. To gain a quick understanding of a term, start at the end of the word, then go to the beginning, and then read the word root. For instance, pericarditis reads inflammation of (itis) the membrane surrounding (peri) the heart (cardi).

        (B) It is not advisable to memorize the meaning of medical terms, due to the large number of medical terms. It is recommended to break apart each component of the term instead.

        (D) There are several rules that make medical terminology easier to understand.

16. Abbreviations

    (A) are to be avoided whenever possible
    (B) are useful in the medical profession
    (C) should be used only if they are from an acceptable abbreviation list
    (D) change meaning, depending on whether they are in capital letters or small letters
    (E) B, C, and D only

        (E) is correct.

17. The combining form hyster/o means

    (A) blood   **(D)** uterus
    (B) liver   **(E)** clot
    (C) intestines

        (D) is correct. Surgical removal of the uterus is called a hysterectomy.

        (A) The combining form for blood is hem/o or hemat/o. Hematology is the study of blood.

        (B) The combining form for liver is hepat/o. An inflammation of the liver is hepatitis.

        (C) The combining form for the intestines is enter/o. Enteritis is an intestinal inflammation.

        (E) The combining form for clot is thromb/o. Thrombophlebitis is an inflammation of a vein in conjunction with the formation of a clot.

18. The combining form cyt/o means

    (A) colon   **(D)** bladder
    (B) cell   **(E)** gallbladder
    (C) cancer

        (B) is correct.

        (A) The combining form for colon is col/o. For instance, colonoscopy is a visual examination of the colon using an instrument.

(C) Carcin/o is the combining form for cancer. For instance, carcinoma is a malignant tumor.

(D) Cyst/o is the combining form for bladder. Cystotomy is cutting into/incision into the bladder.

(E) Cholecyst/o is the combining form for gallbladder. Cholecystectomy is the surgical removal of the gallbladder.

19. The prefix melan/o means

(A) large
(B) white
(C) black
(D) blue
(E) red

(C) is correct.
(A) Macr/o means large. Macrocytes are large blood cells.
(B) Alb- and albumin/o are prefixes meaning white. Albuminuria refers to protein in the urine.
(D) Cyan/o means blue. Cyanosis is a bluish color to the skin due to lack of oxygen.
(E) Erythr/o means red. Erythrocytes are red blood cells.

20. The prefix a- means

(A) both
(B) around
(C) before
(D) against
✓(E) without or not

(E) is correct. The prefix a- means without.
(A) The prefix ambi- means both.
(B) The prefix circum- means around.
(C) The prefix ante- means before.
(D) The prefix anti- means against.

21. The suffix -malacia means

(A) abnormal softening
(B) abnormal enlargement
(C) abnormal drooping
(D) abnormal bleeding
(E) abnormal narrowing

✓(A) is correct. An abnormal softening is the suffix -malacia.
(B) Abnormal enlargement is -megaly.
(C) Abnormal drooping is -ptosis.
(D) Abnormal bleeding is -rrhage.
(E) Abnormal narrowing is -stenosis.

22. The suffix -gram means

(A) picture or recording
(B) instrument to record
(C) the procedure of recording
(D) produced by
(E) A, B, and C

✓(A) is correct. A picture or recording is the suffix -gram.
(B) An instrument to record is the suffix -graph.
(C) A recording is the suffix -graphy.
(D) Produced by is the suffix -genic.

23. Excessive nasal bleeding is

  (A) rhinorrhea

  (B) rhinoplasty

✓**(C)** rhinorrhagia

  (D) rhinorrhexis

  (E) rhinorrhaphy

  (C) is correct. Excessive nasal bleeding is a hemorrhage or rhinorrhage.

  (A) Rhinorrhea is nasal discharge or flow.

  (B) Rhinoplasty is the surgical repair of the nose.

  (D) Rhinorrhexis is a nasal rupture.

  (E) Rhinorrhaphy is to stitch or suture the nose.

24. The medical term for gallstones is

  (A) cholecystectomy

  (B) cholecystotomy

  (C) choledochal

✓**(D)** cholelithiasis

  (E) choledochectomy

  (D) is correct. Cholelithiasis refers to the presence of gallstones.

  (A) Cholecystectomy is the surgical removal of the gallbladder.

  (B) Cholecystotomy is a surgical incision into the gallbladder.

  (C) Choledochal is pertaining to the bile duct.

  (E) Choledochectomy is the excision of a part of the common bile duct.

25. The suffix -stalsis means

  (A) twitch

  (B) to visualize

  (C) the study of

  (D) surgical removal

✓**(E)** constriction

  (E) is correct. Constriction is the suffix -stalsis.

  (A) Twitch is the suffix -spasm

  (B) To visualize is the suffix -scopy.

  (C) The study of is the suffix -ology.

  (D) Surgical removal is the suffix -ectomy.

26. The suffix -lysis means

  (A) stone

  (B) presence of

  (C) pain

✓**(D)** destruction

  (E) surgical puncture to remove fluid

  (D) is correct. The suffix -lysis means destruction.

  (A) Stone is the suffix -lith.

  (B) Presence of is the suffix -iasis.

  (C) Pain is the suffix -algia.

  (E) Surgical puncture to remove fluid is the suffix -centesis.

27. The word root meaning tongue is

  (A) leuk/o

  (B) aden/o

  (C) lingu/o

  (D) gloss/o

  (E) C and D

(E) is correct. Lingu/o and gloss/o both mean tongue.
(A) Leuk/o means white.
(B) Aden/o means gland.

28. The suffix -itis means

(A) disease   ✓**(D)** inflammation
(B) presence of   **(E)** removal of
(C) destruction

(D) is correct. The suffix -itis means inflammation.
(A) Disease is the suffix -pathy.
(B) Presence of is the suffix -iasis.
(C) Destruction is the suffix -lysis.
(E) Removal of is the suffix -ectomy.

29. The prefix inter- means

(A) under   **(D)** above
(B) within   ✓**(E)** between or among
(C) across

(E) is correct. Inter- means between or among.
(A) Under is the prefix infra-.
(B) Within is the prefix intra-.
(C) Across is the prefix trans-.
(D) Above is the prefix supra-.

30. The prefix dorso- means

(A) away from   ✓**(D)** back
(B) middle   **(E)** above
(C) side

(D) is correct. Dorso- means back.
(A) Away from is the prefix ab-.
(B) Middle is the prefix medi- or mes/o.
(C) Side is the prefix later/o.
(E) Above is the prefix supra-.

31. Nephr/o is the word root/combining form meaning

(A) bladder   ✓**(D)** kidney
(B) nerve   **(E)** intestines
(C) liver

(D) is correct. Nephr/o means kidney.
(A) Bladder is cyst/o.
(B) Nerve is neur/o.
(C) Liver is hepat/o.
(E) Intestines is enter/o.

32. Another word root/combining form for kidney is

   (A) rect/o
   ✓**(B)** ren/o
   (C) rhin/o
   (D) onc/o
   (E) ile/o

      (B)   is correct. Ren/o is a word root/combining form meaning kidney.
      (A)   Rect/o means rectum.
      (C)   Rhin/o means nose.
      (D)   Onc/o means tumor.
      (E)   Ile/o means ileum of the small intestine.

33. Arthr/o is the word root/combining form meaning

   (A) disease
   (B) gland
   (C) head
   ✓**(D)** joint
   (E) bone

      (D)   is correct. Arthr/o means joint.
      (A)   Disease is path/o.
      (B)   Gland is aden/o.
      (C)   Head is cephal/o.
      (E)   Bone is oste/o.

34. Oste/o is the word root/combining form meaning

   (A) stomach
   ✓**(B)** bone
   (C) gallbladder
   (D) brain
   (E) heart

      (B)   is correct. Oste/o means bone.
      (A)   Stomach is gastr/o.
      (C)   Gallbladder is cholecyst/o.
      (D)   Brain is encephal/o.
      (E)   Heart is cardi/o.

35. Cerebr/o is the word root/combining form meaning

   (A) brain
   (B) cerebrum
   (C) head
   (D) cerebellum
   ✓**(E)** A and B

      (E)   is correct. Cerebr/o refers to the cerebrum portion of the brain.
      (C)   Head is cephal/o or crani/o.
      (D)   Cerebellum is cerebell/o.

36. Myel/o is the word root/combining form for

   (A) meninges
   (B) muscle
   ✓**(C)** spinal cord
   (D) mucus
   (E) upper jaw bone

      (C)   is correct. Myel/o refers to the spinal cord and bone marrow.
      (A)   Meninges is meningi/o.
      (B)   Muscle is my/o.
      (D)   Mucus is myx/o.
      (E)   Upper jaw bone is maxilla.

37. Ankyl/o is the word root/combining form meaning

 (A) cartilage   ✓(D) stiff joint
 (B) joint   (E) rib
 (C) digit

      (D) is correct. Ankyl/o means a stiff joint.
      (A) Cartilage is chondr/o.
      (B) Joint is arthr/o.
      (C) Digit (finger or toe) is dactyl/o.
      (E) Rib is cost/o.

38. Tars/o is the word root/combining form meaning

 (A) foot   (D) chest
 (B) tendon   (E) tibia
 (C) stretch

      ✓(A) is correct. Tars/o means foot.
      (B) Tendon is ten/o or tendin/o.
      (C) Stretch is tens/o.
      (D) Chest is thorac/o.
      (E) Tibia (the inner bone of the lower leg) is tibi/o.

39. The word root/combining form for kneecap is

 (A) ped/o   (D) orth/o
 (B) pelv/o   (E) oste/o
✓(C) patell/o

      (C) is correct. Patell/o means kneecap.
      (A) Ped/o means foot.
      (B) Pelv/o means pelvic.
      (D) Orth/o means straight.
      (E) Oste/o means bone.

40. Lamin/o means

 (A) lower back   (D) pelvis
 (B) hip   (E) spinal cord
✓(C) vertebra

      (C) is correct. Lamin/o refers to the lamina or part of the vertebra.
      (A) Lower back is lumb/o.
      (B) Hip is ischi/o.
      (D) Pelvis is pelv/o.
      (E) Spinal cord is myel/o.

41. The word root/combining form for the bones of the hand is

 (A) humer/o   (D) fibul/o
✓(B) metacarp/o   (E) phalang/o
 (C) tibi/o

      (B) is correct. The metacarpals are the bones of the hand.
      (A) Humer/o refers to the humerus or upper arm bone.

(C) Tibi/o refers to the tibia or inner bone of the lower leg.
(D) Fibul/o refers to the fibula or the smaller outer bone of the lower leg.
(E) Phalang/o refers to the phalanges or the bones of the toes and fingers.

42. Hard or horny is the word root/combining form

(A) hist/o   ✓(D) kerat/o
(B) hidr/o   (E) cutane/o
(C) lip/o

(D) is correct. Kerat/o means hard or horny.
(A) Hist/o means tissue.
(B) Hidr/o refers to sweat.
(C) Lip/o refers to fat.
(E) Cutane/o refers to skin.

43. The word root/combining form meaning skin is

(A) dermat/o   (D) chrom/o
(B) derm/o   ✓(E) A, B, and C
(C) cutane/o

(E) is correct. Dermat/o, derm/o, and cutane/o all refer to skin.
(D) Chrom/o refers to color.

44. The word root/combining form meaning sugar is

(A) gonad/o   (D) crin/o
(B) gluc/o   ✓(E) B and C
(C) glyc/o

(E) is correct. Both gluc/o and glyc/o mean sugar.
(A) Gonad/o refers to the sex glands.
(D) Crin/o refers to the word secrete.

45. The word root/combining form for the thymus gland is

(A) thyr/o   (D) thyroid/o
(B) toxic/o   (E) kal/i
✓(C) thym/o

(C) is correct. Thym/o is the word root/combining form for the thymus
     gland.
(A) Thyr/o and (D) thyroid/o both refer to the thyroid gland.
(B) Toxic/o refers to toxic.
(E) Kal/i means potassium.

46. Dips/o is the word root/combining form for

(A) double   (D) sodium
(B) two   ✓(E) thirst
(C) sugar

(E) is correct. Dips/o refers to thirst.
(A) Double is dipl/o.
(B) Two is bi- or di-.

(C) Sugar is gluc/o or glyc/o.

(D) Sodium is natr/o.

47. Hemangi/o refers to

   (A) blood clotting   **(D)** vessel

 ✓**(B)** blood vessel   **(E)** vein

   (C) blood color

     (B) is correct. Hemangi/o is the word root/combining form meaning blood vessel.

     (A) Blood clotting is coagul/o.

     (C) Blood (red) color is erythr/o.

     (D) Vessel is vas/o or phleb/o.

     (E) Vein is ven/o.

48. Sangui/o means

   (A) shape   **(D)** clotting

 ✓**(B)** blood   **(E)** clumping

   (C) white cell

     (B) is correct. Sangui/o is the word root/combining form for blood.

     (A) Shape is morph/o.

     (C) White cell is leukocyt/o.

     (D) Clotting is coagul/o.

     (E) Clumping is agglutin/o.

49. Atri/o refers to

   (A) artery   **(D)** joint

   (B) blood vessel   ✓**(E)** atrium

   (C) fatty substance, plaque

     (E) is correct. Atri/o means atrium (of the heart).

     (A) Artery is arteri/o.

     (B) Blood vessel is angi/o.

     (C) Fatty substance or plaque is ather/o.

     (D) Joint is arthr/o.

50. Cost/o means

   (A) lung   **(D)** chest

   (B) air   **(E)** pharynx

 ✓**(C)** rib

     (C) is correct. Cost/o means rib or side.

     (A) Lung is pulmon/o, pneum/o, and pneumon/o.

     (B) Air is pneum/o and pneumon/o.

     (D) Chest is pector/o.

     (E) Pharynx is pharyng/o.

51. Cholangi/o refers to the

    (A) cecum   ✓**(D)** bile duct
    (B) colon   **(E)** lip
    (C) gallbladder

        (D) is correct. Cholangi/o means bile duct.
        (A) Cecum, a portion of the large intestine, is cec/o.
        (B) Colon is col/o.
        (C) Gallbladder is cholecyst/o.
        (E) Lip is cheil/o.

52. Lingu/o refers to the

    (A) lip   **(D)** palate
  ✓**(B)** tongue   **(E)** tooth
    (C) throat

        (B) is correct. Lingu/o means tongue.
        (A) Lip is cheil/o.
        (C) Throat is pharyng/o.
        (D) Palate is palat/o.
        (E) Tooth is dent/o.

53. Proct/o is the word root/combining form for

    (A) sigmoid colon   ✓**(D)** rectum
    (B) pancreas   **(E)** eating
    (C) pylorus

        (D) is correct. Proct/o means rectum.
        (A) Sigmoid colon is sigmoid/o.
        (B) Pancreas is pancreat/o.
        (C) Pylorus is pylor/o.
        (E) Eating is phag/o.

54. Urethr/o is the word root/combining form for

  ✓**(A)** urethra   **(D)** kidney
    (B) urine   **(E)** renal pelvis
    (C) ureter

        (A) is correct. Urethr/o is the combining form for urethra.
        (B) Urine is ur/o.
        (C) Ureter is ureter/o.
        (D) Kidney is nephr/o.
        (E) Renal pelvis is pyel/o.

55. The word root/combining form for bladder is

    (A) glomerul/o   ✓**(D)** cyst/o
    (B) lith/o   **(E)** cyt/o
    (C) urin/o

        (D) is correct. Cyst/o is the word root/combining form for bladder.
        (A) Glomerul/o is glomerulus (of the kidney).

(B)   Lith/o is stone.
(C)   Urin/o is urine.
(E)   Cyt/o is cell.

56. Ov/i or ov/o is the word root/combining form for

(A) ovary   **(D)** uterus
✓**(B)** egg   **(E)** fallopian tube
(C) breast

    (B)   is correct. Ov/i or ov/o is the word root/combining form for egg.
    (A)   Ovary is oophor/o or ovar/o.
    (C)   Breast is mast/o or mamm/o.
    (D)   Uterus is uter/o or hyster/o.
    (E)   Fallopian tube is salping/o.

57. Nat/a is the word root/combining form for

(A) vulva   ✓**(D)** birth
(B) vagina   **(E)** woman or female
(C) pregnancy

    (D)   is correct. Nat/a is the word root/combining form for birth.
    (A)   Vulva is vulv/o.
    (B)   Vagina is vagin/o.
    (C)   Pregnancy is gravid/o.
    (E)   Woman or female is gynec/o.

58. The word root/combining form for uterus is

(A) metr/o   **(D)** cervic/o
(B) uter/o   ✓**(E)** A and B
(C) colp/o

    (E)   is correct. Both metr/o and uter/o mean uterus.
    (C)   Colp/o means vagina.
    (D)   Cervic/o means neck or cervix.

59. Andr/o is the word root/combining form for

(A) gland   **(D)** testes
(B) female   **(E)** semen
✓**(C)** male

    (C)   is correct. Andr/o means male.
    (A)   Gland is aden/o.
    (B)   Female is gynec/o.
    (D)   Testes is test/o.
    (E)   Semen is semin/o.

60. Orch/o is the word root/combining form for

(A) epididymis   ✓**(D)** testes
(B) glans penis   **(E)** seminal vesicle
(C) prostate

(D) is correct. Orch/o refers to testes.
(A) Epididymis is epididym/o.
(B) Glans penis is balan/o.
(C) Prostate is prostat/o.
(E) Seminal vesicle is vesicul/o.

61. Vag/o is the word root/combining form for

(A) vagina

(B) vertebra

✓**(C)** vagus nerve

(D) speech

(E) spinal cord

    (C) is correct. Vag/o means vagus.
    (A) Vagina is vagin/o or colp/o.
    (B) Vertebra is spondyl/o.
    (D) Speech is phas/o.
    (E) Spinal cord is myel/o.

62. Psych/o is the word root/combining form for

(A) speech

(B) nerve root

(C) medulla

(D) mind

(E) meninges

    ✓(D) is correct. Psych/o means mind.
    (A) Speech is phas/o.
    (B) Nerve root is radicul/o.
    (C) Medulla is medull/o.
    (E) Meninges is mening/o.

63. Vitre/o is the word root/combining form for

(A) tears

(B) eyelid

✓**(C)** glassy

(D) retina

(E) iris

    (C) is correct. Vitre/o means glassy.
    (A) Tears is lacrim/o.
    (B) Eyelid is palpebr/o.
    (D) Retina is retin/o.
    (E) Iris is ir/o or irid/o.

64. The word root/combining form for eye is

(A) optic/o

(B) opt/o

(C) ophthalm/o

(D) ocul/o

✓**(E)** all of the above

    (E) All are correct. Optic/o, opt/o, ophthalm/o, and ocul/o all mean eye.

65. Kerat/o is the word root/combining form for

✓**(A)** cornea

(B) iris

(C) conjunctiva

(D) pupil

(E) sclera

(A)   is correct. Kerat/o means cornea.
(B)   Iris is ir/o.
(C)   Conjunctiva is conjunctiv/o.
(D)   Pupil is cor/o.
(E)   Sclera is scler/o.

66. Aur/o and ot/o both mean

(A) stapes

(B) eardrum

✓**(C)** ear

(D) cochlea

(E) mastoid process

(C)   is correct. Both aur/o and ot/o refer to the ear.
(A)   Stapes is staped/o.
(B)   Eardrum is myring/o.
(D)   Cochlea is cochle/o.
(E)   Mastoid process is mastoid/o.

67. The prefix ab- means

(A) toward

(B) away from

(C) against

(D) self

(E) both

✓(B)   is correct. Ab- means away from.
(A)   Toward is ad-.
(C)   Against is anti-.
(D)   Self is auto-.
(E)   Both is ambi-.

68. The prefix retro- means

(A) false

(B) left

(C) together

(D) before

(E) behind

✓(E)   is correct. Retro- means behind.
(A)   False is pseudo-.
(B)   Left is sinistro-.
(C)   Together is syn-.
(D)   Before is pre- or pro-.

69. The prefix dextro- means

(A) painful

(B) left

✓**(C)** right

(D) above

(E) below

(C)   is correct. Dextro- means to the right.
(A)   Painful is dys-.
(B)   Left is sinistro-.
(D)   Above is super-.
(E)   Below is sub-.

70. The prefix for water is

(A) hemi-   ✓(D) hydro-
(B) homo-   (E) hetero-
(C) hypo-

     (D) is correct. Hydro- means water.
     (A) Hemi- is half.
     (B) Homo- means the same.
     (C) Hypo- means under or below.
     (E) Hetero- means different.

71. The prefix circum- means

(A) against   (D) among
(B) around   (E) after
(C) away from

    ✓(B) is correct. Circum- means around.
     (A) Against is contra-.
     (C) Away from is ab-.
     (D) Among is inter-.
     (E) After is post- or retro-.

72. The suffix -emia means

(A) dilation   (D) surgical removal of
(B) displacement   ✓(E) condition of the blood
(C) cut

     (E) is correct. -Emia means a condition of the blood.
     (A) Dilation is -ectasis.
     (B) Displacement is -ectopy.
     (C) Cut is -cise.
     (D) Surgical removal of is -ectomy.

73. The suffix for pertaining to or relating to is

(A) -al   (D) -ia
(B) -ac   (E) all the above
(C) -ic

     (E) is correct.

74. The suffix -rrhaphy means

(A) excessive or abnormal flow   ✓(D) to stitch or suture
(B) rupture   (E) fixation
(C) twitch

     (D) is correct. -rrhaphy means to stitch or suture.
     (A) Excessive or abnormal flow is -rrhage.
     (B) Rupture is -rrhexis.
     (C) Twitch is -spasm.
     (E) Fixation is -pexy.

75. The suffix -ostomy means

(A) to surgically create an opening
(B) cutting into
(C) study of
(D) resembling
(E) disease

(A) is correct. -Ostomy means to surgically create an opening.
(B) Cutting into is -otomy.
(C) Study of is -ology.
(D) Resembling is -oid.
(E) Disease is -pathy.

76. The suffix -ion means

(A) inflammation
(B) resembling
(C) small
(D) condition of
(E) remove

(C) is correct. -Ion means small.
(A) Inflammation is -itis.
(B) Resembling is -oid.
(D) Condition of is -id.
(E) Remove is -ize or -ise.

77. The suffix -derma means

(A) pain
(B) dilation
(C) skin
(D) small
(E) kill

(C) is correct. -Derma means skin.
(A) Pain is -dyne.
(B) Dilation is -ectasis.
(D) Small is -cle.
(E) Kill is -cide.

78. The suffix -blast means

(A) to break
(B) to stabilize
(C) softening
(D) to grow
(E) germ cell

(E) is correct. -Blast means germ cell.
(A) To break is -clast.
(B) To stabilize is -desis.
(C) Softening is -malacia.
(D) To grow is -physis.

79. The suffix -crine means

(A) thirst
(B) stimulate
(C) to secrete
(D) development
(E) a substance

(C) is correct. -Crine means to secrete.
(A) Thirst is -dipsia.
(B) Stimulate is -tropin.
(D) Development is -trophy.
(E) A substance is -in or -ine.

80. The suffix -tension means

(A) instrument to measure pressure   (D) pressure
(B) narrowing   (E) record
(C) enlargement

    (D) is correct. -Tension means pressure.
    (A) Instrument to measure pressure is -manometer.
    (B) Narrowing is measure -stenosis.
    (C) Enlargement is -megaly.
    (E) Record is -gram.

81. The suffix -poiesis means

(A) formation   (D) abnormal condition of cells
(B) standing still   (E) to have an attraction for
(C) destruction

    (A) is correct. -Poiesis means formation.
    (B) Standing still is -stasis.
    (C) Destruction is -lytic.
    (D) Abnormal condition of cells is -cytosis.
    (E) To have an attraction for is -phil.

82. The suffix -phage means

(A) protein   (D) cell
(B) embryonic or primitive germ cell   (E) eat or swallow
(C) blood condition

    (E) is correct. The suffix -phage means to eat or swallow.
    (A) Protein is -globin.
    (B) Embryonic or primitive germ cell is -blast.
    (C) A blood condition is -emia.
    (D) Cell is -cyte.

83. The suffix -prandial means

(A) swallowing   (D) vomit
(B) flow or discharge   (E) pertaining to a meal
(C) formation of

    (E) is correct. -Prandial means pertaining to a meal.
    (A) Swallowing is -phagia.
    (B) Flow or discharge is -rrhea.
    (C) Formation of is -iasis.
    (D) Vomit is -emesis.

84. The suffix -tocia means

(A) pregnancy
(B) labor or childbirth
(C) turning of
(D) to bear
(E) beginning

    (B) is correct. -Tocia means labor or childbirth.
    (A) Pregnancy is -gravida.
    (C) Turning of is -version.
    (D) To bear is -para.
    (E) Beginning is -arch.

85. The suffix -esthesia means

(A) feeling and sensation
(B) movement
(C) pain
(D) strength
(E) paralysis

    (A) is correct. -Esthesia means feeling and sensation.
    (B) Movement is -kinesis.
    (C) Pain is -algia.
    (D) Strength is -sthenia.
    (E) Paralysis is -plegia.

86. The suffix -mycosis means

(A) discharge of pus
(B) hearing
(C) vision
(D) fungal infection
(E) relaxation

    (D) is correct. -Mycosis is a fungal infection.
    (A) Discharge of pus is -pyorrhea.
    (B) Hearing is -cusis.
    (C) Vision is -opia.
    (E) Relaxation is -chalasis.

CHAPTER 2

ANATOMY AND PHYSIOLOGY

1. Anatomy is the

    (A) science of the function of living organisms
    (B) basic unit of all living things
    (C) study of tissue
    ✔(D) study of the structure of an organism
    (E) sum of all physical and chemical changes that take place within an organism

      (D) is correct. Anatomy is the study of the structure of an organism.
      (A) Physiology is the science of the function of all living organisms.
      (B) The cell is the basic unit of all living things.
      (C) Histology is the study of tissue.
      (E) Metabolism is the sum of all physical and chemical changes that take place within an organism.

2. The major categories of tissues are

    (A) striated, smooth, and cardiac
    (B) voluntary and involuntary
    ✔(C) muscle, epithelial, connective, and nerve
    (D) bones, tendons, and fatty
    (E) sagittal, frontal, and transverse

      (C) is correct. The four types of tissue are muscle, epithelial, connective, and nerve.
      (A) Striated, smooth, and cardiac are examples of muscle tissue.
      (B) Voluntary and involuntary are examples of the functions of muscle movement.
      (D) Bones, tendons, and fatty tissue are examples of where connective tissue is found.
      (E) Sagittal, frontal, and transverse are examples of body planes.

3. The study of tissue is

    (A) orthopedics   ✔(D) histology
    (B) hematology   (E) homeostasis
    (C) cardiology

      (D) is correct. The study of tissue is histology.
      (A) Orthopedics is the study of the musculoskeletal systems (bones and joints).
      (B) Hematology is the study of blood.
      (C) Cardiology is the study of the cardiovascular system (heart and circulation).
      (E) Homeostasis is the body's constant state of attempting to maintain a balance or equilibrium.

4. The anatomical position is

   (A) the body position with legs parallel with toes and feet pointing forward
   (B) the body standing erect with the arms at the sides and palms facing forward
   (C) used to describe the positions and relationships of a structure in the human body
   (D) used for descriptive purposes even if the body or body parts are in any other position
   ✓**(E)** all of the above

       (E)   is correct.

5. The frontal, or coronal, body plane

   (A) runs lengthwise and divides the body or any of its parts into right and left components
   ✓**(B)** divides the body into an anterior, or ventral, and a posterior, or dorsal, portion
   (C) is a crosswise plane that runs parallel to the ground
   (D) divides the body or its parts into superior (upper) and inferior (lower) parts
   (E) is also called the horizontal plane

       (B)   is correct.
       (A)   The sagittal plane divides the body into right and left components.
       (C)   The transverse plane is a crosswise plane that runs parallel to the ground.
       (D)   The transverse plane divides the body into its superior and inferior parts.
       (E)   The transverse plane is also called the horizontal plane.

6. A lengthwise body plane running from side to side is the

   (A) frontal plane   ✓**(D)** sagittal plane
   (B) coronal plane   **(E)** transverse plane
   (C) horizontal plane —— SAME

       (D)   is correct. The sagittal plane runs lengthwise and divides the body into right and left components. If the body is divided into two equal parts, this would be called a midsagittal plane.
       (A)   The frontal plane divides the body into anterior and posterior portions.
       (B)   The coronal plane is also called the frontal plane.
       (C)   The horizontal plane is also called the transverse plane.
       (E)   The transverse plane is the same as the horizontal plane.

7. The body planes

   (A) are imaginary cuts slicing through the body
   (B) are useful for describing the body and its parts
   (C) do not have to be equal in size
   (D) have more than one name
   ✓**(E)** all of the above

       (E)   is correct.

8. To move toward the median or midline of the body is called

   (A) adduction
   (B) abduction
   (C) lateral

   (D) inversion
   (E) eversion

   ✓(A) is correct. A movement toward the median is the directional term adduction.
   (B) Abduction is to move away from the median or midline of the body.
   (C) Lateral refers to the side.
   (D) Inversion is to turn inward or inside out.
   (E) Eversion is to turn outward.

9. The body lying horizontally, facing downward, is in what position?

   (A) parietal
   (B) visceral
   (C) supine

   ✓**(D)** prone
   (E) superficial

   (D) is correct. Prone is lying horizontally, facing downward.
   (A) Parietal refers to the wall of an organ or cavity.
   (B) Visceral refers to the covering of the surface of the body or organ.
   (C) Supine refers to the body lying horizontally, facing upward.
   (E) Superficial refers to the outer surface of the body or structure.

10. The cephalic, or superior, position is

   (A) toward the feet or tail
   (B) near or on the front of the body
   (C) near or on the back of the body
   (D) the tip or summit
   ✓**(E)** toward the head, surface of the body, or above

   (E) is correct. The cephalic, or superior, position is toward the head, surface of the body, or above.
   (A) The inferior, or caudal, position is toward the feet or tail or away from the surface of the body.
   (B) The anterior, or ventral, position is near or on the front of the body.
   (C) The posterior, or dorsal, position is near or on the back of the body.
   (D) The apex refers to the tip or summit.

11. The two dorsal cavities of the body contain the

   (A) mediastinum
   (B) diaphragm
   (C) heart and lungs
   ✓**(D)** cranial cavity, including the brain and spinal cavity, and the spinal cord
   (E) abdominopelvic cavity

   (D) is correct. The dorsal cavities include the cranial cavity, containing the brain and spinal cavity, and the spinal cord.
   (A) The mediastinum, which is the area between the lungs, is found in the thoracic cavity.
   (B) The diaphragm is the physical wall between the thoracic cavity and the abdominal cavity.

(C) The heart and lungs are found in the thoracic cavity, which is part of the ventral cavity.

(E) The abdominopelvic cavity contains the organs of digestion, reproduction, and excretion.

12. Which of the following is NOT included in the dorsal cavity?

(A) brain   (D) vertebra
(B) spinal cavity   ✔(E) lungs
(C) spinal cord

(E) is correct. The lungs are included in the thoracic cavity, which is part of the ventral cavity. The brain (A), spinal cavity (B), spinal cord (C), and vertebra (D) are all found in the dorsal cavity.

13. The spleen, lymph vessels, and lymphocytes are considered to be part of what system?

(A) cardiovascular   (D) endocrine
✔(B) lymphatic and hematic (blood)   (E) integumentary
(C) gastrointestinal

(B) is correct. The spleen, lymph vessels, and lymphocytes are all part of the lymphatic and hematic system.

(A) The cardiovascular system contains the heart, blood vessels (including the arteries), veins, and capillaries.

(C) The gastrointestinal system contains the mouth, pharynx, esophagus, small and large intestines, liver, gallbladder, pancreas, and anus (rectum).

(D) The endocrine system contains the thyroid, pituitary, adrenal, pancreas, parathyroid, pineal, and thymus glands, and the testes and ovaries.

(E) The integumentary (skin) system includes the skin, nails, hair, and sweat and sebaceous glands.

14. Which of the following organs and structures is/are NOT found in the endocrine system?

(A) pineal   (D) testes
(B) ovaries   ✔(E) spleen
(C) thymus

(E) is correct. The spleen is part of the lymphatic and hematic systems. The pineal gland (A), ovaries (B), thymus gland (C), and testes (D) are all part of the endocrine system. The ovaries and testes are also part of the reproductive system.

15. Which of the following organs is/are part of the respiratory system?

(A) mouth   ✔(D) A, B, and C
(B) bronchial tubes and lungs   (E) B and C only
(C) pharynx, larynx, and trachea

(D) is correct. The mouth is included as part of the respiratory system. It is also a component of the gastrointestinal system.

16. The special senses include

(A) taste
(B) vision and hearing
(C) smell
(D) touch
✔(E) all of the above

   (E) is correct. The senses of taste (A), vision and hearing (B), smell (C), and touch (D) are all considered special senses.

17. The male reproductive system does NOT include

✔(A) ureters
(B) urethra
(C) vas deferens
(D) prostate
(E) testes

   (A) is correct. The ureters (A), or tubes carrying the urine from the kidneys to the urinary bladder, are part of the urinary system. The urethra (B), or channel for urine to pass from the urinary bladder to outside of the body, is part of the male reproductive system and part of the urinary system. The vas deferens (C), which is severed during the vasectomy procedure, the prostate gland (D), and the two testes (E) are all part of the male reproductive system.

18. The physician who specializes in disorders of the gastrointestinal tract is a/an

(A) urologist
(B) gynecologist
(C) neurologist
(D) proctologist
(E) endocrinologist

   ✔(D) is correct. A proctologist is a physician who specializes in disease and disorders of the gastrointestinal tract and, in particular, the anal canal.
   (A) A urologist specializes in disorders of the urinary system.
   (B) A gynecologist specializes in disorders of the female reproductive system.
   (C) A neurologist specializes in disorders of the nervous system.
   (E) An endocrinologist specializes in disorders of the endocrine system.

19. The dermis layer of the skin contains

(A) keratin
(B) melanin
(C) stratified squamous epithelium
(D) blood vessels
(E) basal layer

   (D) is correct. The dermis layer of skin contains the blood vessels, lymph vessels, sebaceous glands, nerve fibers, and muscle fibers. Keratin (A), melanin (B), stratified squamous epithelium (C), and the basal layer (E) are all found in the epidermis layer.

20. The black pigment that gives skin its color is

(A) basal layer
(B) keratin
(C) melanin
(D) cyano
(E) chloro

   (C) is correct. Melanin is the black pigment that gives skin its color. Melan/o is the combining form meaning black.

(A) The basal layer contains melanocytes, which form melanin.
(B) Keratin is a protein found in the epidermis.
(D) Cyano is a prefix used to describe the color blue.
(E) Chloro is a prefix used to describe the color green.

21. Which of the following is NOT a layer of the skin?

(A) subcutaneous
(B) dermis
(C) epidermis
(D) intramuscular
(E) keratin

(D) is correct. The intramuscular layer is found between muscle layers and is not considered a layer of the skin. The three layers of the skin are subcutaneous (A), dermis (B), and epidermis (C). Keratin (E) is found within the subcutaneous layer.

22. The medical term for a dangerous form of skin cancer caused by an overgrowth of melanin-producing cells is

(A) Kaposi's sarcoma
(B) malignant melanoma
(C) basal cell carcinoma
(D) squamous cell carcinoma
(E) lupus erythematosus

(B) is correct. Malignant melanoma is a dangerous form of skin cancer caused by an overgrowth of melanin-producing cell. This is seen in persons who have had long exposure to the sun.
(A) Kaposi's sarcoma is found in patients with AIDS.
(C) Basal cell carcinoma is an epithelial tumor of the basal cell layer of the epidermis.
(D) Squamous cell carcinoma is a cancer found in the epidermal layer and does not generally metastasize.
(E) Lupus erythematosus is a chronic disease of the connective tissue that may injure joints, kidneys, nervous system, and mucous membranes.

23. Urticaria is the medical term for

(A) ringworm
(B) hives
(C) verruca
(D) furuncle
(E) scabies

(B) is correct. Urticaria is also called hives.
(A) Ringworm, also called tinea, is caused by a fungus.
(C) Verruca, also called warts, is a benign neoplasm.
(D) Furuncle, also called a boil, is caused by a staphylococcus.
(E) Scabies is a contagious skin disease caused by egg-laying mites.

24. A chronic inflammatory condition consisting of crusty, silvery papules forming patches with pink, circular borders is called

(A) eczema
(B) psoriasis
(C) cellulitis
(D) scleroderma
(E) neoplasm

(B) is correct. Psoriasis is a chronic inflammatory condition.

(A)   Eczema is superficial dermatitis accompanied by papules, vesicles, and crusting.

(C)   Cellulitis is an inflammation of the cellular or connective tissue.

(D)   Scleroderma is a skin disorder in which the skin becomes taut, thick, and leatherlike.

(E)   Neoplasm is a tumor, which can be either benign or cancerous.

25. How many bones are in the lumbar vertebra?

(A) 1   **(D)** 7
(B) 3   **(E)** 12
(C) 5

(C)   is correct. There are 5 bones in the lumbar vertebra.

(A)   The sacral vertebra and the coccyx both have 1 bone, which is the result of separate bones becoming fused during childhood (5 in the sacral bone and 3 to 5 in the coccyx).

(B)   There are 5 lumbar vertebra.

(D)   There are 7 cervical bones.

(E)   There are 12 thoracic bones.

26. The end of a long bone is called the

(A) epiphysis   **(D)** mediastinum
(B) diaphysis   **(E)** cartilage
(C) periosteum

(A)   is correct. The epiphysis is the end of a long bone.

(B)   The diaphysis is the middle shaft of a long bone.

(C)   The periosteum is the fibrous membrane that forms the covering of bones.

(D)   The mediastinum is a septum or cavity between two portions of an organ.

(E)   Cartilage is dense connective tissue that forms a part of the skeleton in the adult.

27. Which of the following is NOT one of the os coxae bones?

(A) ilium   **(D)** ischium
(B) ileum   **(E)** all of the above
(C) pubis

(B)   is correct. The ileum is part of the small intestine. The ilium (A), the pubis (C), and the ischium (D) make up the os coxae (also called the innominate bone or hipbone).

28. Which is NOT one of the divisions of the spine?

(A) lumbar   **(D)** cervical
(B) thoracic   **(E)** sacral
(C) parietal

(C)   is correct. The parietal bones (2) are part of the cranial bones. All the other bones listed are divisions of the spine.

29. A deficiency in vitamin D can cause what bone disorder?

(A) gout
(B) scurvy
(C) rickets
(D) scoliosis
(E) lordosis

(C) is correct. Rickets, which results in inadequate bone formation (especially bowed legs), is caused by a lack of vitamin D in the diet.
(A) Gout is an inflammation of the joints caused by excessive uric acid.
(B) Scurvy is caused by a deficiency of vitamin C.
(D) Scoliosis is an abnormal lateral curvature of the spine.
(E) Lordosis is an abnormal increase in the outward curvature of the thoracic spine.

30. The cheekbones are the

(A) mandibular bones
(B) maxillary bones
(C) palatine bones
(D) zygomatic bones
(E) lacrimal bones

(D) is correct. The zygomatic bones are the cheekbones.
(A) The mandibular bone is the lower jaw bone.
(B) The maxillary bone is the upper jaw bone.
(C) The palatine bone forms part of the hard palate.
(E) The lacrimal bones are in the inner corner of each eye.

31. Which of the following is NOT one of the cranial bones?

(A) temporal
(B) vomer
(C) occipital
(D) parietal
(E) sphenoid

(B) is correct. The vomer bone is at the base of the nasal septum.
(A) The temporal bones are at the sides and base of the cranium.
(C) The occipital bone is at the back and base of the skull.
(D) The parietal bones are at the upper sides of the cranium and the roof of the skull.
(E) The sphenoid bone is a bat-shaped bone that forms part of the base of the skull, floor, and sides of eye orbit.

32. Which bone is NOT one of the bones of the upper extremities?

(A) fibula
(B) clavicle
(C) scapula
(D) humerus
(E) radius

(A) is correct. The fibula is the lateral, smaller bone of the lower leg, from the ankle to the knee.
(B) The clavicle is also called the collarbone.
(C) The scapula is also called the shoulder blade.
(D) The humerus is the upper arm bone.
(E) The radius is the bone on the thumb side of the arm.

33. Which bone is NOT one of the lower-extremity bones?

(A) femur   (D) ulna

(B) patella   (E) tarsal

(C) tibia

> (D) is correct. The ulna is the bone on the finger side of the lower arm.
> (A) The femur is the large thigh bone.
> (B) The patella is the kneecap.
> (C) The tibia is the medial bone located in the lower leg.
> (E) The tarsal bones are the ankle bones.

34. A wrist fracture is

(A) comminuted   (D) greenstick

(B) compound   (E) Colles'

(C) transverse

> (E) is correct. A Colles' fracture is a fractured wrist.
> (A) A comminuted fracture is one in which the bone is shattered, splintered, or crushed into fragments.
> (B) A compound fracture is an open fracture in which the skin has been broken through to the fracture.
> (C) A transverse fracture is a complete fracture that is straight across the bone at right angles to the long axis of the bone.
> (D) A greenstick fracture is an incomplete break in which one side of the bone is broken and the other side is bent.

35. Backward bending movement at a joint is called

(A) circumduction   (D) supination

(B) inversion   (E) plantar flexion

(C) dorsiflexion

> (C) is correct. Dorsiflexion is the backward bending of a portion of the body, such as of a hand or foot.
> (A) Circumduction is movement in a circular direction from a central point.
> (B) Inversion is a turning inward movement.
> (D) Supination is turning the palm or foot upward.
> (E) Plantar flexion refers to bending the sole of the foot or pointing the toes downward.

36. An autoimmune disease causing loss of muscle strength and paralysis is

(A) myopathy   (D) rheumatoid arthritis

(B) myasthenia gravis   (E) systemic lupus erythematosis

(C) muscular dystrophy

> (B) is correct. Myasthenia gravis is an autoimmune disorder causing loss of muscle strength and paralysis.
> (A) Myopathy is any disease of the muscles.
> (C) Muscular dystrophy is an inherited disease causing progressive muscle weakness and atrophy.

(D) Rheumatoid arthritis is a chronic form of arthritis with inflammation of joints, swelling, stiffness, pain, and changes in cartilage, which can result in crippling deformities.

(E) Systemic lupus erythematosis is an autoimmune disease that does not result in paralysis.

37. Talipes, or clubfoot, is a congenital deformity of the foot, which has several variations. Which of the following is NOT one of the variations of talipes?

(A) equis   **(D)** varus

(B) valgus   **(E)** planus

(C) vagus

(C) is correct. Vagus is the name of the 10th cranial nerve, which has control over several functions (including heart rate).

(A) Equis occurs when only the front of the foot touches the ground, causing the person to walk on the toes.

(B) Valgus occurs when the foot is everted, with the inner side of the foot resting on the ground.

(D) Varus occurs when the foot is inverted, and the outer side of the foot touches the ground.

(E) Planus occurs when the arch is broken, causing the entire foot to be flat on the ground.

38. Removal of knee cartilage is called

(A) laminectomy   **(D)** arthroplasty

(B) fasciectomy   **(E)** reduction

(C) menisectomy

(C) is correct. A menisectomy is the removal of knee cartilage (meniscus). The word root chondr/o also refers to cartilage.

(A) A laminectomy is the removal of the vertebral posterior arch to correct severe back problems and pain caused by compression of the lamina.

(B) Fasciectomy is the surgical removal of the fascia, which is the fibrous membrane covering and supporting muscles.

(D) Arthroplasty is the surgical reconstruction of a joint.

(E) Reduction is correcting a fracture by realigning the bone fragments. Closed reduction is performed by manipulation without entering the body. Open reduction is the surgical incision at the site of the fracture to do the reduction.

39. Arthrocentesis is the

(A) study of the spinal column after injecting opaque contrast material

(B) visualization of a joint by radiographic study after injection of a contrast medium into the joint space

(C) study and recording of the strength of muscle contractions as a result of electrical stimulation

(D) removal of synovial fluid with a needle from a joint space, such as a knee, for examination

(E) fusion or stiffening of a joint to provide stability

(D) is correct. Arthrocentesis is the removal of synovial fluid with a needle from a joint space, such as a knee, for examination.

(A) Myelography is the study of the spinal column after injecting contrast material.

(B) Arthrography is the radiographic study of a joint.

(C) Electromyography is the study of strength of muscle contractions.

(E) Arthrodesis is the fusion or stiffening of a joint for stability.

40. The measurement of bone density using an instrument for the purpose of detecting osteoporosis is called

(A) computerized axial tomography (CT or CAT scan)

(B) magnetic resonance imaging (MRI)

(C) myelography

(D) bone scan

(E) photon absorptiometry

(E) is correct. Photon absorptiometry is the measurement of bone density using an instrument for the purpose of detecting osteoporosis.

(A) Computerized axial tomography (CT or CAT scan) is a computer-assisted x-ray used to detect tumors and fractures.

(B) Magnetic resonance imaging (MRI) is medical imaging that uses radio-frequency radiation as its source of energy. It is useful for visualizing large blood vessels, the heart, brain, and soft tissue.

(C) Myelography is the study of the spinal column after injecting opaque contrast material.

(D) Bone scan is the use of scanning equipment to visualize bones.

41. The surgical repair of cartilage is

(A) chrondroplasty

(B) periositis

(C) osteopathy

(D) lordosis

(E) kyphosis

(A) is correct. Chrondroplasty is the surgical repair of cartilage.

(B) Periositis is an inflammation of the periosteum.

(C) Osteopathy refers to any bone disease.

(D) Lordosis, also referred to as swayback, is an abnormal increase in the forward curvature of the lumbar spine.

(E) Kyphosis, also referred to as humpback, is an abnormal increase in the outward curvature of the thoracic spine.

42. Glands that secrete a fluid, such as tears, through a duct or another organ are

(A) endocrine

(B) exocrine

(C) thymus

(D) parathyroid

(E) adrenal

(B) is correct. Exocrine glands secrete a fluid through a duct or another organ.

(A) Endocrine glands are ductless glands that produce internal secretions, which are called hormones.

(C) The thymus gland, located in the mediastinal cavity, is an endocrine gland that secretes the hormone thymosin and is essential in the development of T cells.

(D) Parathyroid glands are four tiny glands located on the dorsal or back surface of the thyroid gland.

(E) The adrenal glands (2) are located above each kidney and manufacture steroids.

43. The endocrine gland that is responsible for stimulating growth with the growth hormone (GH) is the

(A) parathyroid
(B) pancreas
(C) pituitary posterior lobe
(D) pituitary anterior lobe
(E) adrenal cortex

(D) is correct. The anterior lobe of the pituitary produces the growth hormone, the adrenocorticotropic hormone (ACTH), the follicle-stimulating hormone (FSH), the luteinizing hormone (LH), the melanocyte-stimulating hormone (MSH), prolactin, and the thyroid-stimulating hormone (TSH).

(A) The parathyroid glands produce parathyroid hormone, which regulates calcium and stimulates bone breakdown.

(B) The pancreas is responsible for the production of insulin and glucagon.

(C) The posterior lobe of the pituitary produces antidiuretic hormone (ADH), which stimulates the reabsorption of water, and oxytocin, which stimulates uterine contractions and releases milk into ducts.

(E) The adrenal cortex produces the sex hormones androgen, estrogen, and progestin. It assists in regulating electrolytes and fluid volume in the body with mineralocorticoids.

44. The result of inadequate secretion of the antidiuretic hormone from the pituitary gland is

(A) diabetes insipidus
(B) diabetes mellitus
(C) tetany
(D) exophthalmos
(E) Addison's disease

(A) is correct. Diabetes insipidus is the result of an inadequate secretion of the antidiuretic hormone by the posterior lobe of the pituitary gland.

(B) Diabetes mellitus is a chronic disorder of carbohydrate metabolism, which results in hyperglycemia and glucosuria.

(C) Tetany, or muscle excitability, is the result of a calcium deficiency caused by a disorder of the parathyroid glands.

(D) Exophthalmos is a condition in which the eyeballs protrude, such as in Graves' disease. This is generally caused by an overproduction of thyroid hormone.

(E) Addison's disease results from a deficiency in adrenocortical hormones. There may be an increased pigmentation of the skin, generalized weakness, and weight loss.

45. A chronic form of thyroiditis is

(A) myasthenia gravis
(B) myxedema
(C) Graves' disease
(D) Hashimoto's disease
(E) ketoacidosis

(D) is correct. Hashimoto's disease is a chronic form of thyroiditis, which is named for a Japanese surgeon.

(A) Myasthenia gravis is a condition in which there is great muscular weakness and progressive fatigue. If due to a thymus tumor, it may be treated with removal of the thymus gland.

(B) Myxedema is a condition resulting from a hypofunction of the thyroid gland. Symptoms include anemia, slow speech, enlarged tongue and facial features, edematous skin, and mental apathy.

(C) Graves' disease is a condition that results in an overactive thyroid gland.

(E) Ketoacidosis is due to an excess of ketone bodies.

46. The inner layer of the heart is the

(A) pericardium
(B) myocardium
(C) apex
(D) endocardium
(E) mediastinum

(D) is correct. The endocardium is the inner layer of the heart.

(A) The pericardium is the outer double-walled sac that contains pericardial fluid between the layers to prevent friction during the heartbeats. The inner layer of the pericardium is the epicardium.

(B) The myocardium is the muscular middle layer of the heart.

(C) The apex is the tip of the heart at the lower edge.

(E) The mediastinum, a septum dividing two cavities, is located in the center of the chest cavity.

47. Another name for the mitral valve of the heart is

(A) tricuspid
(B) pulmonary semilunar
(C) bicuspid
(D) aortic semilunar
(E) intraventricular septum

(C) is correct. The mitral valve is also called the bicuspid valve, indicating that it has two points or cusps. Blood flows through this valve to the left ventricle and cannot go back up into the left atrium.

(A) The tricuspid valve of the heart controls the opening between the right atrium and the right ventricle.

(B) The pulmonary semilunar valve is between the right ventricle and the pulmonary artery.

(D) The aortic semilunar valve is between the left ventricle and the aorta.

(E) The intraventricular septum is the wall of tissue dividing the two sides of the ventricles in the heart.

48. Blood enters the right atrium of the heart through the

(A) pulmonary artery
(B) superior and inferior vena cava
(C) pulmonary veins
(D) descending aorta
(E) coronary artery

(B)   is correct. Blood enters the right atrium from all the tissues of the body through two blood vessels, the superior and inferior vena cava.

(A)   The pulmonary artery receives blood pumped through the pulmonary semilunar valves by the ventricle and carries it to the lungs.

(C)   The pulmonary veins carry blood into the left atrium after it has been oxygenated by the lungs.

(D)   The descending aorta carries blood to the body. The aorta, which is the largest artery in the body, begins from the left ventricle of the heart.

(E)   The coronary artery branches from the aorta and provides blood to the myocardium or heart muscle.

49. The congenital presence of a connection between the pulmonary artery and the aorta that remains after birth is called

(A)   myocardial infarction
(B)   mitral stenosis
(C)   tetralogy of Fallot
(D)   patent ductus arteriosus
(E)   coronary ischemia

(D)   is correct. Patent ductus arteriosus is the congenital presence of a connection between the pulmonary artery and the aorta that remains after birth.

(A)   Myocardial infarction, also called a heart attack, is a condition caused by the partial or complete occlusion or closing of one or more of the coronary arteries.

(B)   Mitral stenosis is the narrowing of the opening (orifice) of the mitral valve, which causes an obstruction in the flow of blood from the atrium to the ventricle.

(C)   Tetralogy of Fallot is a congenital defect present at birth, which is a combination of four symptoms (tetralogy) resulting in pulmonary stenosis, septal defect, abnormal blood supply to the aorta, and hypertrophy of the right ventricle.

(E)   Coronary ischemia is an insufficient blood supply to the heart due to an obstruction.

50. Lymph fluid consists of

(A)   carbon dioxide (CO_2) and oxygen (O_2)
(B)   lymphocytes
(C)   hormones
(D)   salts, water, and nutrients
(E)   all of the above

(E)   is correct.

51. Accessory lymph organs include

(A)   pharynx, larynx, trachea, and bronchi
(B)   liver, gallbladder, and pancreas
(C)   tonsils, spleen, and thymus gland
(D)   lymphatic duct, thoracic duct, and lymph nodes
(E)   ureters, urethra, and kidneys

(C)   is correct. The tonsils, spleen, and thymus assist the lymph organs to maintain the immunity system of the body.

(A) The pharynx, larynx, trachea, and bronchi are organs of the respiratory system.

(B) The liver, gallbladder, and pancreas are accessory organs of the digestive system.

(D) The lymphatic duct, thoracic duct, and lymph nodes are the main organs and structures of the lymphatic system.

(E) The ureters, urethra, and kidneys are organs of the urinary system.

52. Humoral immunity refers to

(A) the binding of an antigen with an antibody
(B) the production of plasma lymphocytes or B cells
(C) the production of lymphocytes or T cells
(D) a severe reaction to an antigen
(E) a hypersensitivity to an allergen

(B) is correct. Humoral immunity results from the production of lymphocytes or B cells.

(A) The binding of an antigen with an antibody to render the toxic antigen harmless is called the immune reaction.

(C) The production of lymphocytes or T cells is called cellular immunity.

(D) A severe reaction to an antigen is called anaphylaxis.

(E) A hypersensitivity to an allergen is called an allergy.

53. An autoimmune viral disease that attacks T4 lymphocytes and destroys them, causing a reduction in the person's ability to fight off infection, is

(A) hepatitis
(B) Epstein-Barr virus
(C) multiple sclerosis
(D) Hodgkin's disease
(E) acquired immune deficiency syndrome (AIDS)

(E) is correct. AIDS is an autoimmune viral disease that attacks T4 lymphocytes.

(A) Hepatitis is an inflammatory disease of the liver caused by the hepatitis B virus.

(B) Epstein-Barr virus is believed to be the cause of infectious mononucleosis.

(C) Multiple sclerosis is an autoimmune disorder of the central nervous system in which the myelin sheath of nerves is attacked.

(D) Hodgkin's disease is a lymphatic system disease that can result in solid tumors in lymphoid tissue.

54. Donut-shaped blood cells that contain no nucleus or central kernel are

(A) erythrocytes   **(D)** neutrophils
(B) leukocytes   **(E)** basophils
(C) monocytes

(A) is correct. Erythrocytes are red blood cells that contain no nucleus.

(B) Leukocytes are white blood cells that provide protection against the invasion of bacteria and other foreign materials.

(C) Monocytes are agranulocytic leukocytes, which are important for phagocytosis (ingest and destroy bacteria).

(D) Neutrophils are granulocytic leukocytes, which are the most numerous leukocytes.

(E) Basophils are granulocytic leukocytes, which release histamine and heparin to damaged tissue.

55. A blood test to determine the rate at which mature blood cells settle out of the blood after the addition of an anticoagulant is

(A) complete blood count (CBC)
(B) differential
(C) erythrocyte sedimentation rate (ESR)
(D) hematocrit (Hct, crit)
(E) hemoglobin (Hg)

(C) is correct. The erythrocyte sedimentation rate (ESR) is a blood test to determine the rate at which mature blood cells settle out of the blood after the addition of an anticoagulant.

(A) A complete blood count (CBC) consists of five tests: red blood cell count (RBC), white blood count (WBC), hemoglobin (Hg), hematocrit (Hct), and white blood cell differential.

(B) A differential blood test is used to determine the number of each variety of leukocytes (WBCs).

(D) A hematocrit (Hct) blood test is used to measure the volume of erythrocytes in a given volume of blood.

(E) The hemoglobin (Hg) blood count measures the amount of iron-containing pigment of red blood cells.

56. Cilia means

(A) lack of oxygen
(B) absence of oxygen in the blood
(C) absence of oxygen in the tissue
(D) hairs
(E) harsh, high-pitched, noisy breathing

(D) is correct. Cilia are small hairs that serve as protection against infectious microorganisms. They are found in the nasal opening and on the eyes as eyelashes.

(A) Lack of oxygen is called anoxia.

(B) The absence of oxygen in the blood is called anoxemia.

(C) The absence of oxygen in the tissue is called hypoxia.

(E) Harsh, high-pitched, noisy breathing is called stridor.

57. A respiratory disease seen mainly in AIDS patients and debilitated children is

(A) paroxysmal nocturnal dyspnea
(B) *Pneumocystis carinii*
(C) Legionnaire's disease
(D) hyaline membrane disease
(E) histoplasmosis

(B) is correct. *Pneumocystis carinii* is a type of pneumonia, with a nonproductive cough, very little fever, and dyspnea, that is seen mainly in AIDS patients.

(A) Paroxysmal nocturnal dyspnea is attacks of shortness of breath (SOB) that occur only at night and awaken the patient.

(C) Legionnaire's disease is a severe, often fatal disease characterized by pneumonia and gastrointestinal symptoms.

(D) Hyaline membrane disease is a condition seen in premature infants whose lungs have not had time to develop properly.

(E) Histoplasmosis is a pulmonary disease from the dust in the droppings of pigeons and chickens.

58. The insertion of a tube into the chest for the purpose of draining off fluid or air is called

(A) tracheotomy
(B) tracheostomy
(C) thoracentesis
(D) thoracostomy
(E) pneumonectomy

(D) is correct. Thoracostomy (or thoracotomy) is the insertion of a tube into the chest for the purpose of draining off fluid or air.

(A) Tracheotomy is a surgical incision into the trachea to provide an airway.

(B) Tracheostomy is a surgical procedure into the trachea to create an airway. A tube is inserted to keep the opening patent.

(C) Thoracentesis is the surgical puncture of the chest wall for the removal of fluids.

(E) Pneumonectomy is the surgical removal of lung tissue.

59. The total volume of air that can be exhaled after a maximum inspiration is called

(A) vital capacity
(B) total lung capacity
(C) residual air
(D) tidal volume
(E) functional residual capacity

(A) is correct. Vital capacity is the volume of air that can be exhaled after a maximum inspiration. This amount will be equal to the sum of tidal air, complemental air, and supplemental air.

(B) Total lung capacity is the volume of air in the lungs after a maximal inhalation or inspiration.

(C) Residual air is the air remaining in the lungs after a forced expiration (about 1500 cc in the adult).

(D) Tidal volume is the amount of air that enters the lungs in a single inspiration or leaves the lungs in a single expiration of quiet breathing (about 500 cc in the adult).

(E) Functional residual capacity is the air that remains in the lungs after a normal expiration has taken place.

60. A small piece of tissue at the back of the pharynx that covers the larynx and trachea so that food cannot enter the lungs is the

(A) fundus
(B) papillae
(C) bolus
(D) cecum
(E) epiglottis

(E) is correct. The epiglottis is a small piece of tissue at the back of the pharynx that covers the larynx and trachea so that food cannot enter the lungs.

(A) The fundus is the upper region, or main portion, of the stomach or uterus.

(B) Papillae, also called taste buds, are raised elevations on the surface of the tongue, which distinguish among bitterness, sweetness, sourness, and saltiness in food.

(C) A bolus is formed material that occurs when saliva mixes with food, which is then ready to swallow.

(D) Cecum is a pouch or saclike area in the first 2 to 3 inches at the beginning of the large intestine.

61. The pyloric sphincter, located in the distal or lower end of the stomach, controls the passage of food into what location?

(A) jejunum of the small intestine
(B) duodenum of the small intestine
(C) cecum of the large intestine
(D) sigmoid colon
(E) appendix

    (B) is correct. The pyloric sphincter controls the passage of food into the duodenum. The duodenum extends from the pylorus of the stomach to the jejunum.

    (A) The jejunum, or middle portion of the small intestine, extends from the middle of the small intestine to the ileum and is about 8 feet long.

    (C) The cecum is a pouch or saclike area in the first 2 to 3 inches at the beginning of the large intestine.

    (D) The sigmoid colon portion of the large intestine is connected above to the descending colon and below to the rectum.

    (E) The appendix, which appears to have no purpose within the body, is a small outgrowth at the end of the cecum.

62. A jejunoileostomy is the surgical

(A) creation of a gastric fistula or opening through the abdominal wall
(B) removal of part or the whole of the stomach
(C) removal of the colon
(D) creation of an opening between the jejunum and the ileum
(E) removal of a lobe of the liver

    (D) is correct. A jejunoileostomy is the surgical creation of an opening between the jejunum and the ileum.

    (A) A gastrostomy is the surgical creation of a gastric fistula or opening through the abdominal wall.

    (B) A gastrectomy is the surgical removal of part or the whole of the stomach.

    (C) A colectomy is the surgical removal of the colon.

    (E) A hepatic lobectomy is the surgical removal of a lobe of the liver.

63. An abdominal operation for the purpose of examining the abdominal organs and tissues for signs of disease or other abnormalities is called a/an

(A) diverticulectomy
(B) fistulectomy
(C) exploratory laparotomy
(D) ileostomy
(E) gastrectomy

(C)   is correct. An exploratory laparotomy is an abdominal operation for the purpose of examining the abdominal organs and tissues for signs of disease or other abnormalities.

(A)   A diverticulectomy is the surgical removal of a diverticulum.

(B)   A fistulectomy is the excision of a fistula.

(D)   An ileostomy is the surgical creation of a passage through the abdominal wall into the ileum.

(E)   A gastrectomy is the surgical removal of part or the whole of the stomach.

64. The genitourinary system includes

(A) brain, spinal cord, and nerves
(B) muscles, tendons, bones, joints, and cartilage
(C) spleen, lymph vessels, and lymphocytes
(D) ureters, urethra, bladder, and kidneys
(E) uterus, fallopian tubes, ovaries, vagina, and mammary glands

(D)   is correct. The genitourinary system, or urinary system, includes the ureters, urethra, bladder, and kidneys.

(A)   The nervous system contains the brain, spinal cord, and nerves.

(B)   The musculoskeletal system contains the muscles, tendons, bones, joints, and cartilage.

(C)   The lymphatic system contains the spleen, lymph vessels, and lymphocytes.

(E)   The female reproductive system contains the uterus, fallopian tubes, ovaries, vagina, and mammary glands.

65. The filtration of waste products takes place in the

(A) ureters   **(D)** bladder
(B) nephrons   **(E)** meatus
(C) urethra

(B)   is correct. The nephrons, located in the outer layer of each kidney, are the functional structures that filtrate the waste products from the body. There are over 2 million nephrons in the body.

(A)   The ureters (2) are narrow tubes, 10 to 12 inches long, that extend from the renal pelvis to the urinary bladder.

(C)   The urethra (1) is a tubular canal that carries the flow of urine from the bladder to the outside of the body.

(D)   The bladder is an elastic muscular sac that lies in the base of the pelvis just behind the pubic symphysis.

(E)   Meatus is a term meaning an opening.

66. The urine is 95 percent

(A) nitrogenous waste products   **(D)** water
(B) toxins   **(E)** hormones
(C) electrolytes

(D)   is correct. Urine is 95 percent water. Nitrogenous waste products (A), toxins (B), electrolytes (C), and hormones (E) are all present in small amounts in the urine.

67. Abnormal urine findings include

(A) protein
(B) glucose
(C) red blood cells

(D) ketones
(E) all of the above

(E) is correct.

(A) The presence of protein in urine may indicate the presence of kidney disease, such as glomerulonephritis, or a condition of preeclampsia in pregnant women.

(B) The presence of small amounts of glucose (sugar) in urine may be the result of eating a high carbohydrate meal, stress, pregnancy, and taking some medications (such as aspirin or corticosteroids). Higher levels of glucose may indicate poorly controlled diabetes, Cushing's syndrome, or infection.

(C) The presence of red blood cells (erythrocytes) may indicate some types of anemias, taking some medications (such as blood thinners), arsenic poisoning, reactions to transfusion, trauma, burns, and convulsion.

(D) The presence of ketones may indicate poorly controlled diabetes, dehydration, starvation, or ingestion of large amounts of aspirin.

68. The surgical fixation of a floating kidney is called

(A) nephromalacia
(B) nephrosclerosis
(C) nephropexy

(D) nephrosis
(E) cystorrhagia

(C) is correct. Nephropexy is the surgical fixation of a kidney.
(A) Nephromalacia is abnormal renal softening.
(B) Nephrosclerosis is abnormal renal hardening.
(D) Nephrosis is kidney disease.
(E) Cystorrhagia is bleeding from the bladder.

69. Removal of part of the urethra is called

(A) ureterectomy
(B) urethrectomy
(C) urethropexy

(D) ureterotomy
(E) urethrostenosis

(B) is correct. Urethrectomy is removal of part of the urethra.
(A) Ureterectomy is removal of the one of the ureters, which connect the kidneys to the bladder.
(C) Urethropexy is surgical fixation of the urethra.
(D) Ureterotomy is an incision into a ureter.
(E) Urethrostenosis is a narrowing of the urethra.

70. A normal bacteria that is found in the intestinal tract is

(A) *Staphylococcus aureus*
(B) *Haemophilus influenzae* type B
(C) hepatitis B

(D) hepatitis A
(E) *Escherichia coli*

(E) is correct. *Escherichia coli (E. coli)* is normally found in the intestinal tract. It can cause a lower urinary tract infection due to improper hygiene after bowel movements.

(A) *Staphylococcus aureus* is not normally found within the body. Staph infections can be serious and usually require antibiotic medication.

(B) *Haemophilus influenzae* type B cause influenza. There is immunization against this organism.

(C) Hepatitis B is a serious contagious disease. There is an immunization to protect against this disease.

(D) Hepatitis A, also referred to as non-A and non-B hepatitis, is the most common form of new hepatitis cases each year. The symptoms and treatments are similar to those of hepatitis B.

71. The upper portion of the uterus is the

(A) fundus
(B) corpus
(C) ovum
(D) cervix
(E) vulva

(A) is correct. The fundus is the upper portion, or rounded edge, of the uterus.

(B) The corpus is the body or central portion of the uterus.

(C) The ovum is a female egg that can become fertilized once it meets the male sperm.

(D) The cervix is the lower portion or neck of the uterus.

(E) The vulva is the external genitalia in the female. It contains the labia majora and the labia minora, which are folds of skin that protect the genital tract and, in particular, the urinary meatus or opening.

72. The normal position of the uterus is

(A) anteversion
(B) retroversion
(C) anteflexion
(D) retroflexion
(E) none of the above

(C) is correct. Anteflexion is the normal position of the uterus. The forward bend is near the neck of the uterus.

(A) Anteversion is a position in which the uterus is actually tipped forward without bending, so that the cervix becomes tipped toward the sacrum and the fundus is tipped toward the pubis.

(B) Retroversion is a position in which the uterus is turned backward with the cervix in an exaggerated direction of the pubis.

(D) Retroflexion is a position in which the uterus is back (retro-) upon itself.

73. The normal period of development for a fetus (of 9 months) is called

(A) the placental stage
(B) effacement
(C) breech position
(D) gestational
(E) lactation

(D) is correct. The gestational period is the period of fetal development, usually lasting 9 months.

(A) The placental stage is the last stage of labor, during which the placenta or afterbirth is delivered.

(B) The effacement period of delivery occurs when the cervix begins its thinning stage.

(C)   The breech position is when the baby's buttocks appear first at the cervical opening, rather than the head. The head, or cephalic, position is normal.

(E)   Lactation is the process of the breast secreting milk for the infant.

74. Surgical removal of the fallopian tube and ovary is called

(A)   panhysterosalpingo-oophorectomy
(B)   oophorectomy
(C)   salpingo-oophorectomy
(D)   panhysterectomy
(E)   laparoscopy

(C)   is correct. The removal of the fallopian (salpingo-) tube and the ovary (oophor-) is called a salpingo-oophorectomy.

(A)   A panhysterosalpingo-oophorectomy is the removal of the entire uterus, cervix, ovaries, and fallopian tubes.

(B)   An oophorectomy is the surgical removal of an ovary.

(D)   A panhysterectomy is the excision of the entire uterus, including the cervix.

(E)   A laparoscopy is an examination of the peritoneal cavity using an instrument called a laparoscope.

75. The male sperm, in the form of semen, are nourished by a fluid in the

(A)   seminal vesicles
(B)   epididymis
(C)   prostate gland
(D)   urethra
(E)   vas deferens

(A)   is correct. The two seminal vesicles are small glands located at the base of the urinary bladder. The vesicles join the ejaculatory duct as it moves in to join the urethra.

(B)   The epididymis is a coiled tubule that lies on top of the testes within the scrotum.

(C)   The prostate gland is located just behind the urinary bladder. It surrounds the urethra and when enlarged can cause difficulty in urination.

(D)   The urethra extends from the urinary bladder to the external opening in the penis in the male. It serves the dual functions of the elimination of urine and the ejaculation of semen containing sperm.

(E)   The vas deferens, also called the ductus deferens, brings the epididymis up into the pelvic cavity of the male and becomes contained within the spermatic cord.

76. The vas deferens in the male reproductive system is also known as the

(A)   vasectomy
(B)   ductus deferens
(C)   spermatic cord
(D)   scrotum
(E)   phimosis

(B)   is correct. The ductus deferens is also called the vas deferens. This is the cord that is cut during a vasectomy, which renders the male sterile.

(A)   A vasectomy is the surgical severing of the vas deferens.

(C) The spermatic cord in the male contains the epididymis, nerves, arteries, veins, and lymphatic tissue.

(D) The scrotum is an external sac located in the groin area of the male that contains the testes.

(E) Phimosis is a narrowing of the foreskin over the glans penis in the male that can result in difficulty with hygiene.

77. The surgical removal of the prostate gland by inserting a device through the urethra and removing prostate tissue is called a/an

(A) vasectomy
(B) circumcision
(C) orchidopexy
(D) castration
(E) transurethral resection of the prostate (TUR)

(E) is correct. A TUR is the surgical removal of the prostate gland by inserting a device through the urethra to remove tissue.

(A) A vasectomy is the removal of a section or all of the vas deferens to prevent sperm from leaving the male body.

(B) Circumcision is the surgical removal of the end of the prepuce or foreskin of the penis.

(C) Orchidopexy is the surgical fixation to move undescended testes into the scrotum, and attaching to prevent retraction.

(D) Castration is excision of the testicles in the male or ovaries in the female.

78. The testes produce

(A) progesterone
(B) estrogen
(C) testosterone
(D) oxytocin
(E) prolactin

(C) is correct. Testosterone, produced in the testes, is the hormone that promotes development of secondary sex characteristics in males.

(A) Progesterone, produced by the ovaries, is a hormone that prepares the female for pregnancy.

(B) Estrogen, produced by the ovaries, stimulates development of secondary sex characteristics in females.

(D) Oxytocin, produced by the posterior lobe of the pituitary, stimulates uterine contractions and releases milk into ducts.

(E) Prolactin, produced by the anterior lobe of the pituitary, stimulates milk production in the lactating female.

79. The portion of the brain controlling motor function is

(A) frontal lobe
(B) parietal lobe
(C) occipital lobe
(D) temporal lobe
(E) none of the above

(A) is correct. The frontal lobe of the brain control controls motor (movement) function.

(B) The parietal lobe receives and interprets nerve impulses from sensory receptors.

(C) The occipital lobe controls eyesight.

(D) The temporal lobe controls hearing and smell.

80. The largest portion of the brain is the

(**A**) brain stem

(**B**) cerebellum

(**C**) cerebrum

(**D**) diencephalon

(**E**) thalamus

(C) is correct. The cerebrum is the largest portion of the brain. It is the area in the upper portion of the brain that processes thoughts, judgment, memory, association skills, and the ability to discriminate between items.

(A) The brain stem contains the pons, medulla oblongata, and the midbrain. The brain stem acts as a pathway for impulses to be conducted between the brain and spinal cord. The 12 pairs of cranial nerves begin in the brain stem. This area of the brain controls respiration, heart rate, and blood pressure.

(B) The cerebellum, the second largest portion of the brain, is located beneath the posterior portion of the cerebrum. It aids in coordinating voluntary body movements and maintaining balance and equilibrium.

(D) The diencephalon, located below the cerebrum, contains two critical parts of the brain: the thalamus and the hypothalamus.

(E) The thalamus is found within the diencephalon.

81. What portion of the brain controls respiration, heart rate, and blood pressure?

(**A**) thalamus

(**B**) hypothalamus

(**C**) medulla oblongata

(**D**) brain stem

(**E**) cerebrum

(D) is correct. The brain stem controls respiration, heart rate, and blood pressure.

(A) The thalamus, in the cerebrum, is composed of gray matter and acts as the center for relaying impulses from the eyes, ears, and skin to the cerebrum.

(B) The hypothalamus, lying just below the thalamus in the cerebrum, controls body temperature, appetite, sleep, sexual desire, and emotions such as fear.

(C) The medulla oblongata, in the brain stem, is the area where the nerve cells cross from one side of the brain to control functions and movement on the other side of the brain.

(E) The cerebrum is the largest section of the brain.

82. The three layers of connective tissue surrounding the brain and spinal cord are

(**A**) vertebra

(**B**) meninges

(**C**) 12 cranial nerves

(**D**) 31 spinal nerves

(**E**) pons

(B) is correct. The meninges are three layers of connective tissue membranes that surround the brain and spinal cord.

(A) The vertebra are individual bones within the 33 bony segments comprising the vertebral column.

(C) The 12 cranial nerves, found within the peripheral nervous system, are the (I) olfactory, (II) optic, (III) oculomotor, (IV) trochlear, (V) trigeminal, (VI) abducens, (VII) facial, (VIII) acoustic, (IX) glossopharyngeal, (X) vagus, (XI) spinal accessory, and (XII) hypoglossal.

(D) The 31 spinal nerves are arranged in identical pairs and are generally named after the artery they correspond to (for example, femoral nerve).

(E) The pons is a portion of the brain stem.

83. The 12 cranial nerves are located within what portion of the nervous system?

(A) central nervous system
(B) peripheral nervous system
(C) autonomic nervous system
(D) voluntary nervous system
(E) none of the above

(B) is correct. The 12 cranial nerves are found within the peripheral nervous system.

(A) The central nervous system, a combination of the brain and spinal cord, controls all basic bodily functions and responds to external changes.

(C) The autonomic nervous system parallels the spinal cord but is separately involved in the control of exocrine glands, blood vessels, viscera, and external genitalia.

(D) The voluntary nervous system, found within the central nervous system, contains the functions within our control, such as muscle movement, taste, smell, and hearing.

84. A physician who specializes in the treatment and prevention of mental disorders is a

(A) psychologist
(B) neurologist
(C) nephrologist
(D) psychiatrist
(E) psychoanalyst

(D) is correct. A psychiatrist is a physician who specializes in the treatment and prevention of mental disorders.

(A) A psychologist is a specialist trained in the study of psychological analysis, therapy, and research.

(B) A neurologist is a physician who specializes in the diagnosis and treatment of disorders of the nervous system.

(C) A nephrologist is a physician who specializes in the diagnosis and treatment of disorders of the kidney.

(E) A psychoanalyst is a specialist trained in the study of mental disorders using detailed accounts of past experiences and repressions.

85. Afferent neurons

(A) carry impulses away from the brain and spinal cord
(B) carry impulses to the brain and spinal cord
(C) are waves of sudden excitement
(D) are knotlike masses of nerve tissue located outside the brain and spinal cord
(E) are a force that activates or excites the nerve and results in an impulse

(B) is correct. Afferent neurons carry impulses to the brain and spinal cord from the skin and sense organs. They are also called sensory neurons.

(A) Efferent neurons carry impulses away from the brain and spinal cord to the muscles and glands. They are also called motor neurons.

(C) Impulses are waves of sudden excitement.

(D) Ganglions are knotlike masses of nerve tissue located outside the brain and spinal cord.

(E) A stimulus is a force that activates or excites the nerve and results in an impulse.

86. The cranial nerve that supplies most organs in the abdominal and thoracic cavity is the

(A) acoustic
(B) glossopharyngeal
(C) vagus
(D) spinal accessory
(E) hypoglossal

(C) is correct. The vagus nerve, cranial nerve X, supplies most organs in the abdominal and thoracic cavity.

(A) The acoustic nerve (VIII) is responsible for impulses of equilibrium and hearing. It is also called the auditory nerve.

(B) The glossopharyngeal nerve (IX) carries sensory impulses from the pharynx (swallowing) and taste on one-third of the tongue.

(D) The spinal accessory nerve (XI) controls the neck and shoulder muscles.

(E) The hypoglossal nerve (XII) controls tongue muscles.

87. The cranial nerve that transports impulses for the sense of smell is the

(A) optic
(B) olfactory
(C) oculomotor
(D) trochlear
(E) trigeminal

(B) is correct. The olfactory nerve, cranial nerve I, carries impulses for the sense of smell.

(A) The optic nerve (II) carries impulses for the sense of vision.

(C) The oculomotor nerve (III) carries motor impulses for eye muscle movement and the pupil of the eye.

(D) The trochlear nerve (IV) controls the oblique muscle of the eye on each side.

(E) The trigeminal nerve (V) carries sensory facial impulses and controls the muscles for chewing.

88. A one-sided facial paralysis is known as

(A) Bell's palsy
(B) Reye's syndrome
(C) Parkinson's disease
(D) Huntington's chorea
(E) tic douloureux

(A) is correct. Bell's palsy is a one-sided facial paralysis with an unknown cause. The patient cannot control salivation, tearing of the eyes, or expression.

(B) Reye's syndrome is a combination of symptoms in which there is acute encephalopathy and various organ damage in children under 15 years of age who have had a viral infection.

(C) Parkinson's disease is a chronic disorder of the nervous system with fine tremors, muscular weakness, rigidity, and a shuffling gait.

(D) Huntington's chorea is a disorder of the central nervous system that results in progressive dementia with bizarre involuntary movements of parts of the body.

(E) Tic douloureux is a painful condition in which the trigeminal nerve is affected by pressure or degeneration.

89. A temporary interference with blood supply to the brain causing neurological symptoms, such as dizziness, numbness, and hemiparesis that may eventually lead to a full-blown stroke (CVA) is called

(A) syncope
(B) subdural hematoma
(C) transient ischemic attack (TIA)
(D) tetraplegia
(E) shingles

(C) is correct. A TIA is a temporary interference with blood supply to the brain that may lead eventually to a full-blown stroke.

(A) Syncope means fainting.

(B) A subdural hematoma is a mass of blood forming beneath the dura matter of the brain.

(D) Tetraplegia is a paralysis of all four limbs. It is the same as quadriplegia.

(E) Shingles is a painful eruption of vesicles on the trunk of the body along a nerve path that is caused by a virus.

90. A recording of the electrical activity of the brain is called

(A) echoencephalogram
(B) cerebral angiography
(C) myelography
(D) pneumoencephalography
(E) electroencephalogram

(E) is correct. An electroencephalogram is a written recording of the electrical activity of the brain.

(A) Echoencephalogram is a recording of the ultrasonic echos of the brain.

(B) Cerebral angiography is an x-ray of the blood vessels of the brain after the injection of a radiopaque dye.

(C) Myelography is the injection of a radiopaque dye into the spinal canal.

(D) Pneumoencephalography is an x-ray examination of the brain following withdrawal of cerebrospinal fluid and injection of air or gas via spinal puncture.

91. The application of a mild electrical stimulation to skin electrodes placed over a painful area, causing interference with the transmission of painful stimuli, is called

(A) Romberg's sign
(B) positron emission tomography
(C) spinal puncture
(D) transcutaneous electrical nerve stimulation
(E) computerized axial tomography

(D) is correct. Transcutaneous electrical nerve stimulation (TENS) is the application of a mild electrical stimulation to skin electrodes placed over a painful area, causing interference with the transmission of painful stimuli.

(A) Romberg's sign is used to establish neurological function in which a person is asked to close the eyes and place the feet together. This test is for body balance and is positive if the patient sways when the eyes are closed.

(B) Positron emission tomography (PET) is the use of radionuclides to reconstruct brain sections. Measurement can be taken of oxygen and glucose uptake, cerebral blood flow, and blood volume.

(C) A spinal puncture is a puncture with a needle into the spinal cavity to withdraw spinal fluid for microscopic analysis. This is also called a spinal tap.

(E) Computerized axial tomography (CT or CAT scan) is the use of x-rays to examine a cross-section of the brain after dye has been injected. The outlines of tumors, blood clots, and hemorrhages can be seen.

92. The layer of the eye that provides the blood supply for the eye is

(A) sclera
(B) pupil
(C) choroid
(D) retina
(E) cornea

(C) is correct. The choroid is the layer of the eye that provides the blood supply.

(A) The sclera is the tough, protective outer layer of the eye. It is also called the "white of the eye."

(B) The pupil is the contractile opening at the center of the iris of the eye.

(D) The retina is the third innermost layer of the eye. It is a delicate 10-layered area composed of nerve endings. The retina receives and transmits light impulses through the optic nerve to the brain.

(E) The cornea is a clear, transparent portion of the sclera that is responsible for allowing light to enter the interior of the eye.

93. The conjunctiva is the

(A) color portion of the eye
(B) tear ducts of the eye
(C) eyelid
(D) mucous membrane lining on the underside of the eye
(E) blood supply for the eye

(D) is correct. The conjunctiva is the mucous membrane lining on the underside of the eye.

(A) The color portion of the eye is the iris.

(B) The tear ducts of the eye are the lacrimal ducts in the corner of each eye.

(C) The eyelid is composed of a protective covering over each eye with cilia or eyelashes to protect the eye from foreign particles.

(E) The blood supply for the eye is in the choroid layer of the eye.

94. Which is NOT one of the layers of the eye?

(A) retina
(B) pupil
(C) sclera
(D) choroid
(E) all of the above

(B) is correct. The pupil is not one of the layers of the eye. It is a hole in the iris. The retina (A), sclera (C), and choroid (D) are the three layers of the eye.

95. The ability of the eye to adjust to variations in distance is called

(A) emmetropia
(B) convergence
(C) accommodation

(D) refraction
(E) achromatopsia

(C) is correct. Accommodation is the ability of the eye to adjust to variations in distance.
(A) Emmetropia is a state of normal vision.
(B) Convergence is the moving inward of the eyes to see an object close to the face.
(D) Refraction is an eye examination performed by a physician to determine and correct refractive errors in the eye.
(E) Achromatopsia is a condition of color blindness that is more common in males.

96. A visual loss due to the aging process is called

(A) hyperopia
(B) myopia
(C) presbyopia

(D) astigmatism
(E) esotropia

(C) is correct. Presbyopia is a visual loss due to the aging process.
(A) Hyperopia, also called farsightedness, is a condition in which a person sees things in the distance but has trouble reading material at close vision.
(B) Myopia, also called nearsightedness, is a condition in which a person can see things close up but not in the distance.
(D) Astigmatism occurs when light rays focus unevenly on the eye, which causes a distorted image due to an abnormal curvature of the cornea.
(E) Esotropia, commonly called "lazy eye," is a turning in of the eye.

97. Anacusis means

(A) hearing loss due to the aging process
(B) middle ear infection
(C) absence of hearing
(D) fungal infection in the ear
(E) rupture of the eardrum

(C) is correct. Anacusis is the absence of hearing.
(A) Presbycusis is hearing loss due to the aging process.
(B) Otitis media is a middle ear infection.
(D) Otomycosis is a fungal infection in the ear.
(E) Tympanorrhexis is a rupture of the eardrum.

98. Which is NOT one of the ossicles (bones) of the ear?

(A) stapes
(B) incus
(C) hyoid

(D) malleus
(E) all of the above

(C) is correct. The hyoid bone is one of the facial bones that assists in holding the tongue.

(A) The stapes is one of the bones in the middle ear and is shaped like a stirrup.

(B) The incus is one of the middle ear bones that lies between the stapes and the malleus. The incus is shaped like an anvil.

(D) The malleus is a middle ear bone that is shaped like a mallet.

99. Surgical reconstruction of the eardrum is called

(A) myringoscopy   **(D)** myringotomy
(B) myringoplasty   **(E)** none of the above
(C) myringectomy

(B) is correct. Myringoplasty is the surgical reconstruction (plasty) of the eardrum.

(A) Myringoscopy is the examination of the eardrum using a myringoscope.

(C) Myringectomy is the removal of a portion of the eardrum.

(D) Myringotomy is the surgical puncture of the eardrum with removal of fluid and pus.

100. An abnormal condition within the labyrinth of the inner ear causing dizziness and tinnitus (ringing in the ears) that can lead to a progressive loss of hearing is called

(A) otosclerosis   **(D)** Meniere's disease
(B) otitis media   **(E)** presbycusis
(C) acoustic neuroma

(D) is correct. Meniere's disease is an abnormal condition within the labyrinth of the inner ear causing dizziness and tinnitus that can lead to a progressive loss of hearing.

(A) Otosclerosis is a progressive hearing loss caused by immobility of the stapes.

(B) Otitis media is a middle ear infection commonly seen in children.

(C) Acoustic neuroma is a benign tumor of the eighth cranial nerve sheath that can cause symptoms from pressure being exerted on tissues.

(E) Presbycusis is a loss of hearing associated with the aging process.

CHAPTER 3

MEDICAL SCIENCE AND TYPE OF MEDICAL PRACTICE

1. The "father of modern anatomy" is

   (A) Galen
   (B) Hippocrates
   (C) Vesalius
   (D) Janssen
   (E) van Leeuwenhoek

   (C)   is correct. Andreas Vesalius is known as the "father of modern anatomy" and is responsible for many of the anatomical terms we use today.
   (A)   Galen founded experimental physiology.
   (B)   Hippocrates, known as the "father of medicine," developed the first scientific system of medicine.
   (D)   Zacharias Janssen invented the microscope.
   (E)   Anton van Leeuwenhoek is the founder of microbiology.

2. The 19th-century surgeon who introduced the antiseptic system in surgery was

   (A) Lister
   (B) Pasteur
   (C) Semmelweiss
   (D) Koch
   (E) Roentgen

   (A)   is correct. Joseph Lister introduced the antiseptic system in surgery.
   (B)   Louis Pasteur, known as the "father of bacteriology," determined that decay was caused by bacteria. He studied the diseases cholera and anthrax.
   (C)   Ignaz Semmelweiss determined the cause of childbed fever (puerperal sepsis) and advocated hand washing.
   (D)   Robert Koch, a bacteriologist, discovered the tubercle bacillus.
   (E)   Wilhelm Roentgen discovered x-rays.

3. Another name for childbed fever is

   (A) cholera
   (B) measles
   (C) anthrax
   (D) puerperal sepsis
   (E) tuberculosis

   (D)   is correct. Childbed fever is also called puerperal sepsis.
   (A)   Cholera is an acute, severe infection caused by a bacillus, *Vibrio cholerae*.
   (B)   Measles is a common, highly communicable childhood disease caused by a virus.
   (C)   Anthrax is an infectious disease caused by *Bacillus anthracis*.
   (E)   Tuberculosis is an infectious disease caused by the tubercle bacillus, *Mycobacterium tuberculosis*.

4. Physicians in ancient Babylon practiced under a code for the practice of medicine that included severe penalties for malpractice. This is known as the Code of

    (A) Hippocrates
    (B) Hammurabi
    (C) Babylon
    (D) American Medical Association
    (E) American Association of Medical Assistants

        (B)   is correct. The Code of Hammurabi is named after Hammurabi, a king of Babylon.

5. The 20th-century physician who accidentally discovered penicillin is

    (A) Sabin   **(D)** Fleming
    (B) Salk   **(E)** Semmelweiss
    (C) Banting

        (D)   is correct. Alexander Fleming is credited with the discovery of penicillin.
        (A)   Albert Sabin and (B) Jonas Salk discovered the polio vaccine.
        (C)   Frederick Banting discovered insulin.
        (E)   Ignaz Semmelweiss discovered the cause of childbed fever and advocated hand washing.

6. The physician who discovered insulin is

    (A) Ehrlich   **(D)** Banting
    (B) Roentgen   **(E)** Harvey
    (C) Jenner

        (D)   is correct. Frederick Banting discovered insulin.
        (A)   Paul Ehrlich discovered the "magic bullet" to treat syphilis.
        (B)   William Roentgen discovered x-rays.
        (C)   Edward Jenner discovered the smallpox vaccine.
        (E)   William Harvey described blood circulation.

7. Dr. Walter Reed helped to conquer the disease

    (A) syphilis   **(D)** polio
    (B) yellow fever   **(E)** childbed fever
    (C) smallpox

        (B)   is correct. Walter Reed helped to conquer yellow fever.
        (A)   Paul Ehrlich discovered a treatment for syphilis.
        (C)   Edward Jenner discovered the smallpox vaccine.
        (D)   Albert Sabin and Jonas Salk discovered the polio vaccine.
        (E)   Ignaz Semmelweiss helped conquer childbed fever.

8. One of the medicinal remedies from very early times that is still used today to treat heart patients is

    (A) sulfur   **(D)** cayenne pepper
    (B) chamomile   **(E)** cranberry
    (C) nitroglycerine

        (C)   is correct. Nitroglycerine is used to treat the heart disease, angina.

9. Clara Barton established what organization when she became aware
   for support services for the Civil War soldiers?

   (A) American Red Cross
   (B) American Medical Association
   (C) Centers for Disease Control (CDC)
   (D) American Nurses Association
   (E) American Association of Medical Assistants

   (A)   is correct. Clara Barton established the American Red Cross.
   (B)   The American Medical Association was founded by a group of physicians.
   (C)   The Centers for Disease Control, located in Atlanta, Georgia, conducts
         disease research, prevention, control, and education programs.
   (D)   The American Nurses Association is a professional organization for
         nurses.
   (E)   The American Association of Medical Assistants, founded in1959, is the
         key association in the field of medical assisting.

10. A New York City physician who founded a school for training persons to work in
    the medical office is

    (A) Läennec   **(D)** Domagk
    (B) Hahnemann   **(E)** Curie
    (C) Mandl

    (C)   is correct. M. Mandl founded a school for training persons to work in
          the medical office. In 1934, this was the earliest known training
          program for the medical assistant.
    (A)   René Läennec invented the stethoscope.
    (B)   Samuel Hahnemann introduced the study of homeopathic medicine.
    (D)   Gerhard Domagk discovered sulfa drugs.
    (E)   Pierre and Marie Curie discovered radium.

11. Who established the science of bacteriology and discovered that decay was
    caused by bacteria?

    (A) Pasteur   **(D)** Freud
    (B) Lister   **(E)** Morton
    (C) Läennec

    (A)   is correct. Louis Pasteur is credited with establishing the science of
          bacteriology. The process of pasteurization is named after him.
    (B)   Joseph Lister developed sterile technique in surgery.
    (C)   René Läennec invented the stethoscope.
    (D)   Sigmund Freud introduced the study of psychiatry.
    (E)   William Morton discovered anesthesia.

12. The analysis of the skills performed by medical assistants is contained in the

    (A) DACUM   **(D)** Code of Ethics of the AAMA
    (B) *Role Delineation Study*   **(E)** CDC
    (C) AMA's Principles of Medical Ethics

    (B)   is correct. The *Role Delineation Study* was released in 1997 by the AAMA,
          detailing the skills performed by medical assistants. It replaced DACUM.

IM was replaced by the *Role Delineation Study* in 1997.

MA's Principles of Medical Ethics sets standards for the ethical r of physicians.

of Ethics of the AAMA is a standard that medical assistants 'ed to follow.

fers to the Centers for Disease Control, located in Atlanta, ich conducts disease research, control, prevention, and ion programs.

type of health insurance offers subscribers, or members, complete medical care in return for a fixed monthly fee?

(A) managed care
(B) fixed payment plans
(C) health maintenance organization (HMO)
(D) preferred provider organization (PPO)
(E) all of the above

> (C) is correct. An HMO is a type of health insurance that offers subscribers complete medical care in return for a fixed monthly fee.

14. An approval, or sanction, that is granted to physician applicants who have successfully passed the National Board Medical Examination is called

(A) licensure
(B) reciprocity
(C) registration

(D) endorsement
(E) examination

> (D) is correct. Endorsement is the approval, or sanction, that is granted to physician applicants who have successfully passed the National Board Medical Examination.
>
> (A) Licensure is the right to practice medicine. It can be granted to a physician in one of three ways: examination, endorsement, or reciprocity.
>
> (B) Reciprocity results when the state in which a physician is applying for a license accepts the state licensing requirements of the state from which the physician already holds a license, and the physician will not have to take another exam.
>
> (C) Registration is a requirement that a physician must periodically submit a registration fee and the required paperwork in order to continue to practice.
>
> (E) Examination is offered by each state board of examiners. A physician must pass the examination in order to practice medicine.

15. The state regulations that direct the practice of medicine in that state are known as the

(A) Hippocratic oath
(B) Code of Hammurabi
(C) Medical Practice Act
(D) United States Medical Licensing Examination
(E) National Board Medical Examination

(C)   is correct. Each state has regulations that direct the practice of medicine in that state.

(A)   The Hippocratic oath is part of the writings of the 5th-century physician, Hippocrates, who admonished physicians to do the patient no harm.

(B)   The Code of Hammurabi, named after an early king in Babylon, had laws relating to the practice of medicine that contained strict penalties for malpractice.

(D)   The United States Medical Licensing Examination (USMLE) provides a single licensing examination for graduates from accredited medical schools.

(E)   The National Board Medical Examination (NBME) is accepted by some states for licensure to practice.

16. A legal arrangement in which physicians agree to share a facility and staff but, as a general rule, do not share responsibility for the legal actions of each other is called a/an

(A)   associate practice   (D)   solo proprietorship
(B)   partnership   (E)   none of the above
(C)   group practice

(A)   is correct. An associate practice is one in which the physicians agree to share a facility and staff but do not share the responsibility for the legal actions of each other.

(B)   A partnership is a legal agreement to share in the business operation of a medical practice. In this arrangement, each of the partners becomes responsible for the actions of all the partners.

(C)   A group practice consists of three or more physicians who share the same facility (office or clinic) and practice medicine together.

(D)   In a solo proprietorship, one physician is responsible for making all the administrative decisions.

17. A group practice has at least how many physicians?

(A)   1   (D)   4
(B)   2   (E)   5
(C)   3

(C)   is correct. A group practice consists of three or more physicians who share the same facility and practice medicine together.

18. The name of the first written source of medical ethics for the first physicians in history is called

(A)   AMA Principles of Medical Ethics   (D)   Code of Ethics of the AAMA
(B)   Hippocratic oath   (E)   none of the above
(C)   Code of Hammurabi

(C)   is correct. The Code of Hammurabi (3000 BC), is the first written source of medical ethics for the physician.

(A)   The AMA Principles of Medical Ethics are a modern-day code of ethical behavior for physicians.

(B)   The Hippocratic oath is part of the writings of the 5th-century physician, Hippocrates, who cautioned the physician to do no harm to the patient.

(D)   The Code of Ethics of the AAMA discusses ethical behavior required for the medical assistant.

19. The "father of medicine" is

(A) Galen

(B) Vesalius

(C) Galileo

(D) Hippocrates

(E) Mandl

(D)   is correct. Hippocrates is called the "father of medicine."

(A)   Galen developed the study of experimental physiology.

(B)   Andreas Vesalius is called the "father of modern anatomy."

(C)   Galileo was the first person to use the telescope and stressed the value of measurement in medicine.

(E)   M. Mandl started the first school to train the office assistant.

20. The type of medical doctor who specializes in the diagnosis and treatment of patients with disorders and diseases of the nervous system is a

(A) physiatrist

(B) psychiatrist

(C) psychologist

(D) neurologist

(E) nephrologist

(D)   is correct. A neurologist treats the nonsurgical patient who has a disorder or disease of the nervous system.

(A)   A physiatrist specializes in physical medicine and rehabilitation.

(B)   A psychiatrist specializes in the diagnosis and treatment of patients with mental disorders.

(C)   A psychologist is one who studies mental health and disorders.

(E)   A nephrologist specializes in pathology of the kidney.

21. A medical specialist who is trained to administer both local and general drugs to induce a loss of feeling is a/an

(A) oncologist

(B) hematologist

(C) pathologist

(D) anesthesiologist

(E) internist

(D)   is correct. An anesthesiologist is one who is trained to administer both local and general drugs to induce a loss of feeling.

(A)   An oncologist specializes in the diagnosis and treatment of cancer.

(B)   A hematologist specializes in the treatment of blood disorders.

(C)   A pathologist specializes in diagnosing the abnormal changes in tissues that are removed during a surgical operation and in postmortem examination.

(E)   An internist is a specialist who treats adult patients with medical problems. This is also referred to as the practice of internal medicine.

22. Another name for an otorhinolaryngologist is a/an

(A) throat specialist

(B) ENT

(C) ophthalmologist

(D) oncologist

(E) orthopedist

(B) is correct. An otorhinolaryngologist is also referred to as an ENT. Oto refers to the study of the ear; rhino refers to the nose, and laryngo refers to the larynx. ENT means ear, nose, and throat.

(A) A throat specialist would be a laryngologist.

(C) An ophthalmologist studies the eye.

(D) An oncologist specializes in the diagnosis and treatment of cancer.

(E) An orthopedist specializes in treatment of disorders and diseases of the bones and joints.

23. CEU means

(A) clinical education units

(B) continual education use

(C) continuing education unit

(D) continuing education use

(E) none of the above

(C) is correct. CEU stands for continuing education unit, which is credit awarded for additional course work beyond certification or licensure in order to remain current in one's field.

24. The American Association of Medical Assistants (AAMA) was founded in

(A) 1934

(B) 1950

(C) 1959

(D) 1968

(E) 1980

(C) is correct. The AAMA was founded in 1959.

25. The role of the certified medical assistant is the same as a

(A) physician's assistant (PA)

(B) nurse (RN)

(C) certified nursing assistant (CNA)

(D) nurse practitioner (NP)

(E) none of the above

(E) is correct. The role of the medical assistant requires knowledge in both the administrative and clinical skills of a medical office and requires certification by the American Association of Medical Assistants (AAMA).

26. The type of health care facility that provides health care to individuals who are not hospitalized is referred to as

(A) hospice

(B) primary care

(C) ambulatory care

(D) proprietary care

(E) intermediate care

(C) is correct. Ambulatory care provides health care to individuals who are not hospitalized.

(A) The hospice movement is an interdisciplinary program of care and supportive services that emphasizes quality care for the terminally ill patient. This can be at home or as an in-patient.

(B) Primary care is the basic care or the first stage of health care a patient receives. This is usually with the patient's personal physician.

(D) Proprietary care is provided on a for-profit basis.

(E) Intermediate care is provided when patients no longer require acute care but are still unable to take care of themselves.

27. The three categories of hospitals are

(A) primary, secondary, and tertiary
(B) general, specialty, and teaching
(C) teaching, ICF, and ECF
(D) ICF, primary, and specialty
(E) general, research, and teaching

(E) is correct. General, research, and teaching are the three main categories of hospitals.

28. The number of individual cases of a disease within a defined population is known as the

(A) mortality rate
(B) morbidity rate
(C) DRG
(D) primary care
(E) terminally ill

(B) is correct. The morbidity rate in a population is the number of individual cases of a disease within a defined population.
(A) The mortality rate is the individual number of deaths within a defined population.
(C) DRG refers to diagnosis-related groups, which are designations used to identify reimbursement per condition in a hospital.
(D) Primary care is the basic or general health care a person receives for common illnesses.
(E) Terminally ill refers to an illness that is expected to result in the death of the patient.

29. In addition to the National Board Medical Examination, a physician can be licensed by passing an examination offered by the

(A) American Medical Association
(B) state government
(C) federal government
(D) specialty boards
(E) AAMA

(B) is correct. The individual states license physicians.
(A) The American Medical Association (AMA) does not license physicians to practice.
(C) The federal government allows the states to supervise the licensing of physicians.
(D) Specialty boards, such as the American Board of Allergy and Immunology, evaluate the candidates who successfully pass an examination in that discipline.
(E) The AAMA (American Association of Medical Assistants) certifies the medical assistant after successful completion of the certification examination.

30. Residency, as a requirement for physicians becoming specialized in a certain area of practice, takes

(A) 1 year
(B) 2–3 years
(C) 3–6 years
(D) 2–6 years
(E) 8–10 years

(D) is correct. Residency in a particular specialty can take from 2 to 6 years, depending on the specialty.

31. The initials "DO" stand for doctor of

(A) chiropractic
(B) osteopathy
(C) optometry
(D) dental medicine
(E) medicine

(B) is correct. DO stands for doctor of osteopathy.
(A) DC stands for doctor of chiropractic medicine.
(C) OD stands for doctor of optometry.
(D) DMD stands for doctor of dental medicine.
(E) MD stands for doctor of medicine.

32. The first female physician in the United States was

(A) Florence Nightingale
(B) Elizabeth Blackwell
(C) Lillian Wald
(D) Marie Curie
(E) Clara Barton

(B) is correct. Elizabeth Blackwell was the first female physician in the United States.
(A) Florence Nightingale is considered the founder of modern nursing.
(C) Lillian Wald, a nurse, established public health nursing.
(D) Marie Curie won the Nobel Prize, along with her husband, Pierre, for the discovery of radium.
(E) Clara Barton, a nurse during the Civil War, established the American Red Cross.

33. Designation used to identify reimbursement per condition in a hospital is

(A) HMO
(B) EPO
(C) PPO
(D) DRG
(E) SNF

(D) is correct. A diagnosis-related group or DRG is used by Medicare to identify reimbursement per condition in a hospital.
(A) A health maintenance organization (HMO) is a type of managed care plan in which a range of health care services are made available to plan members for a predetermined fee (the capitation rate), by a limited group of providers (such as physicians and hospitals).
(B) An exclusive provider organization (EPO) is a relatively new managed care concept, which is a combination of concepts developed by HMOs and PPOs.
(C) A preferred provider organization (PPO) is similar to an HMO but differs in two ways: The PPO is a fee-for-service on a prepayment or capitation program (like the HMO), and the PPO members are not restricted to certain designated physicians or hospitals.
(E) A skilled nursing facility (SNF) provides around-the-clock supervision of patients by skilled nurses assisted by physicians.

34. Which of the following is a fee-for-service insurance program that is not based on prepayment and generally does not restrict the choice of providers?

(A) EPO
(B) HMO
(C) PPO
(D) PCP
(E) DRG

(C)   is correct. PPO is a preferred provider organization, which is a fee-for-service insurance program that is not based on prepayment and generally does not restrict the choice of providers.

(A)   EPO is an exclusive provider organization. This differs from a PPO since no insurance reimbursement is made if there is a nonemergency service provided by a non-EPO provider.

(B)   HMO stands for health maintenance organization, which is a type of managed care plan in which a range of health care services are made available to the plan members for a predetermined fee per member by a limited group of providers.

(D)   PCP refers to a primary care physician, who provides most of the medical care for an individual patient.

(E)   DRG stands for diagnosis-related group.

35. A predetermined fee that a member of a health maintenance organization agrees to pay for health care services is referred to as the

(A) member fee
(B) co-payment
(C) capitation rate
(D) rider
(E) premium

(C)   is correct. Capitation rate is a predetermined fee that a member of a health maintenance organization agrees to pay for health care services.

(A)   Member fee is the amount an individual must pay (usually on a monthly basis) to become a member of an insurance plan.

(B)   Co-payment refers to the sharing of a dollar amount paid by both the member and the insurance plan. This can be as low as $10.

(D)   Rider is a written exception to an insurance contract expanding, decreasing, or modifying coverage of an insurance policy.

(E)   Premium is the amount paid by the member for insurance coverage.

36. A government agency that alerts the medical profession to potential outbreaks of disease such as influenza is

(A) WHO
(B) CDC
(C) AMA
(D) EMT
(E) MLT

(B)   is correct. The Centers for Disease Control (CDC) is a government agency that alerts the medical profession to potential outbreaks of disease, such as influenza.

(A)   The World Health Organization (WHO) is an international agency that oversees the health status of the world.

(C)   The American Medical Association (AMA) oversees the practice of physicians.

(D)   EMT stands for an emergency medical technician or a paramedic. An EMT is trained in providing emergency care and transporting injured patients to a medical facility.

(E)   MLT stands for laboratory technician. An MLT is skilled in testing blood, urine, lymph, and body tissue.

37. Small laboratories that are located in physicians' offices and that conduct routine diagnostic tests are referred to as

(A) POLs   **(D)** MRIs
(B) CLTs   **(E)** CTs
(C) EMTs

    (A)   is correct. A physician's office laboratory (POL) is located in a physician's office and conducts routine diagnostic tests.

    (B)   A CLT, or clinical laboratory technician, is skilled in testing blood, urine, lymph, and body tissues.

    (C)   An EMT, or emergency medical technician, is trained in providing emergency care and transporting injured patients to a medical facility.

    (D)   An MRI, or medical resonance imaging, uses a magnetic field to visualize internal organs, tissues, and structures.

    (E)   A CT, or computerized tomography, is a thin beam of x-ray that penetrates body tissues at angles to produce a film representing a detailed cross-section of tissue structures.

38. How many categories of illness are used with the DRG system?

(A) 200   **(D)** 467
(B) 350   **(E)** 500
(C) 405

    (D)   is correct. The DRG system uses 467 categories of illnesses.

39. A patient-centered interdisciplinary program of care and support services for terminally ill (dying) patients and their families is called

(A) proprietary care   **(D)** inpatient
(B) hospice   **(E)** ambulatory care
(C) primary care

    (B)   is correct. Hospice is a patient-centered interdisciplinary program of care and support services for terminally ill (dying) patients and their families.

    (A)   Proprietary care operates on a for-profit basis.

    (C)   Primary care is the basic or general health care a patient receives, usually from the family physician.

    (D)   Inpatient care occurs when the patient remains within the health care facility, such as a hospital, at least overnight for care and/or treatment.

    (E)   Ambulatory care occurs when health care is provided to patients who are not hospitalized.

40. Medicare is operated by the

(A) Blue Cross and Blue Shield
(B) Social Service Administration and HCFA
(C) state governments
(D) AMA
(E) Medicaid

(B) is correct. The Social Service Administration and the Health Care Financing Administration (or HCFA) oversees and manages Medicare and Medicaid.

(A) Blue Cross and Blue Shield are insurance plans that provide for hospital coverage (Blue Cross) and physician medical and surgical services (Blue Shield).

(C) State governments administer Medicaid (public assistance) programs.

(D) The American Medical Association (AMA) does not operate Medicare.

(E) Medicaid is a type of government-controlled insurance for the indigent patient.

41. Which government agency was established to safeguard health by preventing and controlling disease through research?

(A) ECF
(B) ICF
(C) FDA
(D) HMO
✓(E) CDC

(E) is correct. The Centers for Disease Control was established to safeguard health by preventing and controlling disease through research.

(A) ECF stands for extended-care facility, a type of long-term-care institution.

(B) ICF stands for intermediate-care facility.

(C) FDA stands for the Food and Drug Administration.

(D) HMO stands for health maintenance organization.

42. Which of the following allied health professionals is trained in providing emergency care in the field?

(A) basic EMT
(B) advanced EMT
(C) paramedic
✓(D) all of the above
(E) none of the above

(D) is correct. A basic EMT, advanced EMT, and paramedic are all trained to provide emergency care in the field.

43. A phlebotomist is a technician who is skilled, and possibly certified, in

✓(A) drawing blood
(B) starting IVs
(C) performing clinical laboratory testing
(D) food selection and preparation
(E) physical therapy

(A) is correct. A phlebotomist is skilled, and possibly certified, in drawing blood.

(B) A nurse (RN) is licensed to start IVs.

(C) Laboratory technicians (MLTs and CLTs) and laboratory technologists (ASCPs) are skilled in performing clinical laboratory testing.

(D) Dietitians are skilled in food selection and preparation.

(E) Physical therapists (PTs) are skilled in physical therapy.

44. A trained professional who enters data into the computer, is adept at taking dictation from a tape or recording machine, has an understanding of medical terminology and excellent typing skills, and has the required 2-year associate's degree may be qualified for a position as a

    (A) pharmacy tech   ✓**(D)** health information technologist
    (B) social worker   **(E)** diagnostic-imaging technician
    (C) laboratory technologist MT (ASCP)

    (D) is correct. A health information technologist (also called a medical records technician) is adept at entering data into the computer and taking dictation, has an understanding of medical terminology, and has a 2-year associate's degree.
    (A) A pharmacy tech assists the pharmacist in preparing medications.
    (B) A social worker provides programs and services to meet the special needs of the ill, the physically and mentally challenged, and older adults.
    (C) A laboratory technologist MT (ASCP) must complete a 4-year medical technology program and directs the work of other laboratory staff.
    (E) A diagnostic-imaging technician is trained in the operation of x-ray equipment, such as ultrasound, CT scan, MRI, and many computer-assisted diagnostic machines.

45. A physician's right to practice medicine in a particular hospital or other health care facility is known as

    (A) licensure   **(D)** medical ethics
    (B) professional courtesy   **(E)** solo practice
  ✓**(C)** medical privilege

    (C) is correct. Medical privilege is the physician's right to practice medicine in a particular hospital or health care facility.
    (A) Licensure to practice medicine is granted by states in one of three ways: examination, endorsement, or reciprocity.
    (B) Professional courtesy is courtesy extended by one physician to another.
    (D) Medical ethics is moral conduct based on principles regulating the behavior of health care professionals.
    (E) Solo practice refers to a physician's practice in which he or she practices alone.

46. A health care professional who provides treatment by evaluating the ability for self-care of people who are physically, mentally, developmentally, or emotionally disabled is a/an

    (A) physical therapist   ✓**(D)** occupational therapist
    (B) respiratory therapist   **(E)** x-ray technologist
    (C) ultrasound technologist

    (D) is correct. An occupational therapist (OT) provides treatment by evaluating the ability for self-care of people who are physically, mentally, developmentally, or emotionally disabled.
    (A) A physical therapist (PT) provides treatment to patients with disorders or diseases of the bones and joints by massage, therapeutic exercises, and heat and cold treatments.

(B)   A respiratory therapist (RT) works with patients who have breathing problems.

(C)   An ultrasound technologist (AART) receives training in the uses of inaudible sound waves to outline shapes of tissues and organs.

(E)   An x-ray technologist or radiologic technologist performs radiographic (x-ray) procedures.

47. A member of the health care team who can perform some, but not all, of the clinical nursing tasks of a registered nurse is a

(A) certified medical assistant
(B) licensed practical nurse
(C) certified nursing assistant
(D) nurse practitioner
(E) physician's assistant

(B)   is correct. A licensed practical nurse (LPN) can perform some, but not all, the clinical nursing tasks of a registered nurse.

(A)   A certified medical assistant (CMA) is certified, but not licensed, to perform administrative and clinical functions.

(C)   A certified nursing assistant (CNA) has passed an examination and is qualified to assist nurses in nursing homes.

(D)   A nurse practitioner (NP) is a registered nurse who has completed graduate work.

(E)   A physician's assistant (PA) assists the physician in the primary care of the patient.

48. The CDC has conducted research into the nature and cause of several diseases, including a disease caused by *staphylococcus* bacterium. That disease is

(A) toxic shock syndrome
(B) AIDS
(C) Legionnaire's disease
(D) hepatitis B
(E) hepatitis C

(A)   is correct. Toxic shock syndrome is caused by *staphylococcus* bacterium.

(B)   AIDS (acquired immune deficiency syndrome) is caused by the human immunodeficiency virus (HIV).

(C)   Legionnaire's disease is caused by a bacillus that is inhaled.

(D)   Hepatitis B is caused by a virus.

(E)   Hepatitis C is caused by a virus.

49. A type of health care that emphasizes improved care for the terminally ill patient is

(A) ambulatory care
(B) ICF care
(C) SNF care
(D) hospice care
(E) psychiatric care

(D)   is correct. Hospice care emphasizes improved care for the dying patient.

(A)   Ambulatory care or outpatient care is delivered to patients who can walk into a health care delivery setting. The dying patient may not be able to do this.

(B)   ICF is an intermediate-care facility that is a type of long-term-care institution. A dying patient may be cared for in this type of facility, but it emphasizes caring for persons who cannot live alone but do not require skilled nursing care on a 24-hour basis.

(C)   SNF represents a skilled nursing facility that provides around-the-clock supervision of patients by skilled nurses assisted by physicians, as mandated by law. The dying patient may not need the services of skilled nurses and would, thus, be able to be cared for in a hospice setting.

(E)   Psychiatric care is provided to mentally ill patients in either an in-patient (hospital) or outpatient (clinic) setting.

50. A physician who specializes in disorders and diseases of the lower intestinal tract is a/an

(A)   thoracic surgeon
(B)   orthopedic surgeon
(C)   cardiovascular surgeon
(D)   colorectal surgeon
(E)   neurosurgeon

(D)   is correct. A colorectal surgeon specializes in the surgical treatment of the lower intestinal tract (colon and rectum).

(A)   A thoracic surgeon specializes in treatment of disorders and diseases of the chest with surgical intervention.

(B)   An orthopedic surgeon treats musculoskeletal injuries and disorders, congenital deformities, and spinal curvatures through surgical means.

(C)   A cardiovascular surgeon treats the heart and blood vessels through surgical means.

(E)   A neurosurgeon specializes in surgical intervention for disorders and diseases of the central nervous system.

51. A specialist who treats disorders characterized by inflammation of the joints is a

(A)   pathologist
(B)   nephrologist
(C)   gerontologist
(D)   cardiologist
(E)   rheumatologist

(E)   is correct. A rheumatologist treats disorders characterized by inflammation of the joints, such as arthritis.

(A)   A pathologist specializes in diagnosing the abnormal changes in tissues that are removed during a surgical operation and in postmortem examinations.

(B)   A nephrologist specializes in pathology of the kidneys.

(C)   A gerontologist specializes in the care of the elderly.

(D)   A cardiologist specializes in diseases and disorders of the heart and blood vessels.

52. There are currently how many specialty boards for physicians that are approved by the American Board of Medical Specialists?

(A)   15
(B)   20
(C)   23
(D)   40
(E)   100

(C)   is correct. There are currently 23 approved specialty boards for physicians.

53. Permanently disabled persons receive medical insurance coverage through

(A) Medicare
(B) Medicaid
(C) workers' compensation
(D) Blue Cross and Blue Shield
(E) HMO

    (A) is correct. Medicare is the federally funded program to provide health care to persons over 65 and those who are permanently disabled.

    (B) Medicaid is a state-operated program to provide medical care to persons who are indigent (without funds).

    (C) Workers' compensation provides funding for persons who are injured on the job.

    (D) Blue Cross and Blue Shield are medical insurance plans. They do not provide funds for disabled persons.

    (E) An HMO (health maintenance organization) provides medical coverage for members. It does not provide support for permanently disabled persons unless they are members.

54. The "gatekeeper" mechanism by which an insurance company approves or disapproves all nonemergency care, hospitalization, or tests BEFORE they are provided is called

(A) CDC
(B) FDA
(C) ICF
(D) MCO
(E) DRG

    (D) is correct. An MCO (managed care organization) acts as a "gatekeeper" mechanism in which an insurance company approves or disapproves all nonemergency care, hospitalization, or tests before they are provided.

    (A) The CDC stands for the Centers for Disease Control.

    (B) The FDA stands for the Food and Drug Administration.

    (C) An ICF is an intermediate-care facility.

    (E) DRG stands for diagnosis-related group.

55. A fee-for-service insurance program that is NOT based on prepayment and generally does not restrict the choice of providers is

(A) Medicare part A
(B) Medicare part B
(C) HMO
(D) PPO
(E) EPO

    (D) is correct. A PPO (preferred provider organization) is a fee-for-service insurance program that is not based on prepayment and generally does not restrict the choice of providers.

    (A) Medicare part A covers hospital expenses.

    (B) Medicare part B covers physicians' services.

    (C) HMO stands for health maintenance organization.

    (E) EPO stands for exclusive provider organization.

56. Another term for a phlebotomist is

(A) MT
(B) MLT
(C) venipuncture technician

(D) laboratory technician
(E) blood bank technologist

> (C) is correct. A venipuncture technician and a phlebotomist are the same.
> (A) MT stands for medical technologist or laboratory technologist.
> (B) MLT stands for a medical laboratory technician.
> (D) A laboratory technician (MLT) is the same as a clinical laboratory technician (CLT).
> (E) A blood bank technologist performs routine and specialized tests relating to hematology studies.

57. A type of long-term-care facility that provides living arrangements for older adults in which some meals and services are provided is known as a/an

(A) extended-care facility
(B) intermediate-care facility
(C) assisted-living facility

(D) skilled-nursing facility
(E) hospice

> (C) is correct. An assisted-living facility provides living arrangements for older adults in which some meals and services are provided.
> (A) An extended-care facility (ECF) provides services to patients who no longer need the skilled nursing care of a hospital but are too ill or incapacitated to return home.
> (B) An intermediate-care facility (ICF) is intended for patients who are no longer able to live alone and care for themselves but who do not require skilled nursing care on a 24-hour basis.
> (D) A skilled-nursing facility (SNF) provides around-the-clock supervision of patients by skilled nurses assisted by physicians, as mandated by law.
> (E) A hospice is an interdisciplinary program of care and supportive services for the care of the dying patient.

58. According to state regulations, only a registered nurse (RN) may

(A) administer medications
(B) provide patient education
(C) administer intravenous medications
(D) schedule patients
(E) collect and process specimens

> (C) is correct. Only an RN can administer intravenous medications. The rest of the skills are within the realm of the medical assistant.

59. The certification examination for the registered medical assistant (RMA) is offered by the

(A) AAMA
(B) AMT
(C) AMTIE

(D) CAAHEP
(E) ACCSCT

(B)   is correct. The American Medical Technologists (AMT) offers the certification examination for the registered medical assistant (RMA).

(A)   The American Association of Medical Assistants (AAMA) offers the certification for the certified medical assistant (CMA).

(C)   The AMT Institute for Education (AMTIE) has developed a continuing education (CE) program and recording system for the RMA.

(D)   The Commission on Accreditation of Allied Health Educational Programs (CAAHEP) is recognized by the U.S. Department of Education to accredit medical assistant programs.

(E)   The Accrediting Commission of Career Schools and Colleges of Technology (ACCSCT) is recognized by the U.S. Department of Education to accredit programs for medical assistants.

CHAPTER 4

MEDICAL LAW AND ETHICS

1. The Patient's Bill of Rights

    (A) was developed by the AMA
    (B) was developed by the AHA
    (C) includes the provision that a patient's medical record becomes the domain of the attending physician to distribute as he or she deems necessary
    (D) is designed to inform a patient that a physician has the right, at any time, to discontinue treating the patient.
    (E) is the same as the living will

    (B) is correct. The Patient's Bill of Rights was developed by the American Hospital Association (AHA).

2. Which of the following is in accordance with the Medical Patient's Rights Act?

    (A) complete patient confidentiality, unless directed by a court of law, in regard to their medical record
    (B) all except telephone conversations in regard to patient confidentiality and the medical record
    (C) a promise a medical assistant makes to a patient is never legally binding to the employing physician
    (D) the rules of medical etiquette
    (E) a physician can give patient information to another physician without a patient signature

    (A) is correct. The Medical Patient's Rights Act mandates complete patient confidentiality, unless directed by a court of law, in regard to their medical record.

3. Medical ethics is

    (A) courtesy physicians extend to one another
    (B) an authorization to practice one's profession
    (C) a form of contract that must be honored by law
    (D) moral conduct based on principles regulating the behavior of health care professionals
    (E) the regulations and standards set up by federal, state, and local governments to direct the medical treatment of patients

    (D) is correct. Medical ethics is moral conduct based on principles regulating the behavior of health care professionals.
    (A) Medical etiquette is courtesy physicians extend to one another.
    (B) Licensure is an authorization to practice one's profession.
    (C) A form of contract that must be honored by law is said to be legally binding.

(E) Medical laws are the regulations and standards set up by federal, state, and local governments to direct the medical treatment of patients.

4. The earliest principles of ethical conduct, established to govern the practice of medicine, were known as the

   (A) Code of Hammurabi
   (B) Code of Ethics of the AAMA
   (C) Hippocratic oath
   (D) AMA Principles of Medical Ethics
   (E) Patient's Bill of Rights

   (A) is correct. The Code of Hammurabi (1800 BC) is the earliest known principles of ethical conduct.
   (B) The Code of Ethics of the AAMA is a standard that medical assistants are expected to follow.
   (C) The Hippocratic oath is based on a statement of principles developed by Hippocrates (400 BC), the "father of medicine."
   (D) The AMA Principles of Medical Ethics, developed by the American Medical Association, were formed around 1847. They discuss human dignity, honesty, responsibility to society, confidentiality, the need for continual study, freedom of choice, and a responsibility of the physician to improve the community.
   (E) The Patient's Bill of Rights, developed by the American Hospital Association (AHA), describes the patient-physician relationship.

5. According to the AMA Principles of Medical Ethics, a physician may choose

   (A) regardless of the situation, to treat or not treat a patient
   (B) to refer, rather than treat, a nonemergency patient
   (C) the environment in which to provide medical services
   (D) A and B
   (E) B and C

   (E) is correct. A physician may refer, rather than treat, a nonemergency patient (B) and may choose the environment in which he or she wishes to practice (C).
   (A) is incorrect. A physician must treat a patient experiencing an emergency condition.

6. The Code of Ethics of the AAMA describes

   (A) moral conduct for the medical assistant
   (B) ethical conduct for the medical assistant
   (C) a commitment to patients to maintain their dignity and confidentiality
   (D) a responsibility to improve the health and well-being of the community
   (E) all of the above

   (E) is correct.

7. A courtesy physicians extend to one another is referred to as

(A) medical ethics
(B) fee splitting
(C) professional etiquette
(D) code of ethics
(E) legally binding

    (C) is correct. Professional etiquette is a courtesy that one physician extends to another.

    (A) Medical ethics is moral conduct based on principles regulating the behavior of health care professionals.

    (B) Fee splitting, the practice of one physician accepting payment from another physician for the referral of a patient, is unethical.

    (D) Code of ethics is a statement of principles or guidelines for moral behavior.

    (E) Legally binding means that a form of contract is in place that is honored by law.

8. A person who represents or acts on behalf of another person is called a/an

(A) expert witness
(B) appellant
(C) defendant
(D) minor
(E) agent

    (E) is correct. An agent is a person who represents or acts on behalf of another person.

    (A) An expert witness is a medical practitioner who, through education, training, or experience, has special knowledge about a subject and gives testimony about that subject in court.

    (B) An appellant is a person who appeals a court decision by going to a higher court.

    (C) A defendant is a person or group of persons who is accused in a court of law.

    (D) A minor is a person under the age of 18.

9. A court order or subpoena can require

(A) a person and/or documents to be presented in court
(B) a person to appear in court
(C) written documents only to be presented in court
(D) only a person over the age of 21 to appear in court
(E) none of the above

    (A) is correct. A subpoena is a court order for a person as well as documents to appear in court.

10. Because of unethical behavior, a physician's license to practice medicine may be revoked, meaning

(A) suspended
(B) taken away
(C) required to be reviewed
(D) limited
(E) none of the above

    (B) is correct. A physician's license may be taken away if he or she is found to be guilty of unethical behavior.

11. According to the standards of care of the AMA Principles of Medical Ethics, a physician should

    (A) provide competent care
    (B) participate in activities contributing to an improved community
    (C) expose those physicians deficient in character or competence
    (D) A and B only
    (E) A, B, and C

        (E)   is correct.

12. The unethical practice in which a physician accepts payment from another physician for the referral of a patient is known as

    (A) bait and switch   **(D)** double billing
    (B) ghost billing   **(E)** none of the above
    (C) fee splitting

        (C)   is correct. Fee splitting is the unethical practice of one physician accepting payment from another physician for referral of a patient.

13. Which of the following is TRUE?

    (A) a physician can be found guilty of negligence due to improper performance of a medical assistant
    (B) a medical assistant may only interpret an EKG in the case of an emergency
    (C) a medical assistant may only prescribe non-narcotic medications
    (D) a medical assistant is held to the same standard of care as a physician
    (E) none of the above

        (A)   is correct. A physician can be found guilty of negligence due to improper performance of a medical assistant. (B), (C), and (D) are all false since a medical assistant cannot practice medicine.

14. State statutes that exist in order to allow patients to state, usually in writing, what medical treatment they wish to receive should they develop a terminal disease are known as

    (A) euthanasia   **(D)** death with dignity
    (B) living will   **(E)** none of the above
    (C) life support

        (B)   is correct. A living will is a state statute that exists in order to allow patients to state, usually in writing, what medical treatment they wish to receive should they develop a terminal disease.
        (A)   Euthanasia is the act of willfully ending the life of an individual in a painless way as an act of mercy.
        (C)   Life support includes using medical technology, such as a respirator, to prolong life.
        (D)   Death with dignity refers to honoring a person's desire not to have life prolonged when suffering from a terminal illness.

15. A physician who discontinues treatment of a patient without providing coverage or sufficient notice of withdrawal could be charged with

(A) breach of contract
(B) a misdemeanor
(C) a felony
(D) abandonment
(E) rule of discovery

(D) is correct. Abandonment occurs when a physician discontinues treatment of a patient without providing sufficient notice.

(A) Breach of contract is failure to comply with all the terms of a valid contract.

(B) A misdemeanor is a crime that is less serious than a felony, carrying a penalty of up to 1-year imprisonment and/or a fine.

(C) A felony is a crime more serious than a misdemeanor, carrying a penalty of death or imprisonment.

(E) The rule of discovery refers to the statute of limitations beginning to run at the time the injury is discovered or when the patient should have known of the injury.

16. What are the four types of written laws?

(A) misdemeanor, felony, civil, and tort
(B) felony, misdemeanor, negligence, and contract
(C) civil, tort, multinational, and government
(D) criminal, civil, tort, and military
(E) civil, criminal, international, and military

(E) is correct.

17. Performing surgery on a patient without the proper informed consent of the patient is an example of

(A) intentional tort
(B) battery
(C) assault
(D) A and B
(E) A and C

(D) is correct. The intentional tort of battery has occurred when a patient is operated without the proper informed consent of the patient. Battery is actual bodily harm to another.

(C) Assault is the threat of bodily harm.

18. The doctrine that applies to the law of negligence, which means "The thing speaks for itself," is

(A) *respondeat superior*
(B) *res ipsa loquitur*
(C) standard of care
(D) informed consent
(E) statute of limitations

(B) is correct. *Res ipsa loquitur* means "the thing speaks for itself." This is a doctrine of negligence law and occurs when the cause of an event is so obvious that there can be no other reason for the injury—for instance, if a sponge is left inside a patient during surgery.

(A) *Respondeat superior* means "Let the master answer." This means the physician employer is responsible for acts of the employee.

(C) Standard of care is the ordinary skill and care that medical practitioners, such as physicians, nurses, and medical assistants, use that is commonly used by other medical practitioners when caring for patients.

(D) Informed consent occurs when a patient's consent to undergo surgery or treatment is based on a knowledge and understanding of the risks and benefits provided by the surgeon before the procedure is performed.

(E) Statute of limitations is the maximum time period set by federal and state governments during which certain legal actions can be brought forward.

19. Public duties of the physician would include the reporting of

(A) communicable diseases
(B) births and deaths
(C) injuries such as those that are caused by battery and/or assault
(D) child and elder (or older adult) abuse
(E) all of the above

(E) is correct. The physician must report all communicable diseases, births and deaths, injuries such as those caused by assault and battery, and child and elder abuse.

20. Which of the following actions does NOT require documentation in the patient's medical record?

(A) phone call for medication renewals
(B) office visits and treatments
(C) appointments and appointment cancellations
(D) prescribed medications
(E) all of the above require documentation

(E) is correct.

21. What document, when signed by a patient, allows a representative to act on behalf of the patient in regard to medical treatment and care?

(A) durable power of attorney   **(D)** the Good Samaritan Act
(B) living will   **(E)** none of the above
(C) the Uniform Anatomical Gift Act

(A) is correct. The durable power of attorney (or health care proxy) allows a representative to act on behalf of the patient in regard to medical care and treatment.

(B) A living will allows patients to request that life-sustaining treatments and nutritional support not be used to prolong their life.

(C) The Uniform Anatomical Gift Act allows persons 18 years and older and of sound mind to make a gift of any or all parts of their body for purposes of organ transplantation or medical research.

(D) The Good Samaritan Act protects persons who provide emergency care to injured persons from litigation.

22. The Controlled Substance Act, which requires physicians and their representatives to handle controlled substances in specific ways, includes

(A) storing these substances in a locked cabinet
(B) reporting the theft of any controlled substance to the police
(C) detailed record keeping regarding the administration and dispensing of these substances
(D) A and B
(E) A, B, and C

(E) is correct.

23. What law, also referred to as Regulation Z of the Consumer Protection Act, requires a full written disclosure concerning the payment of any fee that will be collected in more than four installments?

(A) Truth in Lending Act of 1969
(B) Fair Credit Reporting Act of 1971
(C) Fair Debt Collection Practices Act of 1978
(D) Equal Credit Opportunity Act of 1975
(E) none of the above

(A) is correct. The Truth in Lending Act, also known as Regulation Z, requires full written disclosure concerning payment of any fee that will be collected in more than four installments.
(B) The Fair Credit Reporting Act provides guidelines for collecting an individual's credit information. Consumers can correct and update this information.
(C) The Fair Debt Collection Practices Act provides a guide for determining what are considered the fair collection practices for creditors.
(D) The Equal Credit Opportunity Act prohibits discrimination, or unfair treatment, in the granting of credit.

24. According to the laws governing the collection of an accounts receivable, telephone calls must be made only between the hours of

(A) 7 AM and 7 PM
(B) 8 AM and 8 PM
(C) 8 AM and 9 PM
(D) 7 AM and 6 PM
(E) 8 AM and 6 PM

(C) is correct. Telephone calls for the purpose of debt collection can only be made between the hours of 8 AM and 9 PM.

25. Rolling up one's sleeve when asked to do so in order to have blood drawn is an example of

(A) informed consent
(B) implied consent
(C) consent
(D) duty
(E) none of the above

(B) is correct. This is implied consent since the patient may not place consent in writing or state it verbally.

26. A person under the age of 18 who is free of parental care and financially responsible is an example of a/an

  (A) mature minor
  (B) minor
  (C) emancipated minor
  (D) guardian *ad litem*
  (E) appellant

    (C)   is correct. An emancipated minor is one who is still under the age of 18 but is free of parental care and financially responsible.
    (A)   A mature minor is one, usually under the age of 18, who possesses an understanding of the nature and consequences of proposed treatment.
    (B)   A minor is a person under the age of 18.
    (D)   A guardian *ad litem* is a court-appointed guardian who is to represent a minor or unborn child in litigation.
    (E)   An appellant is a person who appeals a court decision by going to a higher court.

27. Another name for professional negligence is

  (A) neglect of duty
  (B) breach of contract
  (C) malpractice
  (D) litigation
  (E) arraignment

    (C)   is correct. Malpractice is another name for professional negligence.
    (A)   Neglect of duty is failure of a physician (or other health care professional) to act as any ordinary and prudent physician (person) within the same community would act in a similar circumstance when treating a patient.
    (B)   Breach of contract is failure to comply with all the valid terms of a contract.
    (D)   Litigation is a lawsuit tried in court.
    (E)   Arraignment is calling someone before a court of law to answer a charge.

28. A person (or group of persons) who brings forth a lawsuit to court is known as the

  (A) defendant(s)
  (B) appellant(s)
  (C) plaintiff(s)
  (D) expert witness(es)
  (E) guardian(s) *ad litem*

    (C)   is correct. The plaintiff brings forth a lawsuit to court.
    (A)   The defendant is a person who is accused in a court of law.
    (B)   The appellant is a person who appeals a court decision by going to a higher court.
    (D)   An expert witness is a medical practitioner who, through education, training, or experience, has a special knowledge about a subject and gives testimony about the subject in court.
    (E)   A guardian *ad litem* is a court-appointed guardian who is to represent a minor or unborn child in litigation.

29. The Latin phrase that means the physician as employer is responsible for the action of the employee is

  (A) *res ipsa loquitur*
  (B) *respondeat superior*
  (C) subpoena *duces tecum*
  (D) proximate cause
  (E) guardian *ad litem*

(B) is correct. *Respondeat superior* means "Let the master answer." This means that the physician/employer is responsible for the actions of his or her employees.

(A) *Res ipsa loquitur* means, "The thing speaks for itself." This is a doctrine of negligence law.

(C) Subpoena *duces tecum* is a court order requiring a witness to appear in court and to bring certain records or other material to a trial or deposition.

(D) Proximate cause is a natural, continuous sequence of events, without intervening cause, which produces an injury. This is also referred to as direct cause.

(E) Guardian *ad litem* is a court-appointed guardian to represent a minor or unborn child in litigation.

30. Case or judicial law is based on

(A) statutes
(B) the U.S. Constitution
(C) precedent
(D) administrative laws
(E) none of the above

(C) Case or judicial law is based on precedent, which is law that was established in a previous case.

31. In order to prove negligence, a patient must prove that there was a continuous, natural sequence of events, without interruption, that produced an injury. This is known as

(A) proximate cause
(B) precedent
(C) contributory negligence
(D) breach of duty (neglect)
(E) deposition

(A) is correct. Proximate cause is the natural, continuous sequence of events, without any intervening cause, which produces an injury.

(B) Precedent is law that is established in a prior case.

(C) Contributory negligence relates to the patient's contribution to the injury that, if proven, would release the physician as the direct cause.

(D) Breach of duty (neglect) is failure to perform an obligation.

(E) A deposition is a written statement of oral testimony that is made before a public officer of the court to be used in a lawsuit.

32. Defamation of character that occurs when the defaming statement is spoken is called

(A) a deposition
(B) libel
(C) slander
(D) consent
(E) abandonment

(C) is correct. Slander is false, malicious spoken words about another person.

(A) A deposition is a written statement of oral testimony that is made before a public officer of the court to be used in a lawsuit.

(B) Libel is a false statement placed in writing about a person.

(D) Consent means to give permission, approve, or allow someone to do something.

(E) Abandonment is to desert or leave a person.

33. The four Ds of negligence include duty, dereliction or neglect of duty, direct cause, and

(A) defamation of character
(B) discovery
(C) direct battery
(D) direct assault
(E) damages

> (E) is correct. Damages is the fourth D of negligence. This refers to compensation for loss or injury.

34. A damage or injury to a patient, whether intentional or not, is known as

(A) breach of duty
(B) damage
(C) tort
(D) neglect
(E) malpractice

> (C) is correct. A tort is a wrongful act (other than a breach of contract) committed against another person or property that results in harm.
> (A) Breach of duty is the neglect or failure to perform an obligation.
> (B) Damage is harm to a person or property.
> (D) Neglect is failure to perform some action.
> (E) Malpractice is professional negligence.

35. A medical assistant may administer medication ONLY

(A) if certified
(B) under the direct supervision of a nurse or physician
(C) under the direct supervision of a physician
(D) to patients who are 18 or older
(E) none of the above

> (C) is correct. A medical assistant may administer medication ONLY under the direct supervision of a physician.

36. When a patient's medical record has been subpoenaed, the patient should be notified by

(A) telephone, as soon as possible
(B) registered mail
(C) next-day mail
(D) certified mail
(E) in person

> (D) is correct. The patient should be notified by certified mail.

37. Errors in documentation on the medical record must be carefully corrected by

(A) using a commercial correcting fluid
(B) erasing completing
(C) using red ink
(D) drawing a line through the error and noting the correction directly above the error, along with the initials of the person making the correction
(E) all of the above

> (D) is correct. An error in documentation is corrected by drawing one line through the error and noting the correction directly above the error, along with the initials of the person correcting the error.

38. The time period during which a patient has the right to file a suit against a physician is known as the

(A) statute of limitations
(B) rule of discovery
(C) *res ipsa loquitur*
(D) *respondeat superior*
(E) precedent

(A) is correct. The statute of limitations is the maximum time period set by federal and state governments during which legal actions can be brought forward.

(B) Rule of discovery states that the statute of limitations begins to run at the time the injury is discovered or when the patient should have known of the injury.

(C) *Res ipsa loquitur* means, "The thing speaks for itself." This is a doctrine of negligence law.

(D) *Respondeat superior* means, "Let the master answer." This means that the physician employer is responsible for the actions of his or her employees.

(E) Precedent refers to law that is established in a prior case.

39. Another name for Regulation Z of the Consumer Protection Act is the

(A) Equal Credit Opportunity Act
(B) Truth in Lending Act
(C) Fair Credit Reporting Act
(D) Fair Debt Collection Act
(E) none of the above

(B) Regulation Z of the Consumer Protection Act is called the Truth in Lending Act.

40. According to the Good Samaritan Law, no one is required by law to offer assistance in the event of an emergency EXCEPT in the state of

(A) Illinois
(B) Connecticut
(C) California
(D) Vermont
(E) Montana

(D) is correct. The only state that requires people to offer assistance in the event of an emergency is Vermont.

CHAPTER 5

QUALITY ASSURANCE AND GOVERNMENT REGULATIONS

1. A formal written description of an accident that has occurred in a medical setting is a/an

   (A) quality assurance report
   (B) incident report
   (C) evaluation
   (D) policy manual
   (E) procedure manual

   (B) is correct. An incident report is a formal written description of an accident that has occurred in a medical setting.

   (A) A quality assurance report, which documents all the quality issues during a certain period of time, is submitted for examination and action to a quality assurance committee.

   (C) An evaluation is an assessment or judgment of what has happened. An evaluation is part of an incident report.

   (D) A policy manual, which describes office policies or protocol, should be available in every medical office.

   (E) A procedure manual, which explains the methods by which procedures will be performed, should be available in every medical office.

2. Data is

   (A) information
   (B) figures
   (C) statistics
   (D) facts
   (E) all of the above

   (E) is correct. Data can be information, figures, statistics, and facts.

3. An example of an organization that continually monitors quality assurance in various health care organizations is the

   (A) American Medical Association
   (B) Joint Commission on Accreditation of Health Organizations
   (C) American Hospital Association
   (D) American Association of Medical Assistants
   (E) Centers for Disease Control

   (B) is correct. The Joint Commission on Accreditation of Health Organizations continually monitors quality assurance in health care organizations, including hospitals.

   (A) The AMA monitors physician quality assurance issues.

   (C) The American Hospital Association (AHA) assists hospitals in developing standards and documents such as the Patient's Bill of Rights.

(D) The American Association of Medical Assistants (AAMA) oversees the practice of medical assisting.

(E) The Centers for Disease Control provides research and education for the prevention and control of disease.

4. A mortality rate is

(A) the cause of death
(B) the prevalence of disease in a given population
(C) the number of deaths in a given population
(D) the norm
(E) regulated by the CDC

(C) is correct. The mortality rate is the number of deaths in a given population.

(A) The cause of death is not the same as the mortality rate. The mortality rate is the total number of deaths in a population.

(B) The prevalence of disease in a given population is the morbidity rate.

(D) A norm is a standard or criterion.

(E) The CDC does not regulate a death rate.

5. The standard, criterion, or ideal measure for a specific group is called the

(A) mean
(B) average
(C) median
(D) norm
(E) all of the above

(D) is correct. The norm is a standard, criterion, or ideal measure for a specific group.

(A) The mean is the average of the values.

(B) The average of the values is obtained by adding all the values and dividing the total by the number of items that were added.

(C) The median is the middle number in a given series.

6. A professional organization that reviews a physician's conduct is the

(A) AAMA
(B) PPO
(C) AMA
(D) PRO
(E) C and D

(E) is correct. Both the American Medical Association (AMA) and a peer review organization (PRO) review a physician's conduct.

(A) The AAMA (American Association of Medical Assistants) reviews the medical assisting profession.

(B) A PPO (preferred provider organization) is a type of managed care insurance plan.

7. A program in which hospitals and medical practices evaluate the services they provide by comparing their services with accepted standards is known as a

(A) peer review organization
(B) quality assurance program
(C) standard of care
(D) CPR
(E) all of the above

(B) is correct. A quality assurance program is one in which hospitals and medical practices evaluate the services they provide by comparing their services with accepted standards.

(A) A peer review organization (PRO) is a professional organization that reviews a physician's conduct.

(C) Standard of care refers to the ordinary skill and care that medical practitioners, such as physicians, nurses, and medical assistants, must use, which is commonly used by other medical practitioners when caring for patients.

(D) Competitive performance reports (CPRs), as mandated by Congress, are reports indicating the types of medical services to Medicare patients that must be filed by physicians on a timely basis.

8. A procedure in which the skin and body are not entered is called a/an

(A) operative procedure
(B) invasive procedure
(C) noninvasive procedure
(D) surgical procedure
(E) none of the above

(C) is correct. A noninvasive procedure is a medical procedure in which the skin and body are not entered. (A), (B), and (D) all require the body to be entered and are, therefore, invasive.

9. A hospital peer review might question a readmission to a hospital, indicating the patient was discharged too quickly, if the patient is readmitted within

(A) 31 days
(B) 40 days
(C) 45 days
(D) 60 days
(E) none of the above

(A) is correct.

10. The Joint Commission on Accreditation of Health Organizations has the authority to

(A) take punitive action against a hospital for poor treatment
(B) take punitive action against an individual physician for poor patient treatment
(C) temporarily close a hospital down
(D) report its findings to the Department of Health and Human Services
(E) none of the above

(D) is correct. The Joint Commission on Accreditation of Health Organizations has the authority to report its findings to the Department of Health and Human Services.

11. The purpose of an incident report is to objectively document an occurrence involving a patient in an effort to

(A) comply with the federal government's standards for reporting accidents
(B) prevent another similar accident
(C) forestall a malpractice claim
(D) document a questionable health care provider
(E) none of the above

(B) is correct. The main purpose of an incident report is to prevent another similar accident.

12. Which of the following would NOT be an example of an issue that may be reviewed by a quality assurance (QA) committee in a physician's office?

(A) use of an incorrect CPT and/or IDC-9 code on insurance forms
(B) a breach of confidentiality
(C) a prolonged waiting time for a physician
(D) an adverse reaction to a prescribed medication
(E) physician accreditation and licensure

(E) is correct. Physician accreditation and licensure are regulated by the Board of Medical Examiners in each state. All the other examples (A through D) are issues that might be addressed by a QA committee.

13. Data gathered by quality assurance programs is used by which of the following to effect quality improvement in patient health care?

(A) standard of care
(B) peer review
(C) quality improvement programs (QIPs)
(D) norms
(E) none of the above

(C) is correct. Quality improvement programs (QIPs) use the data gathered by QA programs to effect quality improvement.
(A) Standard of care refers to the ordinary skill and care that medical practitioners, such as physicians, nurses, and medical assistants, must use, which is commonly used by other medical practitioners when caring for patients.
(B) Peer review occurs when a professional is reviewed by his or her peers (such as when a physician reviews the work of another physician).
(D) Norms are standards or criteria.

14. Under Health Plan Employer Data and Information Set (HEDIS) managed care plans that serve Medicare patients, data relating to how many categories of performance must be collected?

(A) 4   **(D)** 10
(B) 6   **(E)** 12
(C) 8

(C) is correct. Data on 8 categories of performance must be collected under HEDIS.

15. The federal agency that has the power to enforce regulations concerning the health and safety of employees is the

(A) Food and Drug Administration
(B) Department of Health and Human Services
(C) Clinical Laboratory Improvement Amendment
(D) Occupational Safety and Health Administration
(E) all of the above

(D) is correct. The Occupational Safety and Health Administration (OSHA) was established by Congress to ensure safe and healthful working conditions for employees.

(A) The Food and Drug Administration (FDA) is a federal agency that regulates the quality of food and drugs (medications) used by the American consumer.

(B) The Department of Health and Human Services oversees health issues for the general population.

(C) The Clinical Laboratory Improvement Amendment (CLIA) mandates that all laboratories that test human specimens must be controlled.

16. A comprehensive performance report (CPR)

(A) is mandated by Congress
(B) is compiled from a selection of 5,000 physicians
(C) is designed to control the use of medical services by recipients of the Medicare program
(D) may require the use of the medical assistant to gather data
(E) all of the above

(E) is correct.

17. CLIA 88 divides laboratories into how many categories?

(A) 2
(B) 3
(C) 4
(D) 5
(E) 6

(B) is correct. The three divisions under the CLIA 88 regulation are Level I simple testing, Level II intermediate-level testing, and Level III complex-level testing.

18. The CDC guidelines targeted for all patients in health care settings are called

(A) contact precautions
(B) transmission-based precautions
(C) OSHA guidelines
(D) standard precautions
(E) none of the above

(D) is correct. Standard precautions are the guidelines established by the Centers for Disease Control (CDC).

19. When a patient injures himself or herself in a medical facility, the proper procedure is to file a/an

(A) workers' compensation form
(B) OSHA report
(C) incident report
(D) all of the above
(E) none of the above

(C) is correct. An incident report should be completed immediately if a patient is injured in a medical facility.

20. Physicians who administer narcotic medications are required to register with the

(A) FDA
(B) OSHA
(C) DEA
(D) CDC
(E) BNDD

(C) is correct. The Drug Enforcement Agency (DEA) controls and enforces the dispensation of controlled (narcotic) substances.

(A) The Food and Drug Administration (FDA) enforces drug sales and distribution.

(B) The Occupational Safety and Health Administration (OSHA) regulates and controls employee safety.

(D) The Centers for Disease Control provides research, prevention, control, and education programs for the prevention of disease.

(E) The Bureau of Narcotics and Dangerous Drugs (BNDD) is the agency of the federal government that is authorized to enforce drug control.

21. A material safety data sheet (MSDS) contains information about

(A) OSHA guidelines
(B) hazardous chemicals and other substances
(C) office policy
(D) vendor information
(E) none of the above

(B) is correct. A material safety data sheet (MSDS) contains information about hazardous chemicals and other substances.

22. A standard form that provides information about potential hazards of laboratory chemicals is a/an

(A) controlled substances sheet
(B) incident report
(C) office policy
(D) material safety data sheet
(E) all of the above

(D) is correct. The material safety data sheet (MSDS) is a standard form that provides information about potential hazards of laboratory chemicals.

23. Guidelines for handling contaminated materials have been established by

(A) CDC
(B) OSHA
(C) CLIA 88
(D) MSDS
(E) FDA

(B) is correct. The Occupational Safety and Health Administration (OSHA) has established guidelines for handling contaminated materials.

(A) CDC is the Centers for Disease Control in Atlanta, Georgia.

(C) CLIA 88 is the Clinical Laboratory Improvement Act that regulates the type of testing that can take place in various types of laboratories.

(D) A material safety data sheet (MSDS) provides information about potential hazards in laboratory chemicals.

(E) The Food and Drug Administration (FDA) controls drug sales and distribution.

24. OSHA guidelines are available from

(A) U.S. Department of Labor in Washington, D.C.
(B) AAMA
(C) AMA
(D) FDA
(E) BNDD

(A) is correct. The guidelines are available from the U.S. Department of Labor in Washington, D.C.
(B) The AAMA is the American Association of Medical Assistants.
(C) The AMA is the American Medical Association.
(D) The FDA is the Food and Drug Administration.
(E) The BNDD is the Bureau of Narcotics and Dangerous Drugs.

25. The OSHA standard that refers to the visible evidence of blood applies to

(A) urine
(B) stool
(C) sputum and nasal secretions
(D) vomitus and sweat
(E) all of the above

    (E) is correct.

26. An OSHA citation may be issued as a result of failure to

(A) use SOAP charting
(B) affix hazardous waste containers to the wall
(C) remove street clothing before coming to and leaving from work
(D) remove PPE before coming to and leaving from work
(E) all of the above

    (D) is correct. PPE (personal protective equipment, such as clothing) may not be worn out of the laboratory.

27. The Centers for Disease Control (CDC) issued recommendations that became known as

(A) CLIA
(B) OSHA standards
(C) PPE
(D) universal precautions
(E) none of the above

    (D) is correct. The CDC issued universal precautions, which state that all blood and bodily fluid contact is to be treated as if it contains the HIV, HBV, or other blood-borne pathogens.

28. The Fair Debt Collection Practices Act is a federal law that

(A) mandates the collection of blood
(B) regulates the wearing of PPE
(C) controls the administration of controlled substances
(D) protects debtors from harassment
(E) none of the above

    (D) is correct. The Fair Debt Collection Practices Act protects debtors from harassment.

29. The law regulating laboratory safety precautions is

(A) OSHA
(B) FUTA
(C) CLIA
(D) FICA
(E) A and C

(E) Both the Occupational Safety and Health Administration (OSHA) and the Clinical Laboratory Improvement Act (CLIA) address safety in the laboratory.

(B) The Federal Unemployment Tax Act (FUTA) mandates that every employer must contribute to the unemployment tax.

(D) The Federal Insurance Contribution Act (FICA) mandates that Social Security, Medicare, and federal income tax are paid. The employer has an obligation to match the employee payments for Social Security and Medicare.

30. Airborne precautions, issued by the CDC, are designed to reduce the transmission of

(A) droplet-generated diseases, such as *Haemophilus influenzae* type B
(B) contact diseases, such as herpes, scabies, hepatitis A, impetigo, wound infections, and pediculosis
(C) meningitis, pneumonia, diphtheria, and pertussis
(D) tuberculosis, measles, and chickenpox
(E) all of the above

(D) is correct. Tuberculosis (TB), measles, and chickenpox are all caused by infectious microorganisms, which are transmitted via airborne droplet nuclei (smaller than 5 microns).

(A) Droplet-generated precautions are used for patients known or suspected to be infected with microorganisms transmitted by droplets generated during coughing and sneezing.

(B) Contact precautions are used for patients infected with a microorganism that can be transmitted easily between patient and health care worker or from patient to patient.

(C) Meningitis, pneumonia, diphtheria, and pertussis are all caused by droplet infection.

31. Universal precautions mandate that

(A) all blood and bodily fluid contact is to be treated as if it contains HIV, HBV, or other blood-borne pathogens
(B) precautions must be taken only when there is visible blood present
(C) precautions are not necessary if the health care professional practices good hand-washing technique
(D) only medical assistants and nurses must follow the guidelines
(E) none of the above

(A) is correct. Universal precautions mandate that all blood and bodily fluid contact is to be treated as if it contains HIV, HBV, or other blood-borne pathogens. This means that precautions must be taken even if there is NO visible blood present (B), even if good hand-washing technique is present (C), and ALL persons who come into contact with hazardous materials must take precautions (D).

CHAPTER 6

HUMAN RELATIONS AND PSYCHOLOGY

1. Severe mental disorders that interfere with a perception of reality are called

   (A) hysteria   **(D)** psychoses
   (B) anxiety   **(E)** hypochondria
   (C) neuroses

   (D) is correct. Psychoses are severe mental disorders that interfere with a perception of reality.
   (A) Hysteria is a lack of control over emotions that may result in an outburst, amnesia, or symptoms such as sleepwalking.
   (B) Anxiety is a vague feeling of apprehension, worry, uneasiness, or dread. A certain amount of anxiety is normal.
   (C) Neuroses are mild emotional disturbances that impair judgment.
   (E) Hypochondria is an abnormal concern about one's health, with the false belief of suffering from a disease despite being assured otherwise by a physician.

2. A neurotic mental state in which a patient has an uncontrollable desire to dwell on an emotion or idea is known as

   (A) compulsion   **(D)** hysteria
   (B) obsession   **(E)** delusion
   (C) anxiety

   (B) is correct. An obsession is a neurotic mental state in which a patient has an uncontrollable desire to dwell on an emotion or idea.
   (A) A compulsion is a repetitive act that is performed by the patient to relieve fear connected with an obsession.
   (C) Anxiety is a vague feeling of apprehension, worry, uneasiness, or dread.
   (D) Hysteria is a lack of control over emotions, which may result in an outburst, amnesia, or symptoms such as sleep walking.
   (E) Delusion is a persistent, strongly held belief that is most likely wrong.

3. Examples of psychoses are

   (A) hysteria and hypochondriasis
   (B) anxiety, obsessions, and compulsions
   (C) delusions, depression, and a manic-depressive state
   (D) hallucinations and schizophrenia
   (E) C and D

   (E) is correct. Delusions, depression, a manic-depressive state, hallucinations, and schizophrenia are all examples of psychoses.
   (A) Hysteria and hypochondriasis and (B) anxiety, obsessions, and compulsions are examples of neuroses.

4. A mental disorder which is characterized by delusions and hallucinations is

    (A) dissociative disorder   **(D)** schizophrenia
    (B) cognitive disorder   **(E)** personality disorder
    (C) anxiety disorder

        (D) is correct. Schizophrenia is characterized by delusions, hallucinations, disorganized and incoherent speech, severe emotional disorders, and a withdrawal into an inner world.

        (A) A dissociative disorder is a type of amnesia in which important events cannot be remembered after a traumatic event. A dissociative identity disorder, or multiple personality disorder, is one in which two or more personalities are identified.

        (B) A cognitive disorder includes delirium, dementia, amnesia (resulting from brain damage), and degenerative disorders such as found in Alzheimer's disease.

        (C) An anxiety disorder is one in which phobias, panic attacks, and compulsive rituals may be present.

        (E) A personality disorder is one in which there are inflexible behavior patterns that cause stress or the inability to function.

5. The psychopharmaceutical lithium or Lithobid is most often prescribed for

    (A) schizophrenia
    (B) anxiety
    (C) bipolar disorder (manic-depressive disorder)
    (D) depression
    (E) none of the above

        (C) is correct. Lithium or Lithobid is most often prescribed for bipolar disorder (depression alternating with manic excitement).

        (A) Antipsychotic drugs (such as the tranquilizers Thorazine, Haldol, Clozaril, and risperidone) are prescribed for patients with psychoses and schizophrenia.

        (B) "Minor" tranquilizers, such as Valium and Xanax, are prescribed for anxiety.

        (D) Antidepressants, such as monoamine oxidase (MAO) inhibitors, are prescribed for depression.

6. The person best known for the study of death and dying is

    (A) Dr. Benjamin Spock   **(D)** Abraham Maslow
    (B) Dr. Elisabeth Kübler-Ross   **(E)** Dr. Sigmund Freud
    (C) Dr. Jonas Salk

        (B) is correct. Dr. Kübler-Ross, who described the five stages of grief, is best known for her study of death and dying.

        (A) Dr. Benjamin Spock, also known as the "The Baby Doctor," wrote extensively on a commonsense approach to raising babies and children.

        (C) Jonas Salk discovered a vaccine for polio.

        (D) Abraham Maslow developed the hierarchy of needs.

        (E) Dr. Sigmund Freud developed the study of psychoanalysis.

7. Often, the initial or first stage of grief is

   (A) anger
   (B) denial
   (C) bargaining

   (D) acceptance
   (E) depression

   (B) is correct. The initial stage of grief is often denial. The order of the other stages is usually (A) anger, (C) bargaining, (E) depression, and finally (D) acceptance.

8. The hierarchy of needs model, which states that lower-level needs must be satisfied before higher-level needs can be addressed, was developed by

   (A) Dr. Elisabeth Kübler-Ross
   (B) Abraham Maslow
   (C) Dr. Sigmund Freud

   (D) Dr. Albert Sabin
   (E) Hippocrates

   (B) is correct. Abraham Maslow developed the hierarchy of needs.
   (A) Dr. Kübler-Ross developed the five stages of grief.
   (C) Dr. Sigmund Freud developed the study of psychoanalysis.
   (D) Dr. Albert Sabin developed a polio vaccine.
   (E) Hippocrates is known as the "father of medicine."

9. Maslow's hierarchy of needs is based on five levels and includes self-esteem, which is

   (A) Level I
   (B) Level II
   (C) Level III

   (D) Level IV
   (E) Level V

   (D) is correct. Level IV of Maslow's hierarchy of needs is self-esteem. The other levels are (A) Level I, physiological needs; (B) Level II, safety and security needs; (C) Level III, love and social needs; and (E) Level V, self-actualization.

10. When using the five phases of violence while working with abused and abusive patients, the stage in which the person loses control over his or her anger and may resort to physical aggression is the

    (A) triggering stage
    (B) escalation stage
    (C) crisis stage

    (D) recovery stage
    (E) postcrisis

    (C) is correct. The crisis stage occurs when the person loses control over anger and resorts to physical aggression.
    (A) The triggering stage occurs when a stressful situation, or stressor, precipitates threats or verbal aggression attacks.
    (B) The escalation stage occurs when a threat of violence increases as the aggressor becomes more angry and enraged.
    (D) The recovery stage occurs when the aggressor calms down and returns to the first stage (triggering).
    (E) Postcrisis occurs when the aggressor can try to make amends for behavior, rationalize the behavior, or make promises for future peaceful behavior.

11. The final response to depression may be

(A) denial
(B) self-actualization
(C) suicide
(D) self-esteem
(E) security and safety

    (C)   is correct. Suicide may be a response to severe depression. The depressed patient should always be taken seriously.

    (A)   Denial is the first stage of Dr. Kübler-Ross's five stages of grief.

    (B)   Self-actualization is Level V of Maslow's hierarchy of needs.

    (D)   Self-esteem is Level IV of Maslow's hierarchy of needs.

    (E)   Security and safety is Level II of Maslow's hierarchy of needs.

12. Personality disorders include

(A) narcissistic behavior
(B) antisocial reactions
(C) paranoia
(D) sociopathic behavior
(E) all of the above

    (E)   is correct.

    (A)   Narcissistic behavior refers to abnormal self-love and self-admiration.

    (B)   Antisocial reactions are characterized by socially negative actions, such as stealing, lying, and manipulating others.

    (C)   Paranoia occurs when a patient demonstrates intense feelings of persecution and jealousy.

    (D)   Sociopathic behavior is also called antisocial behavior.

13. "Client-centered" or "nondirective" therapy for mental disorders is also called

(A) group therapy
(B) psychoanalysis
(C) humanistic therapy
(D) psychopharmacology
(E) electroconvulsive therapy

    (C)   is correct. Humanistic therapy is "client-centered" or "nondirective" therapy. The therapist does not delve into the patient's past when using this method.

    (A)   Group therapy and/or family therapy is solution-focused. The therapist places minimal emphasis on the patient's past history. A strong emphasis is placed on having the patient state goals and then finding a way to achieve them.

    (B)   Psychoanalysis is a method of obtaining a detailed account of the past and present emotional and mental experiences from the patient in order to determine the source of the problem and eliminate the effects.

    (D)   Psychopharmacology relates to the study of the effects of drugs on the mind and particularly the use of drugs in treating mental disorders.

    (E)   Electroconvulsive therapy (ECT) is a procedure occasionally used for cases of prolonged major depression. It is a controversial therapy in which an electrode is placed on one or both sides of the patient's head, and brief current is turned on, causing a convulsive seizure.

14. Today, mental health care is primarily

    (A) custodial care
    (B) long-term hospital in-patient care
    (C) institutional care
    (D) out-patient care
    (E) none of the above

        (D) is correct. Most mental health care is provided through out-patient or ambulatory means.

        (A) Custodial care, which was widely used at the turn of the century, occurs when the patient is institutionalized with little assistance other than food and shelter.

        (B) Due to the DRG system, hospitals can no longer keep patients in the hospital for long-term care.

        (C) Institutional or custodial care is used only for patients who are unable to manage their illness by remaining in society.

15. According to Freud, of the three divisions of the psyche, the one that controls our instinctual drives is the

    (A) ego   **(D)** libido
    (B) superego   **(E)** none of the above
    (C) id

        (C) The id is the division of the psyche that controls our instincts.

        (A) According to Freud, the ego is the division of the psyche that possesses consciousness and memory and acts to balance the primitive and animal instinct drives of the id and the internal social prohibitions of the superego with reality.

        (B) The superego is the portion of the psyche associated with ethics, self-criticism, and the moral standards of the community.

        (D) The libido is the conscious and unconscious sexual drive of humans.

16. It is proper, when addressing patients, to

    (A) call them by their surname only
    (B) address them by their first name, in order to sound friendly
    (C) ask them how they prefer to be addressed
    (D) avoid all use of names to avoid offending the patient
    (E) none of the above

        (C) is correct. As a courtesy, ask patients how they prefer to be addressed.

17. To protect the physician from legal claims when a patient is angry, the medical assistant should

    (A) tell the patient to keep his or her voice down
    (B) interrupt the patient and ask him or her to return to the office when calm
    (C) do what the patient is asking
    (D) document the incident on the medical record and complete an incident report
    (E) all of the above

(D) is correct. To protect the physician from a later legal claim, the incident should be documented in the patient's medical record and in an incident report. The medical assistant should calmly handle the incident first.

18. When a patient at the reception desk is angry about a bill, the medical assistant should

   (A) not try to explain it since that is not one of the medical assistant's responsibilities
   (B) ask the patient to quiet down
   (C) remain quiet until the patient settles down
   (D) ask the patient to come into another private area or room to discuss this
   (E) refer this immediately to the physician

   (D) is correct. The medical assistant should make an attempt to take the patient to an exam room or area away from the reception room to discuss this matter calmly.

19. When a patient mistakenly refers to a medical assistant as "nurse," the medical assistant should

   (A) remind the patient that he or she is a medical assistant and not a nurse
   (B) ignore the comment so as not to confuse or embarrass the patient
   (C) point to the medical assistant's name tag
   (D) ask the nurse to explain the difference in responsibilities to the patient
   (E) none of the above

   (A) is correct. Always quickly and quietly correct the patient.

20. When assisting a blind patient, the medical assistant should

   (A) speak loudly since blind patients are usually hard of hearing also
   (B) take the patient by the arm to assist him or her
   (C) offer the patient an arm
   (D) explain what is going to be done to or for the patient before doing it
   (E) C and D

   (E) is correct. The medical assistant should offer an arm to the blind patient to guide him or her into the examination room. In addition, everything should be clearly explained to the patient before doing it.
   (A) Blind patients are generally not hard of hearing.
   (B) A blind person is uncomfortable when being pulled by the arm.

PART II

ADMINISTRATIVE KNOWLEDGE

CHAPTER 7

ORAL AND WRITTEN COMMUNICATION

1. A nonverbal form of communication would include

   (A) folding one's arms across one's chest
   (B) frowning
   (C) doing more than one thing at a time
   (D) A and B
   (E) A, B, and C

   (E)   is correct. All are forms of nonverbal communication.

2. Placing your own feelings onto another person is an example of which of the following defensive behaviors?

   (A) rationalization
   (B) projection
   (C) compensation

   (D) displaced anger
   (E) disassociation

   (B)   is correct. Projection is placing your own feelings onto another person.
   (A)   Rationalization is justifying thoughts or behaviors to avoid the truth.
   (C)   Compensation is the substitution of an attitude, feeling, or behavior with its opposite.
   (D)   Displaced anger is expressing angry feelings toward persons or objects that are unrelated to the problem.
   (E)   Disassociation is not connecting one event with another.

3. The ability to imagine how another person is feeling is

   (A) sympathy
   (B) empathy
   (C) defensive behavior
   (D) beyond the domain of a medical assistant
   (E) none of the above

   (B)   is correct. Empathy is the ability to imagine how another person feels without actually experiencing the same situation.
   (A)   Sympathy is feeling sorry for another person. While the medical assistant may have these feelings for patients, the more acceptable attitude is one of empathy.
   (C)   Defensive behavior is a barrier to effective communication. Defensive behaviors include compensation, denial, displaced anger, disassociation, introjection, projection, rationalization, regression, repression, and sublimation.
   (D)   Empathy is one of the skills of the medical assistant.

4. A form of defensive behavior that involves turning back to former behavior in times of stress is called

(A) repression   **(D)** regression
(B) sublimation   **(E)** introjection
(C) rationalization

    (D)   is correct. Regression is turning back to former behavior in times of stress.
    (A)   Repression is keeping unpleasant thoughts or feelings out of one's mind.
    (B)   Sublimation is directing or changing unacceptable drives for security, affection, and/or power into socially or culturally acceptable channels.
    (C)   Rationalization is justifying thoughts or behaviors to avoid the truth.
    (E)   Introjection is adopting the feelings of someone else.

5. Directing the conversation back to the patient by repeating the words is called mirroring or

(A) restating   **(D)** clarification
(B) reflecting   **(E)** all of the above
(C) assessment

    (B)   is correct. Reflecting is directing the conversation back to the patient by repeating the words of the patient.
    (A)   Restating is to state what the patient has said but in different terms.
    (C)   An assessment is an evaluation.
    (D)   Clarification is to request more information in order to better understand what the patient has said or indicated.

6. In terms of the channels of communication, the least amount of information is generally gained from

(A) telephone conversations   **(D)** E-mail
(B) numeric documents   **(E)** face-to-face discussion
(C) written documents

    (B)   is correct. Numeric documents (printouts, budget reports) generally provide the least amount of information. Telephone conversations (A) and direct face-to-face discussion (E) provide the most.

7. The type of long-distance call that might be used to facilitate the consultation of one physician with another is called a/an

(A) operator-assisted call   **(D)** collect call
(B) DDD   **(E)** station-to-station call
(C) conference call

    (C)   is correct. A conference call can facilitate the consultation of one physician with another, particularly if another physician or the patient is the third party on the call.
    (A)   An operator-assisted call is used when a collect call is placed in which the receiver pays for the call, calls charged to a third number, person-to-person calls, station-to-station calls, and some credit card calls.

(B) DDD refers to direct distance dialing. These are calls made outside the caller's area code without the assistance of the operator.

(D) Collect calls are calls for which the charges are reversed. The receiver pays for the phone charges.

(E) Station-to-station calls are made from one location to another without concern for who answers the call. This is the opposite of a person-to-person call.

8. When handling an emergency telephone call from a patient, the FIRST thing a medical assistant should do is

(A) get the caller's name and telephone number
(B) ascertain whether or not it is, in fact, an emergency
(C) gather as much information as possible about the emergency in the shortest amount of time
(D) ask to speak with someone other than the patient if the patient/caller is too hysterical to communicate the details of the situation
(E) ask if an ambulance has been summoned

    (A) is correct. The very first thing to do is get the caller's name and telephone number in case you become disconnected. In some cases, the caller may become unconscious before giving you all the details. As long as you have the name and telephone number, the telephone company can give you the address, and you can summon an ambulance and/or police.

9. Inappropriate affect, such as a patient laughing in response to a very poor prognosis, is a defensive behavior known as

(A) denial
(B) compensation
(C) disassociation
(D) rationalization
(E) regression

    (B) is correct. Compensation is the substitution of an attitude, feeling, or behavior with its opposite.

    (A) Denial is unconsciously avoiding an unwanted feeling or sensation.

    (C) Disassociation is not connecting one event with another.

    (D) Rationalization is justifying thoughts or behaviors to avoid the truth.

    (E) Regression is turning back to former behavior patterns in times of stress.

10. How soon should a patient be greeted after arrival in the office?

(A) immediately
(B) within 1 minute
(C) within 3 minutes
(D) within 5 minutes
(E) within 10 minutes

    (B) is correct. Ideally, a patient should be greeted within 1 minute after arrival in the office.

11. Telephone triage is an example of

(A) passive listening
(B) active listening
(C) evaluative listening
(D) none of the above
(E) all of the above

> (C) is correct. Evaluative listening requires the listener to make a judgment about what they are hearing and to respond quickly, as in telephone triage.
> (A) Passive listening is listening without offering any response.
> (B) Active listening involves participation, such as feedback, from the listener.

12. A man who knowingly does not see his physician because he fears that something might be seriously wrong is experiencing

(A) sublimation
(B) disassociation
(C) repression
(D) denial
(E) introjection

> (D) is correct. Denial is unconsciously avoiding an unwanted feeling or situation.
> (A) Sublimation is directing or changing unacceptable drives for security, affection, or power into socially and culturally acceptable channels.
> (B) Disassociation is not connecting one event with another.
> (C) Repression is keeping unpleasant thoughts or feelings out of one's mind.
> (E) Introjection is adopting the feelings of someone else.

13. A proper initial greeting upon answering the telephone would be

(A) "Gynecology Associates."
(B) "Please hold."
(C) "Good afternoon."
(D) "This is Mary King, may I help you?"
(E) "Gynecology Associates, Ms. King speaking, may I help you?"

> (E) is correct.

14. After a patient is placed on hold, it is proper to check back every

(A) 10 seconds
(B) 20 seconds
(C) 30 seconds
(D) minute
(E) 2 minutes

> (C) is correct. Ideally, the medical assistant should check back every 30 seconds on the patient who has been placed on hold.

15. Which of the following conditions explained over the telephone would NOT be considered an emergency?

(A) asthma
(B) severe pain
(C) high temperature
(D) scarlet fever
(E) premature labor

(D) is correct. Scarlet fever would require the physician's attention and a telephone message. However, it would not be considered an emergency unless there were other conditions present, such as high fever or breathing difficulty.

16. If an emergency is taking place to the person making the telephone call, the first action the medical assistant should take is to

(A) alert the physician immediately
(B) call 911
(C) put the caller on the speaker phone
(D) record the call for liability purposes
(E) tell the person to go to the hospital immediately

(A) is correct.

17. When handling a request for a prescription refill, a medical assistant

(A) may call in the request, but only for a noncontrolled substance
(B) should ask the patient to come into the office to obtain a written prescription
(C) may never call in a refill without the physician's direct order
(D) is certified to call in all prescription refills
(E) should call in the prescription if directed to do so by a nurse

(C) is correct. The medical assistant acts only under the direct supervision of a physician.

18. A ringing telephone should be answered on the

(A) first ring
(B) second ring
(C) third ring
(D) fourth ring
(E) none of the above

(B) is correct. Always try to answer a ringing phone by the second ring.

19. If a medical assistant is already speaking to a patient when another phone line rings, it is best to

(A) call to another medical assistant to answer the other line
(B) let the other line be picked up by voice mail
(C) let the patient finish his or her question and then say, "Would you please hold"
(D) ask the patient if you may place him or her on hold
(E) answer the second caller and handle the problem right away

(C) is correct. As a courtesy, ask the first caller if you can place him or her on hold for a moment.

20. Adopting the feelings of someone else, as when a child is afraid of needles because the mother is afraid, is the defensive behavior of

(A) projection
(B) compensation
(C) regression
(D) introjection
(E) sublimation

(D) is correct. Introjection is adopting the feelings of someone else.

(A) Projection is placing your own feelings onto another person. In the above example, the mother has projected her feelings about needles onto her son.

(B) Compensation is substitution of an attitude, feeling, or behavior with its opposite.

(C) Regression is turning back to former behavior to avoid the truth.

(E) Sublimation is directing or changing unacceptable drives for security, affection, and/or power into socially acceptable channels.

21. Mrs. Sims believes that the appetite suppressant benefit of smoking offsets the risk of developing cancer. This is using the defensive behavior of

(A) projection
(B) compensation
(C) regression

(D) introjection
(E) rationalization

(E) is correct. Rationalization is justifying thoughts or behaviors to avoid the truth.

(A) Projection is placing your own feelings onto another person.

(B) Compensation is substitution of an attitude, feeling, or behavior with its opposite.

(C) Regression is turning back to former behavior to avoid the truth.

(D) Introjection is adopting the feelings of someone else.

22. What is the maximum weight (in pounds) for priority mail?

(A) 100
(B) 150
(C) 70

(D) 50
(E) there is no maximum weight

(C) is correct. The maximum weight for priority mail is 70 pounds.

23. What type of mail is used to send valuables, such as currency and jewelry?

(A) special handling
(B) registered mail
(C) priority mail

(D) special delivery
(E) all of the above

(B) is correct. Registered mail is the preferred route to send valuables since the sender receives a receipt, which can be used to trace the lost item.

(A) Special handling can be requested for third- and fourth-class items.

(C) Priority mail is first-class mail weighing between 11 ounces and 70 pounds.

(D) Special delivery is useful for shipping perishables, such as specimens, since the post office will deliver this type of mail beyond the regular hours of service.

24. The proofreader's mark that means "insert a space" is

(A) #
(B) /=
(C) [

(D) [/]
(E) sp

(A)   is correct. The proofreader's mark # means to insert a space.
(B)   The proofreader's mark =/ means insert a hyphen.
(C)   The proofreader's mark [means to move to the left.
(D)   The proofreader's mark [/] means to insert brackets.
(E)   The proofreader's mark sp means spell out.

25. Which of the following would NOT be used on a memorandum?

(A) writer's name
(B) subject
(C) complimentary close
(D) date
(E) all of the above are used

(C)   is correct. The complimentary close is not used on a memorandum.

26. The two-letter abbreviation for Maryland is

(A) MN
(B) MA
(C) ME
(D) MD
(E) MI

(D)   is correct. The two-letter abbreviation for Maryland is MD.
(A)   MN is the abbreviation for Minnesota.
(B)   MA is the abbreviation for Massachusetts.
(C)   ME is the abbreviation for Maine.
(E)   MI is the abbreviation for Michigan.

27. What type of mail should be used to send contracts, mortgages, deeds, and checks?

(A) priority mail
(B) first class
(C) certified mail
(D) second class
(E) third class

(C)   is correct. Certified mail is used for materials that are not valuable themselves but would be difficult to replace, such as deeds. They are mailed at the first-class rate with a special fee for certified mail, which can be tracked if lost.
(A)   Priority mail is first-class mail weighing more than 11 ounces and less than 70 pounds.
(B)   First-class mail is letters and postcards weighing less than 11 ounces.
(D)   Second-class mail is used for newspapers and periodicals.
(E)   Third-class mail (standard mail A) is used for catalogs, books, photographs, flyers, and other printed materials. Standard mail B is for packages.

28. When the subject of the sentence performs the action, it can be described as

(A) passive voice
(B) active voice
(C) first person
(D) A and C
(E) none of the above

(B)   is correct. In the active voice, the subject of the sentence does the action.
(A)   In the passive voice, the subject receives the action.
(C)   First person refers to the pronoun "I" or the person who is telling the story.

29. The word "its" means

(A) it is
(B) of or belonging to
(C) more than one

(D) the same as it's
(E) none of the above

(B) is correct. "Its" means of or belonging to.
(A) "It's" means it is.

30. The word "complement" means to

(A) praise
(B) flatter
(C) flutter

(D) complete
(E) none of the above

(D) is correct. The word "complement" means to complete. To praise (A) or flatter (B) is a compliment.

31. The medical abbreviation "p.c." means

(A) by mouth
(B) at bedtime
(C) before meals

(D) after meals
(E) as required, as needed

(D) is correct. The abbreviation p.c., or post-prandial, means after meals.
(A) P.O., representing per os, means to take by mouth.
(B) The abbreviation h.s. means to take at bedtime (the hour of sleep).
(C) The abbreviation a.c. means to take before meals.
(E) The abbreviation prn means to take as necessary or as required.

32. Words that sound alike, but that have different meanings and spellings, are

(A) homophones
(B) synonyms
(C) antonyms

(D) eponyms
(E) none of the above

(A) is correct. Homophones are words that sound alike but have different meanings. An example would be there and their.
(B) A synonym is a word that has the same or nearly the same meaning as another word.
(C) An antonym is a word that is opposite to the meaning of another word.
(D) An eponym is a real or mythical person from whose name the name of a nation or race is derived or who has become identified with something. For instance, William Penn's name is the eponym for Pennsylvania.

33. Which of the following is considered to be a proper closing?

(A) Thanks
(B) Truly
(C) Yours Truly

(D) Yours truly
(E) none of the above

(D) is correct.

34. When proofreading a document, it is easiest to spot a typing error by

    (A) looking up each of the difficult words
    (B) reading the document backwards
    (C) having someone else read it
    (D) reading it through very quickly
    (E) none of the above

        (B) is correct. Proofreading, especially for double words such as the the, is easiest when reading a document from the end to the beginning, or backwards.

35. Which of the following must be capitalized?

    (A) single-word expressions used in place of a sentence
    (B) first letter of the first word of each item in a list
    (C) the first letter in the closing of a letter
    (D) a noun that is part of a proper name
    (E) all of the above

        (E) is correct.

36. Which of the following words is misspelled?

    (A) petit mal   **(D)** sphygmomanometer
    (B) illeum   **(E)** stethoscope
    (C) wheal

        (B) is correct. The correct spelling is ileum, meaning a portion of the small intestine.

37. The words you, us, and them are examples of what parts of speech?

    (A) noun   **(D)** adverb
    (B) pronoun   **(E)** preposition
    (C) adjective

        (B) is correct. The words you, us, and them are all examples of pronouns.
        (A) A noun names a person, place, or thing.
        (C) An adjective is a word used to modify a noun or pronoun.
        (D) An adverb is a word used to modify a verb.
        (E) A preposition indicates the relationship between the noun and/or pronoun that follows it and another word in the sentence.

38. The plural form of thorax is

    (A) thoraxes   **(D)** thoraxi's
    (B) thoraxis   **(E)** none of the above
    (C) thoraces

        (C) is correct. The plural form of thorax is thoraces. For a word ending in ax, drop the x and add ces.

39. In the sentence, "Dr. Lopez and Dr. Martinez will be attending the conference," what part of speech is "and"?

(A) conjunction   (D) adjective
(B) interjection   (E) adverb
(C) preposition

    (A)   is correct. A conjunction connects words or word groups. Conjunctions include and, but, nor, for, so, yet, after, and although.
    (B)   An interjection is a word used to express strong feeling. An example would be ouch or hurrah.
    (C)   A preposition indicates the relationship between the noun and/or pronoun that follows it and another word in the sentence. Examples are above, about, across, and after.
    (D)   An adjective modifies a noun or pronoun.
    (E)   An adverb modifies a verb.

40. When using a title in the inside address of a letter, which of the following would be correct?

(A) Dr. Beth Williams   (D) Mrs. Allan Williams, MD
(B) Beth Williams, MD   (E) none of the above
(C) Dr. Beth Williams, MD

    (B)   is correct.

41. PDR stands for

(A) Physician's Drug registry   (D) Physician's Desk Reference
(B) Physician's Drug Recorded   (E) Physical Drug Reference
(C) Physician's Drug Reference

    (D)   is correct. PDR is an acronym for the *Physician's Desk Reference.*

42. First-class letters must not exceed

(A) 7 ounces   (D) 16 ounces
(B) 9 ounces   (E) 70 pounds
(C) 11 ounces

    (C)   is correct. First-class letters and mail must weigh less than 11 ounces.

43. According to the USPS, the last line in an address must not exceed

(A) 20 characters   (D) 30 characters
(B) 25 characters   (E) 35 characters
(C) 27 characters

    (A)   According to the USPS, the last line in an address cannot exceed 20 characters in length.

44. A standard #10 envelope measures

(A) $9^{1/2}'' \times 4^{1/8}''$

(B) $7^{1/2}'' \times 3^{7/8}''$

(C) $6^{1/2}'' \times 3^{5/8}''$

(D) $8^{1/2}'' \times 11''$

(E) none of the above

(A) is correct. A standard #10 envelope measures $9^{1/2}$ inches $\times$ $4^{1/8}$ inches.

45. The synonym for the term larynx is

(A) throat

(B) carcinoma

(C) voice box

(D) white blood cells

(E) otolaryngology

(C) is correct. The synonym (word having the same meaning as another word) for larynx is voice box.

(A) A synonym for throat is pharynx.

(B) Carcinoma means cancer.

(D) White blood cells are leukocytes.

(E) Otolaryngology is the study of the ear and throat.

CHAPTER 8

APPOINTMENT SCHEDULING

1. "Blocking out" the appointment schedule book is called developing

   (A) a double-booking schedule
   (B) a wave schedule
   (C) a matrix
   (D) a modified wave schedule
   (E) open office hours

   (C) is correct. A matrix is a base upon which to build, such as a format or shape for the daily schedule.

   (A) Double booking is assigning two patients to be seen during the same time slot. This is considered to be a poor practice.

   (B) A wave schedule is a type of flexible scheduling in which each hour is divided into segments of time. All patients who will be seen during that hour arrive at the beginning of the hour.

   (D) A modified wave schedule is a form of flexible scheduling in which each hour is divided into segments of time, with each patient arriving within 10 to 15 minutes of each other. Time is allowed at the end of each hour for "catch-up."

   (E) Open office hours scheduling is the least structured of all systems. The hours the medical office is open are posted, and patients may arrive at any time during those hours.

2. Jay Craig is scheduled to have a cast check. He has been given a 15-minute appointment at 2:00 PM. His wife, Jill, has an appointment on the same day at 2:15. What type of scheduling system is the physician using?

   (A) wave scheduling
   (B) open office hours
   (C) double booking
   (D) modified wave scheduling
   (E) none of the above

   (D) is correct. A modified wave schedule is a form of flexible scheduling in which each hour is divided into segments of time, with each patient arriving within 10 to 15 minutes of each other. Time is allowed at the end of each hour for "catch-up."

3. When a patient is given six 15-minute time slots for a complete physical examination requiring 1½ hours, this is called

   (A) wave scheduling
   (B) specified time scheduling
   (C) modified wave scheduling
   (D) open office hours
   (E) double booking

   (B) is correct. Specified time scheduling is an appointment scheduling method in which each patient is given a specific time slot. Every time slot during the day is booked with patient appointments.

(A)   Wave scheduling is a type of flexible scheduling in which each hour is divided into segments of time. All patients who will be seen during that hour arrive at the beginning of the hour.

(C)   A modified wave schedule is a form of flexible scheduling in which each hour is divided into segments of time, with each patient arriving within 10 to 15 minutes of each other. Time is allowed at the end of each hour for "catch-up."

(D)   An open office hours type of scheduling is the least structured of all systems. The hours the medical office is open are posted, and patients may arrive at any time during those hours.

(E)   Double booking is assigning two patients to be seen during the same time slot. This is considered to be a poor practice.

4. With modified wave scheduling, each hour is divided into segments of time, with each patient arriving within

(A) 5 to 10 minutes   (D) every half hour
(B) 10 to 15 minutes   (E) none of the above
(C) 20 to 30 minutes

    (B)   is correct. Using a modified wave scheduling method, each hour is divided into 10- to 15-minute segments of time.

5. The type of scheduling system that may produce the longest patient waiting time is

(A) wave   (D) grouping
(B) specified time   (E) double booking
(C) modified wave

    (A)   is correct. A patient may have to wait an hour, or even longer if the physician is running behind, with the wave method, since all patients come in at the beginning of the hour. Only the first person seen during that hour is seen on time.

    (B)   Specified time scheduling has a patient scheduled during every time slot. There may be delays as the day progresses if the physician begins to get behind. However, the wait is usually not as long as with the wave type of scheduling.

    (C)   The modified wave schedule is a flexible type of schedule in which the patients will come in at various times during the hour, but the scheduler will still leave time open at the end of the hour for the physician to "catch up."

    (D)   Grouping refers to scheduling similar types of appointments (such as well baby visits, cast changes, or school exams) together for greater efficiency.

    (E)   Double booking is not a time-saving method. However, the wait is not as long as with some forms of wave scheduling.

6. The main drawback to specified time scheduling is that

(A) the time waiting for an available appointment is dramatically increased
(B) if not enough information is given to the medical assistant at the time of booking the appointment, the patient may not be booked for and receive the appropriate amount of time

(C) less patients are seen
(D) patients are not permitted to choose appointment times
(E) all of the above

(B) is correct. The greatest difficulty when using a specified time schedule is that patients have not given enough information for the medical assistant to be able to estimate the amount of time that is needed for the appointment.

7. The main purpose of wave scheduling is to

(A) allow the physician to choose the order in which the patients are to be seen
(B) allow for "no-shows"
(C) allow the physician to get caught up with paperwork
(D) begin and end each hour on time
(E) none of the above

(D) is correct. Wave scheduling allows for each hour to begin and end on time since all the patients are scheduled to come in at the beginning of the hour, and the danger of patients coming in toward the end of the hour or even later is diminished.

8. The least structured of all the scheduling systems is the

(A) wave
(B) modified wave
(C) specified time
(D) open office hours
(E) double booking

(D) is correct. Open office hours are the least structured of all the scheduling systems.

9. How far ahead of time should an appointment book be "blocked out"?

(A) 1 year
(B) 3 to 6 months
(C) 2 years
(D) to be done when you make an appointment
(E) should not be done at all

(B) is correct. The appointment should not be "blocked out" more than 6 months ahead of time since the physician's schedule may change.

10. What is the best method to use when a patient cancels 1 hour before an afternoon appointment?

(A) try to move up the last four 15-minute appointments of the day so the physician can leave an hour earlier
(B) do nothing since the physician is always running late
(C) call several patients who have asked to be placed on a waiting list and try to fill the entire hour
(D) move all the rest of the afternoon schedule up 1 hour
(E) leave the time free for the physician to get caught up on paperwork

(C) is correct. Try to fill the time slot with patients who are on a waiting list and can come in with very little prior notice.

11. When a patient requires surgery, the medical assistant would

   (A) provide all the information to the patient so that the patient can schedule surgery at a convenient time for him or her
   (B) ask the surgeon who is performing the surgery to schedule it
   (C) place the surgery request in writing and send it to the surgical center
   (D) call the surgery scheduler where the surgery will be performed to schedule the time
   (E) none of the above

   > (D)   is correct. The medical assistant should schedule the surgery through the surgery scheduler at the surgical site.

12. To assist the physician in avoiding a claim by a patient for abandonment, the medical assistant would

   (A) screen out all patients who really do not need to be seen by the physician
   (B) tell the patient that he or she will have to find another physician for treatment
   (C) call the patient to attempt to reschedule a missed appointment and document the telephone call
   (D) nothing special needs to be done
   (E) A, B, and C all need to be done

   > (C)   is correct. To assist the physician in avoiding a claim by a patient for abandonment, the medical assistant would call the patient to attempt to reschedule a missed appointment and document the telephone call.

13. When a patient does not show up for an appointment, the medical assistant should

   (A) write "N/S" above the scheduled appointment
   (B) record the missed appointment in the patient's record
   (C) record the reason for the missed appointment in the patient's record
   (D) B and C only
   (E) A, B, and C

   > (E)   is correct.

14. The process by which a patient gives a medical assistant demographic information over the telephone prior to an office visit is known as

   (A) precertification
   (B) insurance verification
   (C) preadmission
   (D) preregistration
   (E) none of the above

   > (D)   is correct. Preregistration is the process of collecting demographic information about the patient over the phone.
   > (A)   Precertification or authorization for treatment is obtained by either the patient or the medical assistant from the patient's insurer.
   > (B)   Insurance verification is obtained by calling the insurance company for authorization to treat (see answer B).
   > (C)   Preadmission information is obtained from the patient by the hospital or health facility's admissions clerk.

15. Demographic information includes all of the following EXCEPT

   (A) insurance information
   (B) name, address, and phone number of patient
   (C) patient's consent for treatment
   (D) age of patient
   (E) Social Security number

> (C) is correct. The patient's consent for treatment is obtained in writing from the patient after the physician has thoroughly explained the treatment.

16. Illnesses or injuries that come upon the patient suddenly and require treatment are referred to as

   (A) acute   **(D)** critical
   (B) chronic   **(E)** none of the above
   (C) emergent

> (A) is correct. An acute condition is one that has appeared suddenly and requires treatment.
> (B) A chronic condition is one that has been present for an extended period of time and may never totally be gone.
> (C) An emergent condition is one that has appeared suddenly and requires immediate or emergency treatment.
> (D) A critical condition is a medical condition that may result in death or severe disability if not treated immediately.

17. All of the following are either medical emergencies or acute conditions that require an appointment as soon as possible EXCEPT

   (A) earache
   (B) eye infection
   (C) severe pain
   (D) pain with urination
   (E) fever of 99.8 degrees for the past 2 weeks

> (E) is correct. A fever of 2 weeks' duration is not considered an emergency. However, this patient does need to be seen by the physician.

18. A system of prioritizing patients according to the most severely injured (who have a chance for survival by being treated first) is known as

   (A) classifying   **(D)** mortality rate
   (B) triage   **(E)** morbidity rate
   (C) insurance preapproval

> (B) is correct. Triage is a system of prioritizing patients according to the most severely injured who have a chance for survival by being treated first.
> (A) Classifying is a method of placing people and things in categories according to similarities.
> (C) Insurance preapproval is not needed before administering emergency treatment.
> (D) The mortality rate is the death rate within a particular population.
> (E) The morbidity rate is the rate of illness within a particular population.

19. Facilities that are prepared to handle situations requiring immediate, but not life-threatening, medical care are known as

   (A) surgicenters
   (B) ambulatory care centers
   (C) freestanding urgent care centers
   (D) emergency rooms
   (E) none of the above

   (C) is correct.
   (A) Surgicenters are facilities to handle day-surgery procedures.
   (B) Ambulatory care centers are facilities that handle medical problems of ambulatory patients.

20. Elective surgery is a procedure that

   (A) is necessary for the patient to have but can be postponed until the patient has the time
   (B) is for a life-threatening condition
   (C) does not require a surgical consent
   (D) is not for a life-threatening condition and is often left up to the discretion of the patient as to whether he or she wishes to have the procedure
   (E) C and D

   (D) is correct. Elective surgery is a procedure that is performed for a non–life-threatening condition. It is one that is performed at the patient's request.

21. An example of elective surgery would be

   (A) wisdom teeth extraction
   (B) liposuction
   (C) breast biopsy
   (D) tonsillectomy
   (E) removal of vocal polyps

   (B) is correct. Liposuction is generally performed at the patient's request for purposes of fat removal and weight reduction. All the other examples, although they are not emergencies, relate to surgical procedures that need to be performed.

22. It is unethical for a medical assistant to decide

   (A) a patient's chief complaint
   (B) how much time the patient's appointment requires
   (C) that a patient is lying about the need to be seen by a physician
   (D) if the patient can pay his or her bill
   (E) C and D

   (E) is correct.

CHAPTER 9

COMPUTERS IN MEDICINE

1. The hardware device that converts digital signals to analog signals for transfer over communication lines or links is

   (A) cursor
   (B) mouse
   (C) daisy wheel
   (D) keyboard
   (E) modem

       (E) is correct.
       (A) A cursor is a flashing bar, or symbol, which indicates where the next character will be placed.
       (B) The mouse is a pointing and selection device to input data.
       (C) A daisy wheel printer "strikes" characters onto a page, like a typewriter.
       (D) Keyboard is an input device, similar to a typewriter keyboard.

2. The "brain" or "heart" of the computer is

   (A) ROM
   (B) CPU
   (C) RAM
   (D) DOS
   (E) GIGO

       (B) is correct.
       (A) ROM is read-only memory.
       (C) RAM is random-access memory.
       (D) DOS is disk operating system.
       (E) GIGO means "garbage in, garbage out," which means if you input incorrect information, you will receive incorrect output.

3. Backup means

   (A) a copy of work or software batch data stored for processing at periodic intervals
   (B) to eliminate errors from input data
   (C) time a computer cannot be used because of maintenance or mechanical failure
   (D) entering data into the computer system
   (E) a list of options available to the user

       (A) is correct.
       (B) Data debugging eliminates errors from input data.
       (C) Downtime is when a computer cannot be used.
       (D) Input means to enter data.
       (E) A menu is a list of options available to the user.

4. The speed measurement of printers is in

(A) gigabytes
(B) kilobytes
(C) characters per second

(D) megahertz
(E) RAM

    (C) is correct.
    (A) gigabytes, (B) kilobytes, and (E) RAM are measures of storage capacity within the computer.
    (D) Megahertz is the speed by which the computer can move information from one place to another.

5. A network is another term for

(A) format
(B) input
(C) output

(D) interface
(E) menu

    (D) is correct. A network or interface is technology that allows two or more nonconnected computers to exchange programs and data.
    (A) Format is the method for setting margins, tabs, and line spacing.
    (B) Input refers to entering data into the computer system.
    (C) Output is processed data translated into final form.

6. Another name for a computer monitor is

(A) boot
(B) cursor
(C) modem

(D) disk drive
(E) terminal

    (E) is correct.
    (A) Boot means to start up the computer.
    (B) Cursor is the flashing bar, which indicates where the next character will be placed.
    (C) A modem is a hardware device, which converts digital signals to analog signals for transfer over communication lines or links.
    (D) Disk drive is a container, which holds a read/write head, an access arm, and a magnetic disk for storage.

7. What is NOT recommended to establish computer security?

(A) position screen away from patients
(B) change password frequently
(C) use a password that is unknown to the patient but that you can remember easily
(D) have tiers of security that limit access to patient information to authorized employees
(E) use screen savers to blank out the screen

    (B) is correct. The password should be changed periodically, not frequently. (A), (C), (D), and (E) are recommended to establish computer security. Confidentiality of patient records is a high priority.

8. Computer memory is measured in

(A) DOS
(B) CPUs
(C) kilobytes
(D) RAM
(E) megahertz

(C) is correct.
(A) DOS stands for disk operating system.
(B) CPU stands for central processing unit.
(D) RAM stands for random access memory.
(E) Megahertz is the speed with which the computer can move information from one place to another.

9. Another name for a computer program is

(A) chip
(B) diskette
(C) hardware
(D) software
(E) boot

(D) is correct.
(A) Chip is a small piece of electronic hardware, which allows the processing of information in a very small place.
(B) Diskette is a storage medium for data and software.
(C) Hardware is the actual physical equipment that is used by a computer to process data.
(E) Boot is to start up the computer.

10. Electronic mail is

(A) a process of eliminating errors from input data
(B) physically entering data into the computer system
(C) use of a telephone, modem, or hardware and software to transmit data from computer to computer
(D) a backup copy of work or software
(E) physical equipment used by a computer to process data

(C) is correct.
(A) Data debugging is the process of eliminating errors from input data.
(B) Input is entering data.
(D) Backup is a second copy of work or software.
(E) Hardware is the physical computer equipment.

11. More sophisticated word processing programs allow the user to

(A) check spelling and grammar
(B) create tables, charts, and graphs
(C) have automatic playback of frequently used words, phrases, and letters
(D) generate form letters to every person or to selected individuals in the database
(E) all of the above

(E) is correct. The word processors are used in medical settings to generate and print letters, postcards, newsletters, patient information booklets, and sheets. They also generate (type) patient chart records, history and physical exams, operative reports, and discharge reports.

12. The benefit of electronic claims transmission (ECT) is that it

    (A) corrects grammar and spelling errors
    (B) schedules patient appointments
    (C) posts patient information in the medical record
    (D) posts cash flow received or paid
    (E) allows insurance forms to be sent faster

        (E)   is correct. ECT tremendously speeds the path of an insurance claim and places the money in the bank in 3 working days.

13. Which printer type is the least expensive?

    (A) laser   **(D)** color ink jet
    (B) dot matrix   **(E)** none of the above
    (C) ink jet

        (B)   is correct. These printers use pins against an inked ribbon, and the characters are usually a series of dots. The more pins, the better is the quality of the copy. The more pins, the higher is the cost of the printer.

14. The CD-ROM disc is capable of storing more information than

    (A) 10 floppy disks   **(D)** 500 floppy disks
    (B) 50 floppy disks   **(E)** 1,000 floppy disks
    (C) 100 floppy disks

        (E)   is correct.

15. The special magnetic storage media, contained inside the computer, is the

    (A) D drive   **(D)** A drive
    (B) C drive   **(E)** none of the above
    (C) B drive

        (B)   is correct.

16. The most common operating system is DOS (disk operating system). When loaded, a user will hear a beep and then receive a message called a

    (A) batch   **(D)** password
    (B) program   **(E)** menu
    (C) prompt

        (C)   is correct. A prompt is a reminder to the user that an action must be taken by the user before data processing can continue.
        (A)   Batch is data stored for processing at periodic intervals.
        (B)   A program is a set of instructions that tell the computer hardware what to do.
        (D)   A password is a word or phrase that identifies a person.
        (E)   A menu is a list of options for the user.

17. Some keyboard commands have been completely eliminated by the use of a

    (A) cursor   **(D)** mouse
    (B) hard drive   **(E)** modem
    (C) menu

(D) is correct. The mouse allows the user to point to a picture of the desired function, and click through the program features.

(A) A cursor is a flashing bar, or symbol, which indicates where the next character will be placed.

(B) The hard drive is the internal processing drive of the computer.

(C) A menu is a list of options available to the user.

(E) A modem is hardware that converts computer signals for transfer over communication links, such as telephone lines.

18. Which is NOT a basic component of a computer system?

(A) modem   (D) CPU
(B) monitor   (E) printer
(C) keyboard

    (A) is correct. A modem is not a part on all computers.

19. To protect against a loss of data, a medical assistant should

(A) use E-mail
(B) use word processing whenever possible
(C) handwrite a backup copy for the file
(D) make backup copies on a diskette
(E) change the password frequently

    (D) is correct. A backup of data will prevent losing all data in the event of failure of the computer system, fire, or theft of the computer equipment.

20. The computer program that contains all records and files is

(A) file maintenance   (D) hard copy
(B) catalog   (E) database
(C) batch

    (E) is correct. The database is a computer application that contains the files or records.

    (A) File maintenance is a data entry operation, including additions, deletions, and changes.

    (B) Catalog lists all files stored on a storage device.

    (C) Batch is data stored for processing at periodic intervals.

    (D) Hard copy is a printed copy of data in a file.

21. A desktop personal computer is a

(A) mainframe   (D) supercomputer
(B) minicomputer   (E) none of the above
(C) microcomputer

    (C) is correct. A desktop personal computer is called a microcomputer.

    (A) A mainframe is a large computer that is capable of handling many (even hundreds) of users.

    (B) A minicomputer is a medium-sized computer that is capable of handling several users.

(D)   A supercomputer refers to the large computer system that is capable of performing complex functions at a rapid speed. These computers are used in areas of research and forecasting.

22. The control unit (CU) of the computer performs the following function(s)

(A)   retrieving and storing
(B)   decoding
(C)   executing

(D)   A and B only
(E)   A, B, and C

(E)   is correct. The CU performs retrieving (obtaining data from primary storage), storing (saving instructions in the primary storage unit), decoding (translating instructions into computer language), and executing (carrying out instructions).

23. A peripheral device for communicating between the user and the computer hardware is

(A)   track ball
(B)   mouse
(C)   joystick

(D)   light wand
(E)   all of the above

(E)   is correct. A track ball is a small ball that is imbedded in a base, which, when rolled by the user, will move the cursor on the screen. The mouse is a device held in the user's hand, which, when moved across a flat surface or a mouse pad, will move the cursor to a location on the computer screen. A joystick is a vertical stick or rod that is set in a base of support, which, when moved, will move the cursor in the direction of the stick movement. A light wand, also called a pen, controls the cursor when placed near the computer screen due to the sensitivity to the screen's light.

24. A secondary storage component is a/an

(A)   ASCII
(B)   disk drive
(C)   plotter

(D)   monitor
(E)   digital computer

(B)   is correct. A disk drive is a secondary storage component that is used to store programs and data.
(A)   ASCII refers to American Standard Code for Information Interchange. This is the machine language that is used in microcomputers.
(C)   A plotter is an output device that converts drawings, graphs, and charts into a high-quality type of hard copy.
(D)   A monitor is a piece of hardware that contains a screen or cathode ray tube (CRT) that will display data visually.
(E)   A digital computer processes binary or discrete numerical data.

25. When starting up the computer, you should

(A)   be familiar with the "booting" process
(B)   remove any floppy disks from drive A or B before starting
(C)   place a floppy disk into drive A or B before starting
(D)   A and B
(E)   A and C

(B) is correct. Before "booting" or starting up the computer, remove any floppy disks that were accidentally left in the computer.

26. The "delete" key on the computer keyboard or word-processing keyboard

   (A) allows the cursor to be moved in a direction to the left
   (B) is a toggle key that allows characters to be typed without erasing any of the current characters
   (C) will suspend computer operations
   (D) erases characters wherever the cursor is located
   (E) allows the user to escape the computer program

> (D) is correct. The "delete" key erases characters wherever the cursor is located.
>
> (A) The "backspace" key allows the cursor to be moved in a direction to the left.
>
> (B) The "insert" key allows characters to be typed without erasing any of the current characters.
>
> (C) The "break or pause" key may cause computer operations to become suspended.
>
> (E) The "escape" key allows the user to escape the computer program.

27. The smallest piece of information processed by a computer is called a

   (A) byte
   (B) bit
   (C) kilobyte
   (D) megabyte
   (E) none of the above

> (B) is correct. A bit is the smallest piece of information processed by a computer. A bit takes on the binary value of 1 when it is on, and the binary value of 0 when it is off.
>
> (A) A byte is 8 bits. One byte of memory will be required to form one character.
>
> (C) A kilobyte (K) is 1,024 bytes.
>
> (D) A megabyte (M) is 1,000 kilobytes.

28. Combining two or more files in word processing is referred to as

   (A) default
   (B) sorting
   (C) merging
   (D) an error message
   (E) the menu

> (C) is correct. Merging is when two or more files are combined.
>
> (A) Default refers to a predetermined setting that is automatically loaded with a program unless the user changes it.
>
> (B) The sort function is to organize a list of items in ascending or descending order either numerically or alphabetically.
>
> (D) An error message will come onto the screen when the user has made a mistake either in making a command or in entering data.
>
> (E) The menu is a list of options the user can select that is displayed somewhere on the screen.

29. Security measures refer to

    (A) frequently changing one's password
    (B) properly storing data disks
    (C) the use of a fade-out screen
    (D) A and B only
    (E) A, B, and C

       (E) is correct.

30. A hardware component that connects the user's computer to communication lines is

    (A) E-mail   **(D)** modem
    (B) voice mail   **(E)** network
    (C) facsimile

       (D) is correct. A modem connects the user's computer to communication lines.
       (A) E-mail is electronic mail.
       (B) Voice mail is a verbal message that is stored and transmitted over telephone lines.
       (C) A facsimile or FAX is a machine that can electronically receive and transmit documents using telephone lines.
       (E) A network is a collection of computers and terminals that share information, data, computer hardware, and software.

CHAPTER 10

FEES, BILLING, COLLECTIONS, AND CREDIT

1. A record for each patient of charges, payments, and the current balance is a/an

   (A) medical record
   (B) audit
   ✔**(C)** ledger
   (D) reconciliation
   (E) accounts payable record

       (C)   is correct.
       (A)   The medical record is also known as the chart and contains information regarding the patient, primarily the reason for the visit and treatment.
       (B)   An audit is an examination, usually by an accountant, of the financial records of a medical practice for the purpose of determining the accuracy of the records.
       (D)   Reconciliation is the process of balancing the office account with the bank's statement.
       (E)   Accounts payable record is a record of money owed by the physician/medical practice to companies for services rendered.

2. When an account has been referred for collection, the medical assistant should

   (A) send a reminder letter
   ✔**(B)** not attempt to collect
   (C) discuss payment with the patient
   (D) call the patient's employer
   (E) cancel the balance

       (B)   is correct. When an account has been turned over to a collection agency, the medical office should not attempt to collect.

3. A record of services for billing and insurance processing is a/an

   ✔**(A)** superbill
   (B) ledger
   (C) double-entry bookkeeping
   (D) receipt
   (E) aging account

       (A)   is correct. A superbill is also known as an encounter form or a charge slip.
       (B)   A ledger is a record for each patient of charges, payments, and the current balance.
       (C)   Double-entry bookkeeping is a system in which each transaction is recorded in two different places, which forces a balance of records.
       (D)   A receipt is issued when a payment is made in cash or by check.
       (E)   An aging account refers to the length of time the amount owed has been outstanding.

4. A "skip" is a name for a patient who

    (A) is turned over to a collection agency
    (B) has not paid his or her bill
    (C) was fired from his or her job
    (D) pays his or her bill
    ✔**(E)** has moved and not left a forwarding address

        (E) is correct. "Skips" can be traced by confirming addresses on the registration form, calling telephone numbers, and calling references.

5. Regulation Z, of the Truth in Lending Act, requires the physician to provide disclosure information regarding finance charges when payment arrangements are made in

    (A) one or more installments   ✔**(D)** four or more installments
    (B) two or more installments   **(E)** five or more installments
    (C) three or more installments

        (D) is correct. This act covers agreements between patient and physician to allow the patient to make payments in more than four installments.

6. An effective collection letter is

    (A) a preprinted form letter
    (B) unsigned
    ✔**(C)** simple and encourages the patient to take action
    (D) impersonal
    (E) demands cash

        (C) is correct. Patients who receive a personalized letter feel that his or her account has been reviewed individually. An offer to assist the patient with making payment arrangements should be included.

7. A condition in which a patient is protected by the court and all collection attempts must cease is

    (A) statute of limitations   **(D)** assignment of benefits
    (B) claims against estates   ✔**(E)** bankruptcy
    (C) accounts receivable insurance

        (E) is correct. When all collection attempts must cease due to the patient filing for bankruptcy, the medical office must file a claim for payment.
        (A) Statute of limitations refers to the amount of time a legal collection attempt may be brought against a debtor.
        (B) Claims against estates take place when a patient dies and the bill is sent to the deceased's estate.
        (C) Accounts receivable insurance is purchased to protect against loss of accounts receivable.
        (D) Assignment of benefits is the patient's written authorization allowing the insurance companies to directly pay the physician.

8. Which of the following is NOT a guideline for making collections as presented in the Fair Debt Collection Practices Act?

    (A) do not make threatening statements toward the patient
✔**(B)** use a postcard
    (C) telephone calls should be placed between 8 AM and 9 PM
    (D) avoid calling the place of employment of the debtor
    (E) never place an overdue notice on the outside of an envelope

> (B) is correct. The Fair Debt Collection Practices Act is a federal law that was set up to protect the debtor from harassment. Confidentiality must be maintained. Do not send a collection notice on a postcard.

9. A signed assignment of benefits form is good for

✔**(A)** 1 year   **(D)** 7 years
    (B) 3 years   **(E)** 10 years
    (C) 5 years

> (A) is correct.

10. Which of the following is the most effective method in the collection process?

    (A) telephone call   ✔**(D)** personal interview
    (B) collection agency   **(E)** collection letter
    (C) collection notice

> (D) is correct.

11. The fee that a patient might be expected to pay for similar services is the

    (A) usual fee   **(D)** co-pay fee
    (B) customary fee   **(E)** none of the above
✔**(C)** reasonable fee

> (C) is correct.
> (A) The usual fee is the charge of a physician for his or her private patients.
> (B) The customary fee is the fee for the same procedure charged by a majority of physicians with similar training, geographic location, and socioeconomic area.
> (D) A co-pay fee means that the patient is responsible for payment of a portion of the bill.

12. The process for determining when accounts are overdue is

    (A) accounts receivable insurance
    (B) a collection agency
    (C) the Fair Debt Collection Practices Act
    (D) statute of limitations
✔**(E)** aging of accounts

> (E) is correct. Computerized systems allow the medical assistant to print out aging reports with a 30-, 60-, and 90-day or over analysis.

13. Who makes the final determination as to what fees for services will be charged?

   (A) Medicare
   (B) federal government
   (C) insurance company
   (D) local government
   ✔**(E)** physician

      (E) is correct. The physician takes into consideration the time and services provided, and the community's economic level.

14. Computerized fee schedules should be updated

   (A) every month
   (B) every 2 months
   (C) every 3 months
   (D) every 6 months
   ✔**(E)** when fees change/at least once a year

      (E) is correct. Offices maintain databases that contain codes and fees, which need to be updated periodically.

15. When a physician cancels a patient's debt, it is called

   (A) debt cancellation
   ✔**(B)** write-off
   (C) skip
   (D) assignment of benefits
   (E) accounts receivable reversal

      (B) is correct. Occasionally when there is no hope of collecting the debt, the physician may choose to write off the debt.

16. Which of the following is NOT expected by a collection agency?

   ✔**(A)** no charge for the service
   (B) the medical office not to try to collect the debt
   (C) will discuss its collection methods
   (D) copies of patient information
   (E) copies of itemized statements

      (A) is correct. Collection agencies charge for their services, either a flat rate per account or a percentage of the amount collected.

17. Which of the following is NOT information needed to maintain a current billing file?

   (A) full name
   (B) address
   (C) telephone number
   (D) insurance
   ✔**(E)** diagnosis

      (E) is correct.

18. Which of the following is NOT a collection guideline?

   (A) seek immediate payment
   (B) envelopes should have Address Correction Requested imprinted on them under the postmark
   (C) use change slips or superbills
   (D) outline all fees and finance charges for the patient
   (E) follow up on all commitments by the patient

(B) is correct. The imprint should be placed under the return address.

19. The state statute of limitations should be investigated if you have aging accounts for more than what amount of time?

(A) 6 months
(B) 1 year
(C) 2 years
(D) 3 years
(E) 5 years

(D) is correct. The statute of limitations should be investigated to see if you can still collect on the bill. Each state has its own statute of limitations.

20. The medical assistant must project a professional, but caring, approach when working in collections. Which is NOT a professional question?

(A) How can we help you to work out a suitable payment plan?
(B) We have several payment plans. Which would be suitable for you?
(C) When are you going to pay your bill?
(D) May we set up an appointment with you to discuss payment options that are available to you?
(E) I see from your account that payment is past due. May I discuss payment plans that are available to you?

(C) is correct. This definitely does not project a caring approach, and it is very unprofessional.

21. The back of a check is endorsed or signed by the

(A) payer
(B) payee
(C) maker
(D) signee
(E) all of the above

(B) is correct. The payee is the person or company named as the receiving party to whom the amount on the check is payable.
(A) The payer is the person signing the check to release the money.
(C) The maker of the check is the person who signs the check (or corporation that pays it). This is the same as the payer.
(D) The signee is the person who signs the check or document. This term is used interchangeably with the terms payer and maker.

22. The MICR refers to

(A) the code number on the right upper corner of the printed check to identify the bank
(B) an indication that there is not sufficient money in the account to honor payment of the check
(C) the characters and letters printed on the bottom of the check that are used as routing information to identify the bank and number of the individual account
(D) a blank endorsement
(E) a restrictive endorsement

(C) is correct. Magnetic ink character recognition (MICR) is the characters and letters printed on the bottom of the check that are used as routing information to identify the bank and number of the individual account.

(A) The ABA number is the code number on the right upper corner of the printed check to identify the bank.

(B) Not sufficient funds (NSF) refers to a situation in which there is not sufficient money in the account to honor payment of the check.

(D) A blank endorsement is one in which the check has only the payee's signature present. This allows payment of the check to any bearer. This is an unsafe practice.

(E) A restrictive endorsement is one that specifies to whom money should be paid.

23. A check that contains a date after the date on which it was written is referred to as

(A) an overdraft
(B) a disbursement
(C) a third-party check
(D) postdated
(E) NSF

(D) is correct. A postdated check is dated after the day on which it was written.

(A) An overdraft is issuing a check without having enough funds in the account (NSF). This is illegal.

(B) A disbursement refers to cash payments made to creditors.

(C) A third-party check is a check written to the payment of another payee but presented to you as payment (the third party).

(E) NSF refers to not sufficient funds in the account.

24. To adjust one's banking records against a bank statement so that both are in agreement is called

(A) double-entry bookkeeping
(B) a warrant
(C) debit
(D) credit
(E) reconciliation

(E) is correct. A reconciliation of a bank statement is to adjust one's banking records against a bank statement so that both are in agreement.

(A) Double-entry bookkeeping is a system in which each transaction is recorded in two different places, which forces a balance of records.

(B) A warrant is a written non-negotiable evidence that a debt (money) is due to a person. The warrant can then be used to collect money.

(C) A debit is a charge against an account.

(D) A credit is funds that are added to an account.

25. Liabilities include

(A) land, buildings, and furniture
(B) machinery and equipment
(C) accounts payable
(D) accounts receivable
(E) A, B, and D

(C) is correct. Accounts payable are the vendor/supplier debts that are owed by the medical practice to someone else. (A), (B), and (D) are all assets of the medical practice.

26. When a check is marked by the bank so that it cannot be cashed again, this is referred to as

(A) NSF
(B) MICR
(C) ABA

(D) cancelled
(E) none of the above

(D) is correct. A cancelled check is one in which the bank has stamped or cancelled it after cashing it so that it cannot be cashed again.
(A) NSF stands for "not sufficient funds" in the account.
(B) MICR refers to Magnetic Ink Character Recognition.
(C) ABA refers to the code number on checks that identifies the bank.

27. A law (act) that prohibits discrimination when extending credit is

(A) Regulation Z of the Truth in Lending Act
(B) Fair Debt Collection Practices Act
(C) Equal Credit Opportunity Act
(D) all of the above
(E) none of the above

(C) is correct. The Equal Credit Opportunity Act prohibits discrimination based on race, color, gender, religion, marital status, national origin, or age when extending credit.
(A) Regulation Z of the Truth in Lending Act requires that a written form be completed, which discloses information regarding finance charges if the person will be making payments in four or more installments.
(B) The Fair Debt Collection Practices Act prohibits unfair collection practices and regulates the time during which collection telephone calls can be made (between the hours of 8 AM and 9 PM).

28. What act protects pension funds?

(A) ERISA
(B) ADA
(C) FLSA

(D) Title VII
(E) ADEA

(A) is correct. The Employee Retirement Income Security Act (ERISA) protects pension funds and regulates the operations of pension funds.
(B) The Americans With Disabilities Act (ADA) of 1990 prohibits the unfair employment practices against the handicapped person, including those persons with AIDS.
(C) The Fair Labor Standards Act (FLSA) sets the minimum wage that employers are required to pay their employees. This is also known as the Federal Wage and Hour Act.
(D) Title VII of the Civil Rights Act of 1964 prohibits discrimination based on race, national origin, religion, and gender during the hiring, promoting, or firing process.
(E) The Age Discrimination in Employment Act (ADEA) prohibits unfair employment practices in persons over 40 years of age.

29. Only the employer is required to make payments to

(A) FICA
(B) OASDI
(C) Medicare

(D) FUTA
(E) none of the above

    (D)   is correct. Federal Unemployment Tax Act (FUTA) requires that only the employer make a contribution to pay a tax to support the federal unemployment insurance program to be used in the event that a person becomes unemployed and has met certain requirements.

    (A)   Federal Insurance Contributions Act (FICA) payments are withheld from the employee's paychecks by the employers.

    (B)   Old-Age Survivors and Disability Insurance (OASDI) is a component of FICA.

    (C)   Medicare, which provides supplemental medical benefits for persons over 65 years of age, is a component of FICA.

30. What income tax form is mandated by law to be given to every employee at the end of each year?

(A) W-4 form
(B) W-2 form
(C) Form 941
(D) all of the above need to be given to the employee
(E) none of the above

    (B)   is correct. The W-2 form is the record of earnings and taxes withheld (or already paid) by the employee. The employee uses this form when computing the yearly personal tax return.

    (A)   A W-4 form is given to the new employee for a declaration of the number of exemptions the employee claims that should be used when calculating the withheld tax money.

    (C)   Form 941 is the quarterly report that employers must file before the last day of the first month after the end of the quarter. This is called the Employer's Quarterly Federal Tax Return.

CHAPTER 11

HEALTH INFORMATION TECHNOLOGY (MEDICAL RECORDS)

1. Active medical files are those of patients that may cover the period from

   (A) 1 to 2 years   **(D)** 1 to 5 years
   (B) 1 to 3 years   **(E)** 5 to 10 years
   (C) 1 to 4 years

   (C) is correct. Active medical files cover the period from 1 to 4 years.

2. Records that are no longer needed, such as when a patient dies, are

   (A) inactive   **(D)** closed
   (B) archives   **(E)** active
   (C) terminal digit filing

   (B) is correct. Archived records are no longer needed but must be kept for legal purposes.
   (A) Inactive medical files relate to patients who have not been seen, according to the time period set by the office (generally 1 to 5 years).
   (C) Terminal digit filing is a filing system for records based on the last digits of the ID number.
   (D) Closed files are medical files of patients who have indicated they are no longer patients.
   (E) Active files are medical files of patients who are currently being seen by a physician.

3. Miniaturized photographs of records are known as

   (A) numeric   **(D)** microfiche
   (B) microfilms   **(E)** none of the above
   (C) archives

   (B) is correct. Microfilms are miniaturized photographs of records.
   (A) A numeric system is one method used for filing medical records.
   (C) Archives are records that are no longer needed.
   (D) Microfiche are sheets of microfilm.

4. In a standard medical record, the reason for the doctor's visit by the patient is known as the

   (A) relevant past history   **(D)** diagnosis
   (B) chief complaint   **(E)** none of the above
   (C) consultation report

(B) is correct. The chief complaint in a medical record is the reason for the doctor's visit by the patient.

5. The most commonly used filing system is based on what method?

   (A) alphabetic
   (B) color coding
   (C) numeric
   (D) unit numbering
   (E) straight numbering

   (A) is correct. The alphabetic filing system is still the most commonly used method.

6. In a numeric filing system, the number assigned generally has

   (A) 4 digits
   (B) 5 digits
   (C) 6 digits
   (D) 7 digits
   (E) none of the above

   (C) is correct. Six digits are usually assigned when using a numeric filing system.

7. The filing system that assigns a number to patients the first time they are seen or admitted to a hospital is known as

   (A) straight numerical filing
   (B) middle digit filing
   (C) serial numbering
   (D) unit numbering
   (E) none of the above

   (D) is correct. A unit numbering system is used to assign a number to patients the first time they are seen or admitted to a hospital.

8. With a serial numbering filing system, the patient receives

   (A) a different medical record for each hospital visit
   (B) a number of different account numbers filed within their own systems
   (C) multiple records, which are stored at different locations
   (D) all of the above
   (E) none of the above

   (D) is correct.

9. In filing correspondence for Janelle Louise Daniels (Mrs. Kevin Masters), 123 Valley Drive, Kalispell, MT 59999, which of the following would NOT be used as an indexing unit?

   (A) Kevin
   (B) Daniels
   (C) Janelle
   (D) Masters
   (E) ZIP code

   (E) is correct. The ZIP code is not used for filing purposes.

10. What is the third indexing unit in Mr. Richard Allan Richards, Jr.?

   (A) Richards
   (B) Richard
   (C) Allan
   (D) Jr.
   (E) all of the above

(C)   is correct. Allan is the third indexing unit in this example. (A) Richards is the first indexing unit, and (B) Richard is the second.

11. Dr. Gemma Reingold is filed as

(A) Reingold, Dr. Gemma
(B) Dr. Gemma Reingold
(C) Reingold, Gemma
(D) Reingold, Gemma (Dr.)
(E) none of the above

(D)   is correct. Titles are disregarded for filing purposes but placed in parentheses after the name.

12. Maura Fitzpatrick has been assigned the patient ID number 239431. To search for her file, you will look under 94, then 23, then 31. What system are you using?

(A) unit numbering
(B) middle digit filing
(C) terminal digit filing
(D) straight numbering
(E) serial numbering

(B)   is correct. Middle digit filing is using the middle two digits of the ID number for filing purposes.
(A)   Unit numbering filing refers to a number that is assigned to patients the first time they are seen.
(C)   Terminal digit filing is based on the last digits of the ID number.
(D)   Straight numbering is the simplest numerical filing system in which each record is filed sequentially.
(E)   Serial numbering is used when a patient receives a different medical record number for each visit.

13. Filing by subject matter is

(A) always done in conjunction with an alphabetic system
(B) used for specific files only
(C) adequate as long as the files are relatively small
(D) all of the above
(E) none of the above

(C)   is correct. Filing by subject matter is adequate as long as the files are relatively small.

14. The Alpha-Z color-coded system method of filing using an alphabetical system is based on

(A) 4 colors
(B) 10 colors
(C) 12 colors
(D) 13 colors
(E) 15 colors

(D)   is correct. The Alpha-Z color-coded system is based on using a combination of 13 colors and a white stripe.

15. Adrian Washington has been assigned a color using the Alpha-Z color-coded system. Under what color would you find his chart?

   (A) lavender with white stripe   **(D)** yellow

   (B) light brown   **(E)** yellow with white stripe

   (C) dark brown with white stripe

     (E) is correct.

16. David Jesse Montgomery III's file would be filed in what relation to David Jesse Montgomery, Jr.'s file?

   (A) before

   (B) after

   (C) with David Jesse Montgomery, Jr.'s file

   (D) the designation III and Jr. are ignored when filing

   (E) none of the above

     (A) is correct. Numeric seniority terms (such as III) are filed before alphabetic terms (such as Jr.).

17. The method that alerts the medical assistant that a file may be found under another name is known as

   (A) cross-referencing   **(D)** editing

   (B) alphabetic filing   **(E)** archiving

   (C) numerical filing

     (A) is correct. Cross-referencing is a method that alerts the medical assistant that a file may be found under another name.

     (B) Alphabetic filing is a filing system based on the letters of the alphabet.

     (C) Numerical filing is a filing system that assigns an identification (ID) number to each person's name.

     (D) Editing involves a rearrangement or restatement of a word or group of words in a document.

     (E) Archiving is placing records that are no longer needed into a safe storage area.

18. Legally, from the time of the last entry, medical records must be stored for

   (A) 1 year   **(D)** 7 years

   (B) 3 years   **(E)** forever

   (C) 5 years

     (D) is correct. Medical records should be kept for 7 years.

19. VRT is an example of a/an

   (A) synonym   **(D)** phonetics

   (B) acronym   **(E)** eponym

   (C) antonym

     (B) is correct. Acronyms are words that are structured by taking the first letter of each word in a group of words.

     (A) Synonyms are words with like meanings, such as fever and pyrexia.

(C) Antonyms are words having opposite meanings, such as supine and prone.

(D) Phonetics is the key to pronunciations that is found in all standard dictionaries.

(E) Eponyms are names of diseases based on the physician or patient who first documented the disease, such as Bright's disease.

20. A report containing information about the tissue removed during a surgical procedure is called a/an

(A) consultation report   **(D)** additional report
(B) operative note   **(E)** history report
(C) pathology report

(C) is correct. A pathology report is a report containing information about the tissue removed during a surgical procedure.

(A) A consultation report is written by the consulting physician and contains his or her findings (impressions) regarding the patient's condition.

(B) The operative note is a detailed account of the surgical procedure including the exact area of an incision, type of suture used, and what specimen (or organ) was removed.

(D) Additional reports come from a variety of sources, such as autopsy, pathology, etc.

(E) History report is the medical history of the patient as told to the physician.

21. The newest transcription technology, which allows the physician to speak into a microphone connected to a computer program that then translates the dictation into a typed report, is known as

(A) TDD   **(D)** all of the above
(B) VRT   **(E)** none of the above
(C) TActile CONverter

(B) is correct. Voice recognition technology (VRT) recognizes the voice of the physician dictating a medical record.

(A) Telecommunication device for the deaf (TDD) will place information onto paper for the deaf and hearing-impaired transcriptionist.

(C) TActile CONverter is a device that allows the blind person to read printed material by placing one hand inside the converter holding a printed document and "reading" the material with the index finger resting on the transmitter plate.

CHAPTER 12

INSURANCE AND CODING

1. The amount of eligible charges each patient must pay each calendar year before the plan pays benefits is called the

   (A) claim
   (B) coinsurance
   (C) deductible

   (D) premium
   (E) co-payment

   (C) is correct.
   (A) A claim is a written and documented request for insurance reimbursement.
   (B) Coinsurance requires the insured to assume a portion of the cost of covered services.
   (D) A premium is the amount paid monthly or annually for insurance coverage.
   (E) Co-payment is the amount specified by an insurance plan that the patient must pay before the plan pays.

2. A written authorization by the patient giving the insurance company the right to pay the physician directly for billed services is called a/an

   (A) co-payment
   (B) assignment of benefits
   (C) preauthorization

   (D) deductible
   (E) premium

   (B) is correct.
   (A) A co-payment is an amount specified by an insurance plan that the patient must pay before the plan pays.
   (C) Preauthorization is a requirement by some insurance companies to obtain prior approval for a procedure.
   (D) A deductible is an amount of eligible charges the patient pays each calendar year before the insurance plan begins to pay benefits.
   (E) A premium is an amount paid for insurance coverage.

3. The amount specified by an insurance plan that the patient must pay before the plan will pay is the

   (A) insured's fee
   (B) premium
   (C) deductible

   (D) co-payment
   (E) preauthorization

   (D) is correct. The co-payment is the amount of the service that the patient must pay "up front," and that insurance does not cover. It must be paid before the insurance company will make payment. (B), (C), and (E) are explained in the previous answer.

4. A person who holds a health benefit plan is the

    (A) insured   **(D)** dependent
  ✓**(B)** subscriber   **(E)** medically indigent
    (C) rider

      (B) is correct.
      (A) An insured is an individual who is covered under an insurance plan, not necessarily the person the plan is issued to.
      (C) A rider is a written exception to an insurance contract that increases, decreases, or modifies coverage of the plan.
      (D) A dependent is an individual who is covered under the insurance plan of a subscriber due to age, marital status, or certain long-term disabilities.
      (E) Someone who is medically indigent is without insurance and with no funds.

5. A list of determined amounts to be paid for specific services by the insurance carrier on behalf of the insured is called

    (A) assignment of benefits   **(D)** preauthorization
    (B) fee schedule   ✓**(E)** indemnity schedule
    (C) crossover claim

      (E) is correct.
      (A) Assignment of benefits is the patient's written authorization giving the insurance company permission to pay directly to the physician.
      (B) A fee schedule is a schedule of the amount paid by a specific insurance company for each procedure or service.
      (C) A crossover claim is when a patient is eligible for Medicare and Medicaid.
      (D) Preauthorization is a requirement of Medicare and some other insurance companies to obtain prior approval for surgery and other procedures in order to receive payment by the insurance company or Medicare.

6. A military medical insurance plan that is part of the government is

    (A) CHAMPUS   **(D)** HMO
    (B) Medicare   **(E)** Blue Cross and Blue Shield
    (C) Medicaid

    ✓(A) is correct.
      (B) Medicare is a government program, but not a military program.
      (C) Medicaid is a plan for those of low income.
      (D) HMO is a managed care option whereby the patient is assigned a physician as his or her primary care provider.
      (E) Blue Cross and Blue Shield is a prepayment medical insurance system and is not part of the military.

7. The process of turning verbal descriptions into numerical designations is called

    (A) rider   **(D)** modifying
  ✓**(B)** coding   **(E)** classifying
    (C) grouping

(B) is correct.
(A) A rider is a written exception to an insurance contract.
(C) Grouping is placing like procedures together in a group.
(D) Modifying means making changes.
(E) Classifying is the process of naming a group by looking for similar characteristics.

8. In ICD-9 coding guidelines, E codes

(A) stand alone
(B) should never be used with V codes
(C) are required for all diagnoses
✓**(D)** give external causes or factors for an illness or injury
(E) are the same as CPT codes

(D) is correct. E codes are used as additional information regarding a diagnosis.
(B) V codes are visits not directly related to an illness or injury.

9. Which coding convention is used in coding procedures?

(A) ICD-9   **(D)** PPO
✓**(B)** CPT   **(E)** none of the above
(C) HMO

(B) is correct. The medical assistant needs to be familiar with the convention of CPT coding in order to maximize reimbursements for a particular practice.
(A) ICD-9 coding provides numeric codes for the patient's diagnosis.
(C) HMO is a managed care system.
(D) PPO is another managed care system.

10. The HCFA-1500 insurance claim form

(A) must be filled out by the patient
(B) must be filled out by the physician's billing staff
(C) is accepted by every insurance company within the United States
(D) is never used
✓**(E)** is commonly accepted by most carriers

(E) is correct. The HCFA-1500 insurance form is the most commonly used and was designed by the Health Care Financing Administration.

11. ICD-9 codes used in the medical office

(A) may be coded directly from Volume III
✓**(B)** may require a fifth digit
(C) never require a fifth digit
(D) always require a V code to support the diagnosis
(E) always require an E code to support the diagnosis

(B) is correct. Diagnoses are given a 3-digit code; a fourth and fifth code may be needed when certain conditions are present.

12. When payment is being determined for a provider, insurance companies consider

   (A) fee schedules
   (B) any riders on the contract
   (C) relative value studies and resource-based relative value scales
   (D) all of the above
   (E) none of the above

   > (D) is correct. Fee schedules, riders on contracts, relative value studies, and resource-based relative value scales are all considered before payment is made by the insurance companies.

13. Most disability insurance companies require a waiting period of

   (A) 1–2 weeks   **(D)** 6–8 weeks
   (B) 2–4 weeks   **(E)** no waiting period
   (C) 4–6 weeks

   > (B) is correct.

14. The special report that the provider must complete in workers' compensation cases is the

   (A) doctor's report   **(D)** attending physician's report
   (B) injury report   **(E)** daily report
   (C) surgeon's report

   > (C) is correct. The provider must provide a surgeon's report and further reports at specified intervals.

15. Which is the patient eligible for if he or she has a crossover claim?

   (A) Medicare and Blue Cross
   (B) Medicare and Blue Shield
   (C) Medicare and Blue Cross and Blue Shield
   (D) Medicare and Medicaid
   (E) Medicare and supplemental insurance

   > (D) is correct. Being eligible for Medicare does not mean the patient is eligible for Medicaid. In some states, if the patient is eligible for both (Medi/Medi), a crossover claim can be filed.

16. Medicare pays for what percent of the approved amount of a service provided?

   (A) 10 percent   **(D)** 80 percent
   (B) 20 percent   **(E)** 100 percent
   (C) 50 percent

   > (D) is correct. After the deductible is met, Medicare pays 80 percent of the approved amount, and the patient pays a 20 percent co-payment.

17. Assignment of lifetime benefits is available with

    (A) Medicare   **(D)** CHAMPUS
    (B) Medicaid   **(E)** CHAMPVA
    (C) workers' compensation

      (A) is correct. There are two parts to Medicare coverage. Part A, covering the hospital expenses, is automatically started when the insured becomes eligible for Social Security benefits. A patient must qualify and pay a monthly premium to receive part B.

18. The first cost-containment measure, implemented when Congress amended the Social Security Act of 1972, was

    (A) ICD-9-CM   **(D)** CPT
    (B) HMO   **(E)** DRGs
    (C) PRO

      (C) is correct. PRO refers to peer review organization.
      (A) ICD-9-CM refers to the International Classification of Diseases.
      (B) HMO refers to health maintenance organization.
      (D) CPT refers to current procedural terminology.
      (E) DRGs refers to diagnosis-related groups.

19. What percent of a physician's income is paid by some sort of medical insurance?

    (A) 80 percent   **(D)** 95 percent
    (B) 85 percent   **(E)** 100 percent
    (C) 90 percent

      (B) is correct. As the cost of medical care increases, new and different types of health care plans are being promoted. In today's medical office, approximately 85 percent of the physician's income is paid by a medical insurance system.

20. The "birthday rule" is used when both parents have individual insurance plans and a dependent needs to be covered. According to this "rule," the insurance plan that would be designated the primary plan is that belonging to the parent

    (A) who obtained insurance first
    (B) who is the youngest
    (C) who is the oldest
    (D) whose birthday falls earliest in the year
    (E) whose birthday falls earliest in the month

      (D) is correct. The parent whose birthday falls earliest in the year has the primary insurance plan, not necessarily the oldest parent.

CHAPTER 13

OFFICE MANAGEMENT

1. Which of the following is a purpose of the procedure manual?

    (A) standardization of procedures
    (B) listing of job descriptions
    (C) listing of tasks to perform within the office
    (D) marketing tool
    (E) only A, B, and C

    (E) is correct. The procedure manual contains a standardization of procedures, a listing of job descriptions, and a listing of tasks to be performed.

2. A real or imaginary wrong regarded as the cause for a complaint is known as a/an

    (A) citation
    (B) judgment
    (C) grievance
    (D) fault
    (E) illegal action

    (C) is correct. A grievance is a real or imaginary wrong that is regarded by the employee as a cause for complaint.

3. An employee policy describing the grievance process should be contained in the

    (A) general policy manual
    (B) personnel policy manual
    (C) employee handbook
    (D) patient information booklet
    (E) A, B, and C only

    (E) is correct. The grievance policy would be found in (A) the general policy manual, (B) the personnel policy manual, and (C) the employee handbook. In some smaller medical offices, all policies are found in a general policy manual.

4. What law affects the hiring of a new employee?

    (A) OSHA
    (B) EEOA
    (C) Title VII of the Civil Rights Act
    (D) EEOC
    (E) none of the above

    (B) is correct. The Equal Employment Opportunity Act (EEOA) of 1972, which is an amendment of Title VII of the earlier 1964 Civil Rights Act, prohibits asking applicants questions about their race, color, sex, religion, and national origin during the application process.

5. Which of the following questions could be ruled discriminatory?

(A) "What is the least amount of money you would accept if offered this position?"
(B) "May we inquire about your job performance from past employers?"
(C) "Can you reassure us that finding a reliable baby-sitter will not be a problem?"
(D) "I notice you are wearing an engagement ring. What are your wedding plans?"
(E) C and D only

> (E) is correct. According to the Equal Employment Opportunity Act (EEOA) of 1972, questions that refer to marriage and children are considered to be discriminatory. These questions are said to be discriminatory against women (gender).

6. A systems approach to office management is

(A) using outside consultants for all financial and business operations
(B) performing individual office functions in isolation
(C) integrating functions
(D) not advisable in the office setting
(E) none of the above

> (C) is correct. A systems approach to office management involves integrating all the management functions performed within the office.

7. The personnel management function includes

(A) selection
(B) firing
(C) probation
(D) salary review
(E) all of the above

> (E) is correct. Personnel management includes the employee selection, firing, probation, and salary review process.

8. Arranging staff vacation coverage is usually the responsibility of the

(A) physician
(B) individual who is going on vacation
(C) office manager
(D) medical assistant
(E) nurse

> (C) is correct. The office manager is usually the person designated to handle vacation coverage, to conduct interviews and performance evaluations, to arrange work schedules, and to hire, terminate, and train employees.

9. The purpose of a performance evaluation is to

(A) positively encourage the continued improvement of the employee's performance
(B) negotiate a salary increase
(C) find any fault(s) in an employee's performance
(D) provide a document to compare one employee's performance with another employee's performance
(E) all of the above

(A) is correct. The primary purpose of a performance evaluation is to positively encourage the continued improvement of the employee's performance.

10. Employee records must be kept for all of the following EXCEPT

(A) Social Security number
(B) net salary
(C) gross salary
(D) number of claimed exemptions (W-4 form)
(E) deductions

(B) is correct. The net salary is calculated by subtracting the deductions from the gross salary.

11. Patient instruction booklets should be used

(A) in place of individual instruction
(B) to avoid contact with difficult patients
(C) to prevent lawsuits
(D) to standardize instruction
(E) only with hearing-impaired patients

(D) is correct. The purpose of patient instruction booklets is to standardize instruction.

12. Which of the following would be included in an employee handbook?

(A) salary amounts
(B) OSHA guidelines
(C) protocol for attire
(D) A, B, and C
(E) only B and C

(E) is correct. (B) OSHA guidelines and (C) attire are addressed in employee handbooks, but (A) salary amounts are not.

13. An employee handbook would contain job descriptions for all employees EXCEPT the

(A) office manager
(B) medical assistants
(C) physician
(D) custodian
(E) C and D

(C) is correct. The employee handbook would not contain a job description for the physician.

14. A small payment for a professional service, such as giving a speech, would be a/an

(A) draft
(B) honorarium
(C) royalty
(D) all of the above
(E) none of the above

(B) is correct. An honorarium is a small payment for a professional service other than providing medical care.

15. A to-do list includes

(A) nonprioritized items
(B) daily duties such as emptying the trash
(C) completed tasks
(D) tasks done in the order they appear on the list
(E) none of the above

(E)   is correct. A to-do list contains nonroutine tasks, which have been listed and prioritized.

16. A new employee's probationary period is usually

(A) 30 days
(B) 2 months
(C) 3 months
(D) 6 months
(E) none of the above

(C)   is correct. A new employee's probationary period is usually 3 months (90 days).

17. A probationary period for a new employee is a time frame during which

(A) the employee can be dismissed without cause
(B) the employee can determine if the position is right for him or her
(C) the employer can determine if the position and the employee are a good match
(D) both the employer and employee can make adjustments
(E) all of the above

(E)   is correct.

18. Seniority refers to the person in the organization who

(A) is the oldest
(B) is in the highest position of power
(C) has been recognized the most for achievement
(D) has been with the company the longest
(E) none of the above

(D)   is correct. Seniority refers to the person who has been with the company the longest.

19. In a typical medical office, the in-basket, containing mail and laboratory reports, is emptied

(A) once a day
(B) twice a day
(C) twice a week
(D) every Friday
(E) whenever there is something in it

(A)   is correct. The in-basket is usually emptied after the mail delivery once every day.

20. Patient information booklets are designed to

(A) decrease liability in case of a malpractice suit
(B) replace the need for time-consuming personal instructions to the patient
(C) give a satisfied patient a means of referring friends and family to the office
(D) augment patient education
(E) be used as a marketing tool

(D)   is correct. Patient information booklets are designed to augment patient education. They are not intended to (A) decrease liability, (B) replace individualized personal instructions, or (E) be a marketing tool.

PART III

CLINICAL KNOWLEDGE

Examination Room Techniques— Medical and Surgical

CHAPTER 14

INFECTION CONTROL: ASEPSIS

1. What famous surgeon discovered that germs could be killed using carbolic acid and would clean surgical wounds by spraying the surrounding tissue with carbolic acid?

   (A) Louis Pasteur
   (B) Joseph Lister
   (C) Ignaz Semmelweiss
   (D) Robert Koch
   (E) Andreas Vesalius

   (B) is correct.
   (A) Louis Pasteur was a French chemist who discovered that many diseases are caused by bacteria that could be killed by excess heat. He also perfected a treatment that prevented rabies and discovered a means for controlling anthrax; he is known as the father of bacteriology and for the process of pasteurization.
   (C) Ignaz Semmelweiss taught his medical students to wash their hands before delivering babies, which dramatically decreased the deaths from childbed fever in new mothers.
   (D) Robert Koch, a German physician, developed the culture plate method for isolation of bacteria, discovered the cause of cholera, and isolated the tuberculin bacteria.
   (E) Andreas Vesalius, a Belgium anatomist, is known as the father of modern anatomy.

2. What physician perfected the treatment for rabies?

   (A) Louis Pasteur
   (B) Joseph Lister
   (C) Ignaz Semmelweiss
   (D) Robert Koch
   (E) Andreas Vesalius

   (A) is correct.

3. What man is known as the father of modern anatomy?

   (A) Louis Pasteur
   (B) Joseph Lister
   (C) Ignaz Semmelweiss
   (D) Robert Koch
   (E) Andreas Vesalius

   (E) is correct.

4. This is a thick-walled reproductive cell so strong that it can withstand exposure to many harmful chemicals and extreme temperatures. It is known as a/an

   (A) spore
   (B) normal flora
   (C) aerobe
   (D) anaerobe
   (E) nosocomial

(A)   is correct. A spore can withstand exposure to chemicals and extreme temperatures. A spore is the dormant stage of some bacteria.

(B)   Normal flora are microorganisms that normally reside within certain areas of the body. Their function is to protect the body from harmful microorganisms. They are nonpathogenic if they stay within the region of the body where they normally reside.

(C)   Aerobes are pathogens that thrive in oxygen-rich environments.

(D)   Anaerobes are pathogens that thrive in oxygen-free environments.

(E)   Nosocomial refers to an infection that is acquired after a person has entered a hospital.

5. What microorganisms are harmless to certain areas of the body in which they reside and work to protect the body from pathogenic microorganisms?

(A) spore
(B) normal flora
(C) aerobe
(D) anaerobes
(E) nosocomial

(B)   is correct. Normal flora are microorganisms that are harmless to certain areas of the body in which they reside and protect the body from pathogenic microorganisms.

6. Pathogens that grow in oxygen-rich environments are known as

(A) spores
(B) normal flora
(C) aerobes
(D) anaerobes
(E) nosocomial

(C)   is correct. Aerobes are pathogens that grow in oxygen-rich environments.

7. In order for the chain of infection to occur, a pathogen must find a means of exit from its reservoir host, and then it must

(A) find a means of transmission
(B) find a means of entrance
(C) have a susceptible host
(D) find a reservoir host
(E) none of the above

(A)   is correct. A pathogen must find a means of transmission after exiting its reservoir host. This is how the organism spreads. It does this by either direct transmission, which is contact with an infected person (as with cough or sneeze droplets from an infected person), or contact with the infected person's bodily fluids (as in HIV).

(B)   After a means of transmission has been found, the pathogen must find a means of entrance (mouth, nose, eyes, intestines, urinary tract, or an open wound).

(C)   Once the pathogen has gained entrance, it must have a susceptible host (one that can support growth and reproduction).

(D)   With the right environment, the pathogen can reach infectious levels. When this occurs, the susceptible host becomes a reservoir agent.

8. In order for a pathogen to reproduce and grow within the host, it must

    (A) find a means of transmission
    (B) find a means of entrance
    (C) find a susceptible host
    (D) find a reservoir host
    (E) none of the above

> (C) is correct. In order for a pathogen to reproduce and grow within a host, it must find a susceptible host.

9. Human immunodeficiency virus (HIV) is transmitted by

    (A) indirect transmission
    (B) contact with droplets
    (C) direct contact
    (D) droplets produced by sneezing
    (E) none of the above

> (C) is correct. HIV is transmitted by direct contact with an infected person or infected bodily fluids.

10. During the inflammatory response, white blood cells overpower and consume the pathogenic microorganisms in a process called

    (A) suppuration
    (B) septicemia
    (C) specific defense
    (D) phagocytosis
    (E) nonspecific defense

> (D) is correct. Phagocytosis is the process in which white blood cells (phagocytes) overpower and consume pathogenic microorganisms.
>
> (A) Suppuration is the process of pus formation. Another term for suppuration is pyopoiesis.
>
> (B) Septicemia is the spread of infection to the bloodstream.
>
> (C) Specific defense is a term used to describe immunity. Immunity is a means of protection from disease due to the production of antibodies. Antibodies are specific predators, that is, antibody A can only kill antigen B. It cannot kill other antigens; therefore, it is specific in its nature of defense.
>
> (E) Nonspecific defense mechanisms can protect the body from many different kinds of antigens. Some examples of nonspecific defense mechanisms are skin, mucous membranes, hair, saliva, tears, stomach acid, and the lymphatic system.

11. The skin can protect the body from many different types of disease by simply not allowing a pathogen to enter the body. What type of defense is this?

    (A) antigen
    (B) antibody
    (C) nonspecific defense
    (D) specific defense
    (E) inflammation

> (C) is correct. Nonspecific defense can protect the body from many different types of disease by not allowing a pathogen to enter the body.

12. The entrance of a disease-producing organism into a cell or organism is referred to as a/an

    (A) disease
    (B) infection
    (C) pathogen
    (D) microorganism
    (E) infestation

(B) is correct. The entrance of a disease-producing organism into a cell or organism is an infection. It may or may not alter the normal structure, function, or metabolism of a cell or organism.

(A) A disease occurs when any sustained harmful alteration of the normal structure, function, or metabolism of a cell or organism comes about.

(C) A pathogen is a disease-producing organism.

(D) A microorganism is a tiny living organism that is not visible to the naked eye.

(E) An infestation is the presence of parasites in the environment.

13. Which is a disease-producing microbe?

(A) asepsis
(B) infestation
(C) pathogen
(D) germicide
(E) antiseptic

(C) is correct. A pathogen is a disease-producing microbe or microorganism.

(A) Asepsis is a condition free of germs or infection.

(B) Infestation refers to the presence of parasites.

(D) A germicide is a chemical used to kill pathogenic microorganisms, but it is too harsh to be used on people.

(E) An antiseptic is a substance that prevents the growth of microorganisms without necessarily killing them and is generally safe to use on people.

14. A substance that can kill many organisms but is not effective on spores is

(A) an antiseptic
(B) a disinfectant
(C) a germicide
(D) formaldehyde
(E) a bactericide

(B) is correct. A disinfectant is not effective on spores and, in most cases, is not used on people. The exceptions are alcohol and betadine, which are classified as both antiseptic and/or disinfectant. An antiseptic does not single out and kill bacteria, as a bactericide does, or pathogens, as a germicide does.

(A) An antiseptic is a substance that prevents the growth of microorganisms without necessarily killing them and is generally safe to use on people.

(C) A germicide is a chemical used to kill pathogenic microorganisms, but it is too harsh to be used on people.

(D) Formaldehyde is used as a disinfectant, fixative, or preservative.

(E) A bactericide is destructive to bacteria and too harsh to be used on people.

15. A substance that prevents the growth of microorganisms without necessarily killing them and is generally safe for use on people is

(A) a bactericide
(B) a germicide
(C) disinfectant
(D) an antiseptic
(E) formaldehyde

(C) is correct.

16. A mixture of 1:10 bleach and water is a substance that can kill microorganisms but not spores and is not used on people. It can be classified as

(A) a bactericide
(B) a germicide
(C) a disinfectant
(D) an antiseptic
(E) formaldehyde

(C)   is correct. A solution of 1:10 bleach and water is a disinfectant.

17. What is a form that is resistant to heat, drying, and chemicals, but that can be killed by steam under pressure (as in autoclaving)?

(A) virus
(B) spore
(C) HIV
(D) TB
(E) ARC

(B)   is correct. A spore is the dormant form assumed by some bacteria that acts as a protective environment for the bacteria. Under the right conditions, the spore may revert back to an active form of bacteria.

(A)   A virus is not resistant to heat, drying, or chemicals. It is, however, resistant to antibiotics. It is a very small parasitic microorganism that can only duplicate if within a living cell of an organism.

(C)   Human immunodeficiency virus (HIV) is the virus that causes acquired immune deficiency syndrome (AIDS).

(D)   Tuberculosis (TB) is caused by a bacteria that is not resistant to heat, drying, or chemicals.

(E)   AIDS-related complex (ARC) is a less serious condition than AIDS. It occurs when the HIV has seriously damaged the immune system but before the final stage of an HIV infection (AIDS).

18. What type of bacteria usually forms grape-like clusters of pus-producing organisms (as seen in boils, wound infections, impetigo, and osteomyelitis)?

(A) staphylococci
(B) streptococci
(C) diplococci
(D) bacilli
(E) spirilla

(A)   is correct. Staphylococci is a type of bacteria that forms grape-like clusters of pus-producing organisms. They stain gram-positive, which appears purple or blue in color.

(B)   Streptococci form chains of round cells, as seen in strep throat, rheumatic heart disease, scarlet fever, or glomerulonephritis. They stain gram-negative, which appears reddish/pink in color.

(C)   Diplococci form in pairs in chains of round cells, such as seen in gonorrhea, pneumonia, and meningitis. They stain gram-negative.

(D)   Bacilli are rod-shaped bacteria, as seen in tuberculosis (TB), tetanus, diphtheria, and gas gangrene. These are all examples of gram-positive bacilli (*Escherichia coli* or *E. coli*).

(E)   Spirilla are spiral-shaped bacteria, as seen in syphilis and cholera. They usually stain gram-negative.

19. This type of bacteria form pairs and stain gram negative. It is seen in gonorrhea and pneumonia.

   (A) streptococci
   (B) staphylococci
   (C) diplococci

   (D) bacilli
   (E) spirilla

       (C)   is correct.

20. Which of the following are examples of diseases caused by fungi?

   (A) amebic dysentery, malaria, trichomonas, and giardiasis
   (B) Rocky Mountain spotted fever, typhus, rickettsial pox, trench fever, and Brill's disease
   (C) thrush, athlete's foot, jock itch, ringworm, and candidiasis
   (D) tetanus, diphtheria, whooping cough, UTI, syphilis, pneumonia, strep throat, boils, and meningitis
   (E) herpes I and II, HIV, common cold, influenza, hepatitis A and B, MMR, polio, and warts

       (C)   is correct. Thrush, athlete's foot, jock itch, ringworm, and candidiasis are all caused by a fungus.

       (A)   Amebic dysentery, malaria, trichomonas, and giardiasis are examples of diseases caused by single-celled organisms called protozoa.

       (B)   Rocky Mountain spotted fever, typhus, rickettsial pox, trench fever, and Brill's disease are examples of rickettsiae diseases, which are transmitted by insects.

       (D)   Tetanus, diphtheria, whooping cough, UTI, syphilis, pneumonia, strep throat, boils, and meningitis are examples of diseases caused by bacteria, which are unicellular and can be treated with antibiotics. Note that both pneumonia and meningitis can be caused by either bacteria or virus.

       (E)   Herpes I and II, HIV, common cold, influenza, hepatitis A and B, MRR (mumps, measles, rubella), polio, and warts are examples of diseases caused by viruses, which are the smallest microorganisms and are not susceptible to antibiotics.

21. Which of the following conditions is NOT favorable for the growth of bacteria?

   (A) moisture
   (B) temperature of 98.6°F
   (C) direct sunlight

   (D) oxygen
   (E) dampness

       (C)   is correct. Direct sunlight can kill bacterial growth. (A), (B), (D), and (E) are all examples of conditions that are favorable for the growth of bacteria (aerobic bacteria require oxygen, and anaerobic bacteria thrive without oxygen).

22. What type of immunity would one have if given tetanus immune serum globulin (TIG)?

(A) passive acquired natural immunity (PANI)
(B) passive acquired artificial immunity (PAAI)
(C) active acquired natural immunity (AANI)
(D) active acquired artificial immunity (AAAI)
(E) all of the above

    (B) is correct. TIG (tetanus immune serum globulin) and TAT or TA (tetanus antitoxin) are examples of temporary protection against tetanus and are acquired through the process of passive acquired artificial immunity (PAAI).

    (A) PANI is naturally acquired from someone else's antibodies, such as from mother to fetus through the placenta or through breast milk.

    (C) AANI occurs by having the disease, which results in production of antibodies and "memory cells" that respond when the antigen reappears again.

    (D) AAAI is acquired by the administration of a vaccine, which actively stimulates production of one's own antibodies and "memory cells" to prevent that disease from occurring.

23. The first tier of the Centers for Disease Control (CDC) 1994 isolation guidelines focuses on

(A) standard precautions (SPs)
(B) airborne precautions (APs)
(C) droplet precautions (DPs)
(D) contact precautions (CPs)
(E) transmission-based precautions

    (A) is correct. These precautions are used when caring for all patients, regardless of the patient's diagnosis or whether or not the patient has a known infectious disease. Major features of universal precautions are stated under Tier I.

    (B) Airborne precautions (APs) are part of Tier II, which focuses on patients who either are suspected of carrying an infectious disease or are already infected. It requires extra precautions in addition to the standard precautions and is known as transmission-based precautions. APs are used to reduce the transmission of diseases like TB, measles, or chickenpox. Precautions include isolation if hospitalized, mask and protective gown worn by health care workers, washing hands before gloving and after removing gloves, transporting patients with a mask, and limiting transportation.

    (C) Droplet precautions (DPs) are part of Tier II. Droplet precautions (DPs) are used to reduce the transmission of diseases such as meningitis, pneumonia, sepsis, diphtheria, pertussis, streptococcal pneumonia, scarlet fever, mumps, and rubella. Precautions include isolation if hospitalized, washing hands before gloving and after removing gloves, gloves and gowns being worn if coming into contact with bodily fluids or blood of the patient, wearing a mask if within 3 feet of the patient, and limiting transport of patients. All reusable equipment should be cleaned and disinfected.

(D) Contact precautions (CPs) are part of Tier II. These precautions are used for patients known to be infected with a microorganism that is not easily treated with antibiotics or that is easily transmitted to others. Examples of these diseases are intestinal infections; respiratory, skin, or wound infections; diphtheria; herpes simplex virus; impetigo; hepatitis A; scabies; pediculosis; and herpes zoster. Precautions include isolation if hospitalized, gloves and gown worn when in contact with the patient, and mask and eyewear worn when there is potential for exposure to infectious body materials and fluids. When possible, patient care equipment should not be used on other patients.

(E) Transmission-based precautions is the descriptive title given to the second tier (Tier II) of the CDC guidelines.

24. Caring for patients who have meningitis or pneumonia requires what type of precautions?

(A) standard precautions
(B) airborne precautions
(C) droplet precautions
(D) contact precautions
(E) transmission-based precautions

(C) is correct. Droplet precautions are required when caring for patients with meningitis or pneumonia.

25. Universal precautions (Ups) under the Occupational Safety and Health Administration (OSHA) are

(A) guidelines
(B) suggestions
(C) recommendations
(D) law
(E) bills

(D) is correct. Ups are the law and must be observed by employers of health care personnel.

26. Which of the following is appropriate when hand washing?

(A) use hot water and hold hands upward
(B) use cool water and hold hands downward
(C) use cold water and hold hands upward
(D) use tepid or lukewarm water and hold hands downward
(E) use hot water under pressure and hold hands outward

(C) is correct.

27. The destruction of organisms after they leave the body is called

(A) incubation
(B) phagocytosis
(C) medical asepsis
(D) surgical asepsis
(E) opportunistic infections

(C) is correct. Medical asepsis is the destruction of organisms after they leave the body.
(A) Incubation refers to a period of time during which a disease develops after the person is exposed.
(B) Phagocytosis is the process of engulfing, digesting, and destroying pathogens.

(D) Surgical asepsis is a technique practiced to maintain a sterile environment.

(E) Opportunistic infections, such as pneumonia, occur in a body when there is a reduced immune system (for example, as seen in AIDS).

28. Sterilization time requirements in the autoclave for surgical instruments that are double-thickness wrapped are

(A) 10 minutes
(B) 15 minutes
(C) 20 minutes

(D) 30 minutes
(E) 1 hour

(D) is correct.

29. The symptoms of HBV are

(A) slow onset of symptoms, fever, loss of appetite, jaundice, nausea, vomiting, malaise, dark urine, and whitish stools
(B) rapid onset of symptoms, fever, chills, diarrhea with clay-colored stools, orange-brown urine, anorexia, enlarged liver, and jaundice
(C) T-cell count less than 200, unexplained weight loss, swelling or hardening of lymph nodes, discolored or purplish growths and spots on the skin and inside the mouth, and an altered state of consciousness
(D) A and C
(E) B and C

(B) is correct. HBV (hepatitis B or serum hepatitis) generally has a rapid onset of symptoms with an incubation period of 60 to 90 days.

(A) Hepatitis A (acute infective hepatitis) has a very slow onset of symptoms with an incubation period of 14 to 50 days.

(C) The symptoms of AIDS include a T-cell count of less than 200, unexplained weight loss, swelling or hardening of lymph nodes, discolored or purplish growths and spots on the skin and inside the mouth, and an altered state of consciousness.

CHAPTER 15

VITAL SIGNS AND MEASUREMENTS

1. What part of the brain controls <u>body temperature?</u>

   (A) medulla oblongata   ✔**(D)** hypothalamus
   (B) midbrain   **(E)** cerebrum
   (C) thalamus

       (D)   is correct. The hypothalamus is a portion of the brain located just below the thalamus. It controls autonomic nervous system functions, and it is able to adjust the body temperature, appetite, sleep, sexual desire, and emotions such as fear.
       (A)   The medulla oblongata, located in the base of the brain, contains the respiratory, cardiac, and vasomotor centers.
       (B)   The midbrain is located in the base of the brain in what is commonly referred to as the brain stem. It serves as a two-way conduction pathway, and a relay for visual and auditory impulses.
       (C)   The thalamus is located just above the hypothalamus. It acts as a center for relaying impulses from the eyes, ears, and skin to the cerebrum. Perception of pain is controlled by the thalamus.
       (E)   The cerebrum is the largest section of the brain. It is located in the upper portion of the brain and is the area that processes thoughts, judgment, memory, association skills, and the ability to discriminate between items.

2. The part of the brain that controls respiratory, cardiac, and vasomotor functions is the

   ✔**(A)** medulla oblongata   **(D)** hypothalamus
   (B) midbrain   **(E)** cerebrum
   (C) thalamus

       (A)   is correct. The medulla oblongata, located in the base of the brain, contains the respiratory, cardiac, and vasomotor centers.

3. Which of the following statements is FALSE?

   (A) the highest body temperature usually occurs in the evening between 5:00 PM and 8:00 PM
   ✔**(B)** infants and children normally have a lower body temperature than adults
   (C) pregnancy may cause body temperature to rise
   (D) pyrexia is a body temperature above 100.4°F
   (E) hyperpyrexia develops when the body temperature exceeds 105.8°F

       (B)   is false. Infants and children normally have a higher body temperature, due to immature heat regulation.

4. Which of the following temperatures is considered normal?

(A) oral, 98.6°F/37°C

(B) rectal, 99.6°F/37.6°C

(C) axillary, 97.6°F/36.4°C

(D) aural, 98.6°F/37°C

✓**(E)** all of the above.

(E)   is correct. All are normal temperatures.

5. Which of the following statements is FALSE?

(A) the oral method of temperature measurement is the most commonly used

(B) one of the newest technologies for temperature measurement involves the aural site

✓**(C)** the axillary method has proven to be the most accurate method for temperature measurement

(D) the rectal route is more reliable than the oral method

(E) patients who have just eaten, smoked, drunk liquids, or come in from the cold or hot outdoors should not have their temperature taken for a period of at least 10 minutes

(C)   is correct.

6. A temperature of 101 degrees F is equal to how many degrees Celsius?

✓**(A)** 38.3°C

(B) 24.1°C

(C) 88.1°C

(D) 39.0°C

(E) 37.6°C

(A)   is correct. To convert Fahrenheit (F) to Celsius (C), subtract 32, then multiply by 5/9. To convert Celsius (C) to Fahrenheit (F), multiply by 9/5 and then add 32.

7. A temperature of 37 degrees Celsius is equal to how many degrees Fahrenheit?

(A) 70.3°F

(B) 98.0°F

(C) 99.0°F

✓**(D)** 98.6°F

(E) 101.2°F

(D)   is correct. (See question 6 for the rationale.)

8. When reading a mercury thermometer, each short line represents

(A) a degree

(B) two degrees

(C) one-tenth of a degree

✓**(D)** two-tenths of a degree

(E) three-tenths of a degree

(D)   is correct. Each short line represents two-tenths of a degree (0.2). A whole degree is marked with a long line. The even numbered degrees are printed on the thermometer.

9. When taking a rectal temperature on a pediatric patient, insert the thermometer into the anal canal approximately

(A) 2 to 2½ inches

(B) ¼ of an inch

✓**(C)** ½ to 1 inch

(D) 1 to 1½ inches

(E) no more than 3 inches

(C)   is correct. For an adult, you may insert the thermometer approximately 1 to 1½ inches into the anal canal.

10. An accurate axillary temperature registers approximately how many degrees lower than a rectal temperature?

  ✔**(A)** one degree
    (B) two degrees
    (C) three degrees
    (D) four degrees
    (E) it registers the same as a rectal temperature

    (A)   is correct. The average normal temperature orally is 98.6 degrees F, and the average normal rectal temperature is 99.6 degrees F, which equals one degree difference.

11. The average normal rectal temperature is

  (A) 99°F
  (B) 97.6°F
  (C) 98.6°F
    (D) 101°F
  ✔**(E)** 99.6°F

    (E)   is correct. (See question 10 for the rationale.)

12. The gradual drop of a fever is termed

  ✔**(A)** lysis
    (B) crisis
    (C) intermittent
    (D) remittent
    (E) continuous

    (A)   is correct.
    (B)   Crisis is a sudden drop of a high body temperature to or below a normal level.
    (C)   Intermittent describes a fever that is elevated at certain times within a 24-hour period but that falls to normal or subnormal levels during the same period of time.
    (D)   Remittent describes a fever that fluctuates frequently but does not fall to normal.
    (E)   Continuous describes a fever that remains elevated and does not fluctuate.

13. Which of the following statements is FALSE?

    (A) when taking an aural temperature on an adult, the MA must gently pull upward on the patient's outer ear
  ✔**(B)** when taking an aural temperature on a pediatric patient, the MA must not pull the child's ear in any direction
    (C) an electronic thermometer has probes for both oral and rectal temperature measurements
    (D) the term afebrile means without fever
    (E) the term sublingual means under the tongue

    (B)   is correct. The MA must gently pull downward on an infant's or child's ear when taking an aural temperature.

14. Which of the following statements is TRUE?

(A) keep a glass/mercury thermometer in place orally for at least 3 minutes
(B) keep a glass/mercury thermometer under the axilla for at least 10 minutes
(C) keep a glass/mercury thermometer within the anal opening for 5 minutes
(D) keep a tympanic thermometer in the aural till it beeps
✓ (E) all of the above are true

   (E)   is correct. It is critical for accuracy to allow the thermometer enough time to register the patient's true temperature. Not keeping a glass/mercury thermometer in place for the appropriate time can lead to inaccurate readings that are below the patient's actual temperature.

15. Which of the following statements is FALSE?

(A) activity may increase a pulse rate by 20 to 30 beats per minute
✓(B) as age increases, pulse rate increases
(C) female pulse rate is about 10 BPM higher than a male of the same age
(D) athletes and people in good physical condition tend to have a slower pulse rate
(E) increased pulse rate in thyroid disease, fever, and shock is due to an increased metabolism

   (B)   is correct. As age increases, pulse rate decreases. Remember, infants and children have a faster pulse rate than adults. Pulse rate is proportionate to the size of the body. Heat loss is greater in a small body, resulting in the heart pumping faster to compensate.

16. A child less than 1 year old may have a pulse rate that ranges between

(A) 50 and 65
(B) 60 and 80
(C) 70 and 90
(D) 80 and 120
✓(E) 120 and 160

   (E)   is correct.
         2–6 yrs. = 80–120
         6–10 yrs. = 80–100
         11–16 yrs. = 70–90
         Adult = 60–90
         Older adult = 50–65

17. The force or strength of the pulse is commonly referred to as the

(A) condition of the arterial wall
(B) rhythm
✓(C) volume
(D) pulse pressure
(E) pulse deficit

   (C)   is correct. Volume is noted as full, normal, bounding, weak, feeble, or thready (barely perceptible). Volume is influenced by the forcefulness of the heartbeat, the condition of the arterial walls, and dehydration. A variance in intensity of the pulse may indicate heart disease.
   (A)   The condition of the arterial wall should be felt as elastic and soft. A pulse taken in a blood vessel that feels hard and rope-like is considered abnormal and may indicate heart disease, such as arteriosclerosis

(narrowing of the artery with loss of elasticity), whereas atherosclerosis refers to hardening of the arteries (note the h when discriminating between arteriosclerosis and atherosclerosis).

(B)   Rhythm refers to the regularity, or equal spacing of all the beats, of the pulse. It is not considered abnormal for the heart to occasionally skip a beat. This is referred to as an intermittent pulse. Exercise or caffeine may cause this to occur. An arrhythmia is a pulse lacking in regularity and should be brought to the physician's attention.

(D)   Pulse pressure is the difference between the systolic and diastolic readings. This is found by subtracting the diastolic reading from the systolic reading. A p.p. that is greater than 50 mm Hg or less than 30 mm Hg is considered to be abnormal. Extremes of pulse pressure can result in stroke or shock.

(E)   Pulse deficit is the difference between the apical and radial pulse rate, taken at the same time by two MAs (or by taking the apical first and then taking the radial immediately after if only one MA is available). A pulse deficit is said to be present if the radial pulse beat is less than the apical. This condition is seen in patients with atrial fibrillation.

18. Hardening of the arteries is referred to as

✓**(A)** arteriosclerosis   **(D)** pulse deficit
  (B) atherosclerosis   **(E)** pulse pressure
  (C) arthrosclerosis

(A)   is correct.
(B)   Atherosclerosis is a form of arteriosclerosis in which yellowish plaques of cholesterol form in the arteries.
(C)   Arthrosclerosis is hardening of a joint.
(D)   A pulse deficit is the difference between the apical and the radial pulse.
(E)   Pulse pressure is the difference between the systolic and diastolic blood pressure.

19. The most common site for taking a pulse on infants and young children is

  (A) brachial   **(D)** apical
  (B) pedis   **(E)** carotid
  (C) radial

✓(D)   is correct. The apical pulse is found at the apex of the heart, which is located on the left side of the chest at the fifth intercostal space.
(A)   The brachial site is only used on an infant in an emergency and is more typically used when taking blood pressure. It is located on the inner antecubital space of the arm.
(B)   Pedis, as in dorsal pedis, refers to the foot (specifically, the top of the foot slightly lateral to the midline). This site should always be checked on patients with diabetes in order to detect adequate circulation in the feet.
(C)   A radial pulse on the thumb is the most frequently used site for counting pulse rate in adults.
(E)   The carotid site is located between the larynx and the sternocleidomastoid muscle in the side of the neck. This site is used during CPR.

20. When taking a pulse, the medical assistant should count the pulse for at least

(A) 10 seconds

(B) 15 seconds

(C) 20 seconds

(D) 30 seconds

✓(E) 60 seconds

(E) is correct. Although one may take a pulse for 15 seconds and multiply it by 4, or take a pulse for 30 seconds and multiply it by 2, to get an estimate of BPM, neither allows enough time to adequately evaluate for arrhythmias.

21. What term describes a pulse rate above 100 BPM?

✓(A) tachycardia

(B) pulse deficit

(C) pulse pressure

(D) thready

(E) bradycardia

(A) is correct. See question 18 for the rationale to (B) and (C). Thready (D) indicates that a pulse rate is barely perceptible. Bradycardia (E) is a term that describes a pulse rate below 60 BPM.

22. Which of the following statements is FALSE?

(A) fear, anxiety, and anger may cause the pulse rate to rise

(B) depression, hypothyroidism, or brain injuries that cause intracranial pressure may lower the pulse rate

(C) it is normal if the heart occasionally skips a beat

✓(D) a fever may lower the pulse rate

(E) shock may increase the pulse rate

(D) is correct. A fever will cause the pulse rate to increase, due to an increased metabolism.

23. During the process of inspiration, the diaphragm

✓(A) moves downward

(B) moves upward

(C) moves inward

(D) moves outward

(E) does not move

(A) is correct. The diaphragm moves downward, the intercostal muscles move outward, and the lungs expand in order to take oxygen into the lungs.

24. The minute air sacs of the lungs are termed

✓(A) alveoli

(B) diaphragm

(C) medulla oblongata

(D) aural

(E) croup

(A) is correct. Alveoli are minute air sacs in the lungs.

(B) The diaphragm is a musculofibrous partition that separates the thoracic and abdominal cavities.

(C) The medulla oblongata is a vital part of the brain that controls the respiratory, cardiac, and vasomotor centers.

(D) Aural pertains to the ear or hearing.

(E) Croup is an acute viral infection of the upper and lower respiratory tract in children that may result in difficult, noisy breathing.

25. The average respiratory rate in adults ranges between

(A) 30 and 50   **(D)** 18 and 24
(B) 20 and 40   **(E)** 14 and 20
(C) 20 and 30

    (E)   is correct. The adult range for respiratory rate is 14 to 20.
    (A)   30 to 50 is the average range for newborns.
    (B)   20 to 40 is the average range for 1-year-olds.
    (C)   20 to 30 is the average range for 2- to 10-year-olds.
    (D)   18 to 24 is the average range for 11- to 18-year-olds.

26. The average respiratory rate in newborns ranges between

(A) 120 and 160   **(D)** 30 and 50
(B) 80 and 120   **(E)** 50 and 65
(C) 60 and 80

    (D)   is correct. The average respiratory rate for newborns ranges between 30 and 50.

27. Difficult breathing when lying down is termed

(A) tachypnea   **(D)** bradypnea
(B) orthopnea   **(E)** apnea
(C) dyspnea

    (B)   is correct. Orthopnea is seen in patients suffering from emphysema or congestive heart failure.
    (A)   Tachypnea is characterized by rapid breathing (above 40 RPMs), as seen in patients suffering from high fever or pneumonia.
    (C)   Dyspnea is difficulty breathing, as seen in patients suffering with asthma or pneumonia.
    (D)   Bradypnea is slow breathing (an adult below 10 RPMs), as seen in patients who are near death.
    (E)   Apnea is temporary cessation of breathing, as seen in sleep apnea patients.

28. Which of the following ratios is accurate for the proportion of respiratory rate to pulse rate?

(A) 10:1   **(D)** 5:1
(B) 20:1   **(E)** 1:5
(C) 1:4

    (C)   is correct. The proportion 1:4 means that for each respiration the heart will generally beat 4 times. (Example: if a patient's respiration rate is 20, the pulse rate will be 4 times greater [20 × 4 = 80 BPM].) This method for estimating a pulse rate is not an acceptable practice for determining a patient's pulse rate. It is simply a general gauge. Since there is a definite correlation between respirations and pulse rates, it is safe to say that the situations that cause the pulse rate to rise or fall will typically cause the respiration rate to rise or fall.

29. Which of the following will cause a decreased respiratory rate?

(A) allergic reactions
(B) epinephrine
(C) morphine
(D) asthma
(E) fever

    (C) is correct. All of the other situations will cause an increase in respiratory rate. In addition, heart disease, exercise, excitement, anger, hemorrhage, high altitudes, shock, and pain will also increase the respiratory rate. However, a decrease of carbon dioxide, a stroke, coma, sleep, and injuries that cause pressure on the brain will decrease the respiratory rate.

30. Cyanosis is due to a/an

(A) increase in carbon dioxide
(B) decrease in carbon dioxide
(C) increase in oxygen
(D) rich oxygen levels
(E) poor carbon dioxide levels

    (A) is correct. Typically when this occurs there is a decrease in oxygen and the patient's skin and/or nail beds may appear bluish in color.

31. Which breath sound resembles the crackling sound of crushing tissue paper and is caused by fluid accumulated in the airways?

(A) stridor
(B) rales
(C) stertorous sounds
(D) rhonchi
(E) wheezes

    (B) is correct. Rales occur with some types of pneumonia.
    (A) Stridor is a shrill, harsh sound that is heard more clearly during inspiration. It may be heard in children with croup and in patients with laryngeal obstruction.
    (C) Stertorous sounds are noisy breathing sounds, such as snoring.
    (D) Rhonchi, or gurgles, are rattling, whistling sounds made in the throat. It is heard in patients with tracheostomies or those requiring suctioning of mucous.
    (E) Wheezes are high-pitched, whistling sounds made when airways become obstructed or severely narrowed, as in asthma or chronic obstructive pulmonary disease (COPD).

32. Which of the following statements is FALSE?

(A) prior to measuring a patient's respirations, explain the procedure to him or her
(B) don't take respiration measurements immediately after the patient has experienced exertion
(C) count each inhalation and expiration as one respiration
(D) Cheyne-Stokes respiration is a breathing pattern characterized by a period of apnea for 10 to 60 seconds, followed by increased depth and frequency of respirations
(E) the depth of respiration refers to the volume of air being inhaled and exhaled; it may be described as either shallow or deep

(A) is correct. One should attempt to keep the patient unaware that respirations are being measured since the patient may alter the breathing pattern. Therefore, the MA should appear to be taking the pulse while he or she is actually taking respirations.

33. The pressure against the walls of the arteries when the heart contracts is considered to be

(A) hypertension
(B) diastolic pressure
(C) pulse pressure
(D) cardiac cycle
(E) systolic pressure

(E) is correct. Systolic pressure is the highest pressure that occurs as the heart is contracting.
(A) Hypertension is simply defined as high blood pressure.
(B) Diastolic pressure is the lowest pressure level that occurs when the heart is relaxed (the ventricle is at rest).
(C) Pulse pressure is the difference between the systolic and diastolic readings.
(D) Cardiac cycle is considered to be the two phases of heart activity—contraction and relaxation. It is identified by two heart sounds (lubb and dubb) occurring during the cardiac cycle.

34. During which of the Korotkoff phases might an auscultatory gap occur?

(A) I
(B) II
(C) III
(D) IV
(E) V

(B) is correct. During this phase, the sound has a swishing quality. An auscultatory gap is said to have occurred if there is a total loss of sound at this stage, which then reoccurs later. It may be an indication of heart disease and/or hypertension. Due to this phenomenon, it is advisable to get an estimated systolic reading prior to taking a patient's blood pressure.
(A) Phase I is the first faint sound heard as the cuff is deflated.
(C) Phase III sound will become less muffled and develop a crisp tapping sound.
(D) Phase IV sound will now begin to fade and become muffled. The American Heart Association, which believes Phase IV is the best indicator of the diastolic pressure, recommends the reading at this phase be recorded as the diastolic pressure for a child.
(E) Phase V sound will disappear at this phase. Some physicians want both Phase IV and Phase V recorded for the diastolic pressure reading (for example, 120/78/74).

35. The average blood pressure reading in children between the ages of 6 and 9 is

(A) 138/86
(B) 120/80
(C) 118/76
(D) 100/65
(E) 95/65

(E) is correct.
(A) 138/86 is the average normal reading for older adults.
(B) 120/80 is the average normal reading for adults.
(C) 118/76 is the average normal reading for age 16 to adulthood.
(D) 100/65 is the average normal reading for 10- to 15-year-olds.

Newborns tend to have an average normal reading of 50/25. However, blood pressure readings are not generally taken on infants.

36. Which of the following physiological factors may affect blood pressure?

   (A) volume of blood   **(D)** elasticity of vessels
   (B) peripheral resistance   **(E)** all of the above
   (C) condition of the heart

     (E) is correct. All may affect blood pressure.
     (A) An increase of blood volume increases the BP, and a decrease of blood volume decreases BP. For example, polycytopenia increases BP; hemorrhage causes blood volume and BP to drop.
     (B) Peripheral resistance relates to the size of the lumen within blood vessels and amount of blood flowing through them. For example, the smaller the lumen, the greater is the resistance to blood flow, and thus, a high BP.
     (C) The condition of the heart, the strength of heart muscle, affects the volume of blood flow. For example, a weak heart muscle can cause an abnormal increase or decrease in BP.
     (D) Elasticity of vessels allows them to expand and contract easily. Elasticity decreases with age, and with this an increase in BP is seen.

37. Which is a primary hypertension of unknown cause?

   (A) renal   **(D)** malignant
   (B) essential   **(E)** secondary
   (C) benign

     (B) is correct.
     (A) Renal hypertension is seen with an elevated blood pressure as a result of kidney disease.
     (C) Benign hypertension is characterized by a slow onset of elevated blood pressure without symptoms.
     (D) Malignant hypertension is a rapidly developing hypertension that may become fatal if not treated immediately.
     (E) Secondary hypertension is elevated blood pressure associated with other conditions, such as renal disease, pregnancy, arteriosclerosis, and obesity. Essentially, if you correct the primary condition, such as renal disease, the hypertension will dissipate.

38. Which is a temporary fall in blood pressure that occurs when a patient rapidly moves from a lying to a standing position?

   (A) hypotension   **(D)** Korotkoff
   (B) postural hypotension   **(E)** none of the above
   (C) orthostatic

(C) is correct.
(A) Hypotension is abnormally low blood pressure, which may or may not be caused by shock, hemorrhage, and/or central nervous system disorders.
(B) Postural hypotension is a temporary fall in blood pressure from standing motionless for extended periods of time.
(D) Korotkoff refers to the Korotkoff sounds heard in auscultation of blood pressure.

39. Which of the following statements is FALSE?

   (A) hypertension has many noticeable symptoms
   (B) blood pressure is measured in millimeters of Hg
   (C) a patient's BPs are usually tested at least twice before being placed on medication
   (D) women generally have lower blood pressure than men
   (E) blood pressure tends to increase with age

   (A) is correct. Hypertension is often called the silent killer because it is usually asymptomatic, or without any symptoms.

40. Which of the following conditions will cause an increased BP?

   (A) anemia   **(D)** hypothyroidism
   (B) approaching death   **(E)** infection and fever
   (C) exercise

   (C) is correct. Exercise will cause an increase in BP. Anger, nicotine, caffeine, hyperthyroidism, fear, excitement, liver disease, renal disease, late pregnancy, smoking, and rigidity of blood vessels can also cause an increase in BP. The other conditions can cause a decrease in BP.

41. Which artery is most commonly used for taking a patient's BP?

   (A) carotid   **(D)** dorsalis pedis
   (B) brachial   **(E)** apical
   (C) popliteal

   (B) is correct. The brachial artery, located at the inner aspect of the antecubital space of the elbow, is the most common artery used in taking BPs.
   (A) The carotid artery, located between the larynx and the sternocleido-mastoid muscle in the side of the neck, is most commonly used to detect a pulse during cardiopulmonary resuscitation.
   (C) The popliteal artery is located behind the knee.
   (D) Dorsalis pedis, located on top of the foot slightly lateral to midline, is used to determine adequate circulation to the feet (especially in diabetics).
   (E) The apical artery, located on the left side of the chest by the fifth intercostal space at the midclavicular line, is found just below the nipple.

42. Which of the following statements is FALSE?

(A) the mercury sphygmomanometer is considered to be the most accurate
(B) BP is usually higher in the right arm than the left if the patient is right-handed
(C) when taking a blood pressure, the patient's arm should be just below the level of the heart
(D) the BP cuff should be placed 1 to 2 inches above the antecubital space
(E) BP is measured in mm Hg

   (C) is correct. The patient's arm should be level with his or her heart.

43. Which of the following statements is FALSE?

(A) when getting an estimated systolic pressure, one should feel the radial pulse while the blood pressure cuff is being inflated
(B) when taking a BP, one should inflate the cuff 30 mm Hg above the estimated systolic pressure reading
(C) the mercury column should be calibrated to 1
(D) a BP that is too small for a patient may give an abnormally high reading
(E) if you are unsure about the BP reading, wait at least 1 minute before taking a second reading

   (C) is correct. The mercury column should be calibrated to zero.

44. Which of the following will NOT cause an error in blood pressure readings?

(A) improper cuff size
(B) a loosely applied cuff
(C) rapid deflation
(D) nervous patient
(E) inflating the cuff 30 mm Hg above the previous BP

   (E) is correct. Inflating the cuff 30 mm Hg above the previous BP will generally not cause an error in BP reading.

45. One kilogram (kg) is equal to how many pounds?

(A) 0.45 lb.   (D) 4.2 lbs.
(B) 2.2 lbs.   (E) 5.4 lbs.
(C) 3 lbs.

   (B) is correct. One kilogram is equal to 2.2 pounds.

46. One pound (lb.) is equal to how many kilograms?

(A) 0.45 kg.   (D) 4.5 kg.
(B) 0.4 kg.   (E) 5.4 kg.
(C) 3.0 kg.

   (A) is correct. One pound is equal to 0.45 kilogram.

47. Mr. Duffy weighs 220 lbs. How many kilograms does he weigh?

(A) 48.40 kg.   (D) 99.00 kg.
(B) 26.40 kg.   (E) 136.08 kg.
(C) 102 kg.

(D) is correct. 220 lbs. × 0.45 kg. = 99.00 kg.

48. Ms. DeBeir weighs 52.00 kg. How many pounds does she weigh?

(A) 114 lbs.   (D) 195 lbs.
(B) 144 lbs.   (E) 123 lbs.
(C) 23.40 lbs.

(A) is correct. 52.00 kg. × 2.2 lbs. = 114 lbs.

49. Which decimal is equal to 1/4 of a pound?

(A) 0.25   (D) 1.25
(B) 0.75   (E) 1.50
(C) 0.50

(A) is correct. 0.25 is 1/4 of a pound.
(B) 0.75 is 3/4 of a pound.
(C) 0.50 is 1/2 of a pound.
(D) 1.25 is 1 1/4 of a pound.
(E) 1.50 is 1 1/2 of a pound.

50. Which of the following statements is FALSE?

(A) set all weights to zero and check if the scale is calibrated before weighing a patient
(B) a scale must be calibrated by a trained scale technologist
(C) ″ is the symbol for inch
(D) there are 12 inches to 1 foot
(E) when measuring height, the patient's back should face the scale

(B) is correct. A medical assistant can calibrate a scale. Set all weights to zero and balance the scale by adjusting the small screw-like knob at one end until the balance bar pointer floats in the center of the frame. (A coin or paper clip can be used if a screw driver is not available to make this adjustment.)

51. Which of the following statements is FALSE?

(A) an infant's head circumference is usually measured during each checkup until the age of 36 months
(B) there are 12 ounces to 1 pound
(C) a small child may be weighed by weighing the mother and then weighing the mother holding the child; subtracting the two weights will give you the weight of the small child
(D) when weighing an infant, keep one hand over the infant's body as a safety precaution
(E) never raise the height bar in an opened position

(B) is correct. There are 16 ounces in 1 pound.

CHAPTER 16

ASSISTING WITH PHYSICAL EXAMINATIONS

1. Which section of the patient history is considered to be the reason for the office visit?

   (A) assessment of body systems (review of symptoms)
   (B) personal history
   (C) family medical history
   (D) past medical history
   (E) chief complaint

   (E)   is correct. The chief complaint (CC) is referred to as the presenting problem. It is usually stated in the patient's own words in quotes.

   (A)   Assessment of body systems is performed just before the physical examination. It may also be referred to as the review of systems, which is a systematic review of all body systems.

   (B)   Personal history would include the following: lifestyle patterns that affect the health status of the patient (i.e., smoking, drinking, occupation, marital status, sexual preferences, diet, exercise, and sleep habits).

   (C)   Family medical history covers the dates of major illnesses, hospitalizations, and surgeries. Also, it records the health problems of the patient's blood relatives.

   (D)   Past medical history should include all diseases and medical problems the patient has experienced in the past: dates of major illnesses, hospitalizations, allergies, childhood diseases, injuries, immunizations, and surgeries.

2. When using the problem-oriented medical record (POMR) method for medical recording, which of the following areas is the patient's history housed in?

   (A) objective findings   **(D)** initial plan
   (B) database   **(E)** progress notes
   (C) problem list

   (B)   is correct. The database houses the patient's history, physical examination, and initial laboratory findings.

   (A)   Objective findings are located in the progress notes. They are signs that are perceptible to others, such as those found by the physician upon examination.

   (C)   The problem list is found at the front of the patient's chart. It is a numerical, dated listing of all medical problems. As each problem is resolved, the date of resolution is documented next to the problem.

   (D)   The initial plan is a written plan for each identified problem.

(E)   Progress notes are used to further document each problem on the problem list. It is made up of SOAP notes: subjective data, objective data, assessment, and plan.

3. Which of the following would be considered to be a symptom?

(A)   hypertension   **(D)**   arthritis
(B)   diabetes   ✔**(E)**   dizziness
(C)   pregnancy

    (E)   is correct. Dizziness would be considered a symptom. A symptom, also referred to as a subjective finding, is perceptible only to the patient. (A), (B), (C), and (D) are all considered signs.

4. In which part of the SOAP charting system can the diagnosis be found?

(A)   subjective   **(D)**   plan
(B)   objective   **(E)**   problem list
✔**(C)**   assessment

    (C)   is correct.
    (A)   Subjective findings are symptoms provided by the patient and/or family.
    (B)   Objective findings are signs identified by the physician through physical examination.
    (D)   The plan includes the recommended treatments, further tests, medications, consultation, surgery, and physical therapy.
    (E)   The problem list is not included as a part of SOAP notes. The problem list is used with the problem-oriented medical record (POMR).

5. Which of the following is NOT a recommended guideline when charting?

(A)   double-checking to make sure that you have the correct patient chart
(B)   using black ink
✔(C)   lengthy, superfluous entries
(D)   the patient's name should appear on each page of the record
(E)   dating and initialing each entry

    (C)   is correct. Lengthy, superfluous entries should be avoided. Entries should be brief but to the point. (A), (B), (D), and (E) are all recommended guidelines to use when charting. Furthermore, the medical assistant should also: sign his or her full name, either in the medical record or on file in the physician's office; use only accepted medical abbreviations; never erase, use white-out, or in any way remove information from a medical record; document all telephone calls relating to the patient in the medical record as well as other correspondence; document any action(s) taken as a result of telephone conversations; and document all missed appointments.

6. Which of the following is NOT an acceptable practice for the medical assistant when preparing the patient for an examination?

✓ **(A)** have the patient undress from the waist up
   (B) take the patient's height, weight, vital signs, temperature, pulse, respirations, and blood pressure
   (C) have the patient empty his or her bladder
   (D) the medical assistant remaining in the room with an elderly patient
   (E) the removal of all clothing, including underwear and stockings

   (A) is correct. Having the patient only undress from the waist up would not be an acceptable practice. All of the other practices listed are acceptable.

7. Which position is used for patients having difficulty breathing?

   (A) Sims'   **(D)** Trendelenburg
   (B) supine   **(E)** knee-chest
✓ **(C)** Fowler's

   ✓(C) is correct.
   (A) Sims' position is used for rectal examination or vaginal examination. The patient lies on left side, left arm behind body for support, left leg bent slightly, and right leg bent sharply.
   (B) Supine position is used to examine the abdomen, chest, and legs. The patient lies flat on back.
   (D) Trendelenburg is used to treat shock and in abdominal surgery. The patient is supine with his or her head lower than the feet.
   (E) Knee-chest position is used for rectal examinations. The patient kneels on the table with buttocks raised, head and chest on exam table. The head is turned to side, with knees slightly apart.

8. Which position is used for pelvic examinations?

   (A) proctologic   **(D)** prone
   (B) knee-chest   **(E)** semi-Fowler's
✓ **(C)** lithotomy

   (C) is correct.
   (A) Proctologic is used in sigmoidoscope examinations. A special exam table, which bends in the center, is used to correctly position the patient. The patient is placed in the prone position (flat on stomach) on the exam table.
   (B) Knee-chest is used to examine the rectum. The patient should kneel on the table with buttocks raised, head and chest on the exam table. Head is turned to the side, with knees slightly apart.
   (D) Prone position is used to examine the back, spine, or legs. The patient is instructed to lie on the abdomen with head to one side.
   (E) Semi-Fowler's is used for patients having difficulty breathing. The patient is instructed to sit but with his or her back resting at a 45-degree angle.

9. Which method of examination is used to gauge the growth of the body or to determine size?

   (A) mensuration
   (B) inspection
   (C) palpation
   (D) percussion
   (E) auscultation

   ✓(A) is correct. Mensuration measures the growth of the body.
     (B) Inspection is the visual examination of the body.
     (C) Palpation is the application of the hands or fingers to the external surface of the body.
     (D) Percussion refers to using the fingertips to tap the body lightly but sharply to determine the presence or absence of fluid or pus and to gain information about the position and size of an organ.
     (E) Auscultation is examination based on listening to sounds.

10. What instrument is used to examine the interior eye?

    ✓**(A)** opthalmoscope
    (B) percussion hammer
    (C) otoscope
    (D) stethoscope
    (E) tuning fork

      (A) is correct. The opthalmoscope is used to examine the interior eye.
      (B) A percussion hammer is used for testing neurological reflexes.
      (C) The otoscope is used to inspect the outer ear and tympanic membrane.
      (D) A stethoscope is used to amplify sounds (heart, lungs, bowel) within the body.
      (E) A tuning fork is used to test the patient's hearing ability.

11. Which of the following pieces of equipment is NOT typically used in a CPX?

    (A) sphygmomanometer
    (B) syringe
    ✓**(C)** fixative
    (D) penlight
    (E) nasal speculum

      (C) is correct. A syringe is not typically used in a CPX.
      (A) The sphygmomanometer is used to take blood pressure.
      (B) A fixative is used to spray slides.
      (D) The penlight is used to illuminate.
      (E) A nasal speculum is used to inspect the lining of the nose, nasal membranes, and internal septum.

12. Which of the following diagnostic or laboratory tests may be ordered for a CPX?

    (A) blood chemistry profile and complete blood count
    (B) pulmonary function test
    (C) electrocardiogram
    (D) visual acuity
    (E) all of the above

      (E) is correct. All of the above may be ordered for a CPX. The following may also be ordered for a CPX: SMA-12, SMAC, differential, sedimentation rate, vital signs, weight and height, and x-rays.

13. What instrument is used to test the reflexes of the body?

- **(A)** tuning fork
- **(B)** laryngeal mirror
- ✓**(C)** percussion hammer
- **(D)** proctosigmoidoscope
- **(E)** emesis basin

  (C) is correct. The percussion hammer is used to test reflexes.
  (A) A tuning fork is used to test the patient's hearing ability.
  (B) The laryngeal mirror is used to visualize the larynx.
  (D) A proctosigmoidoscope is used to view the interior sigmoid colon.
  (E) An emesis basin is a kidney-shaped receptacle for body drainage.

14. Which of the following represents an item that would be documented under past medical history?

- **(A)** vomiting
- ✓**(B)** tonsillectomy
- **(C)** sleeps 8 hours a night on average
- **(D)** mother deceased
- **(E)** respirations regular

  (B) is correct.
  (A) Vomiting would be documented under present illness.
  (C) Sleeps 8 hours a night on average would be documented under personal history.
  (D) Mother deceased would be documented under family history.
  (E) Respirations regular would be documented under review of systems.

15. Which of the following would be correct for the medical assistant to document in a patient's chart?

- ✓**(A)** cc: "I have pain on the right side of my stomach"
- **(B)** Cc: The patient c/o pain in the RLQ of the abdomen
- **(C)** B/P: 120:70, R: 16, T: 99.6
- **(D)** Allergies: none, Meds: none
- **(E)** The pts. Throat appears to be infected with strep

  (A) is correct. Always use the patient's own words to explain the chief complaint and use quotes.
  (B) Always use the patient's own words to explain the chief complaint and use quotes.
  (C) B/P should be written 120/70, and the patient's pulse should also be documented.
  (D) If the patient states he or she is not allergic to anything, the medical assistant should document NKA (no known allergies).
  (E) This statement is an attempt at diagnosing. It is not within the medical assistant's duties to diagnose.

16. Which term refers to blood in the stool?

- **(A)** hemoptysis
- **(B)** tinnitus
- **(C)** laryngitis
- **(D)** leukoplakia
- ✓**(E)** hematuria

(E) is correct.
(A) Hemoptysis means to cough up blood.
(B) Tinnitus means ringing of the ears.
(C) Laryngitis is inflammation of the larynx.
(D) Leukoplakia is white patches on mucous membranes.

17. The area of flexation in the groin area between the hips and legs is referred to as

(A) hernia
(B) axilla
(C) renal colic
(D) inguinal
(E) orifice

(D) is correct.
(A) Hernia refers to a protrusion of an organ through the wall of a cavity in which it is usually located.
(B) Axilla refers to the armpit.
(C) Renal colic is a pain in the kidney area, usually due to kidney stones.
(E) Orifice refers to an opening of a body part, such as the mouth.

18. An itchy skin rash, commonly called hives, is also referred to as

(A) urticaria
(B) leukorrhea
(C) cyanosis
(D) rosacea
(E) oliguria

(A) is correct.
(B) Leukorrhea is a white discharge.
(C) Cyanosis is a bluish coloration of the skin.
(D) Rosacea is a chronic skin disease.
(E) Oliguria is a reduced production of urine.

19. The intraocular pressure of the eye is measured with a/an

(A) otoscope
(B) opthalmoscope
(C) tonometer
(D) penlight
(E) Titmus II

(C) is correct.
(A) An otoscope is used to inspect the outer ear and tympanic membrane (eardrum).
(B) The opthalmoscope is used to examine the interior of the eye, especially the retina.
(D) A penlight is used for illumination of an area.
(E) Titmus II is a machine used to measure visual acuity (both far and near).

CHAPTER 17

ASSISTING WITH MEDICAL SPECIALTIES

1. The initial exposure a person has to an allergen recognized as foreign by the body's immune system is known as

   (A) inoculation
   (B) sensitization
   (C) anaphylactic shock

   (D) PKU
   (E) metastasis

   > (B)   is correct. Sensitization is the initial exposure a person has to an allergen or substance (antigen) recognized as foreign by the body's immune system.
   >
   > (A)   An inoculation is the injection of serum, microorganisms, or viral organisms for the purpose of creating immunity to disease in a person.
   >
   > (C)   Anaphylactic shock is a life-threatening reaction to certain foods, drugs, and insect bites in some people.
   >
   > (D)   Phenylketonuria (PKU) is a recessive hereditary disease caused by a lack of an enzyme, phenylalanine hydroxylase, which results in severe mental retardation in children if not detected and treated soon after birth.
   >
   > (E)   Metastasis occurs when cancerous cells or tumors spread to another location or organ.

2. Anaphylactic shock can result in

   (A) edema and rash
   (B) convulsions
   (C) unconsciousness and death

   (D) A, B, and C
   (E) B and C only

   > (D)   is correct. Anaphylactic shock can result in edema, rash, convulsions, unconsciousness, and death if untreated.

3. The round, raised skin lesions with itching that are a positive sign of reaction to allergy testing are called

   (A) papules
   (B) wheals
   (C) nodules

   (D) macules
   (E) vesicles

   > (B)   is correct. A wheal is a round, raised skin lesion with itching that is a positive sign of reaction to allergy testing.
   >
   > (A)   A papule is a small, solid, circular raised spot on the surface of the skin.
   >
   > (C)   A nodule is a solid, raised group of cells.
   >
   > (D)   A macule is a small, flat, discolored area that is flush with the skin surface.
   >
   > (E)   A vesicle is a small, fluid-filled raised spot on the skin.

4. A test consisting of placing allergens on the patient's anterior forearm to determine sensitivity and then covering this with a plastic covering is called a/an

(A) acuity test
(B) sweat test
(C) patch test
(D) dermatome
(E) dermabrasion

(C) is correct. A patch test is a test consisting of placing allergens on the patient's anterior forearm to determine sensitivity and then covering this with a plastic covering.
(A) An acuity test is a visual eye test.
(B) A sweat test is performed to determine the level of chloride.
(D) A dermatome is an instrument for cutting the skin or taking thin transplants of the skin.
(E) Dermabrasion is rubbing the skin using wire brushes or sandpaper.

5. The skin is also called the

(A) integument
(B) integumentary system
(C) dermal layer
(D) all of the above
(E) none of the above

(D) is correct.

6. A discomforting uneasiness that is often a sign of infection is

(A) metastasis
(B) acuity
(C) benign
(D) malaise
(E) contagious

(D) is correct. Malaise is a discomforting uneasiness that is often a sign of infection. It is noncontagious.
(A) Metastasis occurs when cancerous cells or tumors spread to another location or organ.
(B) Acuity is a sharpness. This term is usually associated with visual acuity.
(C) Benign is a nonthreatening, noncancerous condition.
(E) Contagious diseases are those that can be transmitted from one person to another.

7. The branch of medicine that deals with diseases and disorders of the female reproductive system is

(A) pediatrics
(B) gynecology
(C) urology
(D) nephrology
(E) neurology

(B) is correct. Gynecology is the branch of medicine that deals with diseases and disorders of the female reproductive tract.
(A) Pediatrics is the branch of medicine that involves the development, diagnosis, and treatment of disorders and diseases of children.
(C) Urology is the branch of medicine that involves disorders and diseases of the urinary and male reproductive tract.

(D) Nephrology is the branch of medicine that deals with the disorders and diseases of the kidney.

(E) Neurology is the branch of medicine that treats the nonsurgical patient who has a disorder or disease of the nervous system.

8. A fungal infectious skin disease that can be detected through use of a Wood's light is

(A) tinea
(B) herpes zoster
(C) impetigo
(D) scabies
(E) herpes simplex

    (A) is correct. Tinea is a fungal infectious skin disease that can be detected through use of a Wood's light.

    (B) Herpes zoster is a painful, infectious disease that attacks the nerve endings.

    (C) Impetigo is an inflammatory skin disease with pustules that become crusted and rupture.

    (D) Scabies is a contagious skin disease caused by an egg-laying mite.

    (E) Herpes simplex is an infectious disease caused by the herpes simplex virus 1 and characterized by thin vesicles that tend to recur in the same area, such as the lips or conjunctiva.

9. A benign neoplasm that results in enlarged blood vessels is

(A) melanoma
(B) nevus
(C) hemangioma
(D) keratosis
(E) lipoma

    (C) is correct. A hemangioma is a benign neoplasm that results in enlarged blood vessels.

    (A) A melanoma is a malignant, darkly pigmented mole or tumor of the skin.

    (B) A nevus is a pigmented congenital skin blemish.

    (D) Keratosis is an overgrowth and thickening of the epithelium.

    (E) A lipoma is a fatty tumor that generally does not metastasize.

10. A cardiovascular condition that results in death of tissue from lack of blood supply is a/an

(A) aneurysm
(B) angioma
(C) murmur
(D) infarct
(E) Reynaud's phenomenon

    (D) is correct. An infarct is a cardiovascular condition that results in death of tissue from lack of blood supply.

    (A) An aneurysm is an abnormal dilation of a blood vessel, usually an artery, due to a congenital weakness or defect in the wall of the vessel.

    (B) An angioma is a tumor, usually benign, consisting of blood vessels.

    (C) A murmur is a soft blowing or rasping sound heard upon auscultation of the heart.

    (E) Reynaud's phenomenon is intermittent attacks of pallor or cyanosis of the fingers or toes associated with cold or emotional distress.

11. The most common symptom/s of cardiovascular disorders is/are

(A) edema and cyanosis
(B) irregular heartbeat
(C) diaphoresis and dyspnea

(D) crushing chest pain
(E) all of the above

    (E) is correct.

12. Dyspnea is difficulty

(A) swallowing
(B) urinating
(C) breathing

(D) performing a function
(E) menstruating

    (C) is correct. Dyspnea is difficulty breathing.
    (A) Difficulty swallowing is called dysphagia.
    (B) Difficulty urinating is called dysuria.
    (D) Difficulty performing a function is called dysfunction.
    (E) Difficulty menstruating is called dysmenorrhea.

13. A tuberculin skin test is a

(A) Mantoux test
(B) tine test
(C) culture for tuberculosis

(D) A and B
(E) none of the above

    (D) is correct. The Mantoux test is a tuberculosis antibody test using an interdermal injection. The tine test is a test for tuberculosis using a small multipuncture device.

14. What disease results in edema, slowed speech, enlarged facial features and tongue, drowsiness, and mental apathy?

(A) myasthenia gravis
(B) myxedema
(C) von Recklinghausen's disease

(D) Graves' disease
(E) Cushing's syndrome

    (B) is correct. Myxedema is a disease that results in edema, slowed speech, enlarged facial features and tongue, drowsiness, and mental apathy.
    (A) Myasthenia gravis is a condition in which there is great muscular weakness and progressive fatigue.
    (C) von Recklinghausen's disease is an excessive production of parathyroid hormone, which results in degeneration of the bones.
    (D) Graves' disease results from an overactivity of the thyroid gland and can result in a crisis.
    (E) Cushing's syndrome is a set of symptoms, including weakness, edema, excessive hair growth, and osteoporosis, that is caused by hypersecretion of the adrenal cortex.

15. A group of symptoms and signs that are related to one another through some anatomic, physiological, or biochemical connection is called a

(A) prognosis
(B) diagnosis
(C) treatment

(D) syndrome
(E) syncope

(D) is correct. A syndrome is a group of symptoms and signs that are related to one another through some anatomic, physiological, or biochemical connection.

(A) A prognosis is the prediction of the course and end of a disease.

(B) Diagnosis is the disease or condition a person has.

(C) Treatment consists of the course of medical and surgical procedures prescribed to correct or cure a disease or condition.

(E) Syncope is fainting.

16. A procedure in which contrast medium is used to visualize the bile ducts is called

(A) endoscopic retrograde cholangiopancreatography (ERCP)
(B) cholecystogram
(C) intravenous cholangiogram
(D) peritoneoscopy laparoscopy
(E) choledocholithotripsy

(C) is correct. An intravenous cholangiogram is a procedure in which contrast medium is used to visualize the bile ducts

(A) Endoscopic retrograde cholangiopancreatography (ERCP) is the use of an endoscope to x-ray the bile and pancreatic ducts.

(B) A cholecystogram is an x-ray taken to visualize the gallbladder as dye enters it.

(D) A peritoneoscopy laparoscopy is a procedure in which an instrument or scope is passed into the abdominal wall through a small opening in order to examine the abdominal cavity for tumors and other conditions.

(E) A choledocholithotripsy is using lithotripsy equipment to crush gallstones located in the common bile duct.

17. The crushing of a stone located within the gallbladder is called

(A) cholecystectomy
(B) proctoplasty
(C) colostomy
(D) cholelithotripsy
(E) lithotripsy

(D) is correct. A cholelithotripsy is the crushing of a stone located within the gallbladder.

(A) A cholecystectomy is surgical removal of the gallbladder.

(B) A proctoplasty is plastic surgery of the anus or rectum.

(C) A colostomy is the surgical creation of an opening of some portion of the colon through the abdominal wall to the outside surface.

(E) Lithotripsy refers to crushing a kidney stone.

18. A musculoskeletal disorder in which a softening of bone occurs that may result from a deficiency in vitamin D is

(A) osteoporosis
(B) osteomalacia
(C) osteoarthritis
(D) talipes
(E) scoliosis

(B) is correct. Osteomalacia is a musculoskeletal disorder in which a softening of bone occurs that may result from a deficiency in vitamin D.

(A) Osteoporosis is a decrease in bone mass that results in a thinning and weakening of the bone with resulting fractures.

(C) Osteoarthritis is a noninflammatory type of arthritis resulting in degeneration of the bones and joints.

(D) Talipes is a congenital deformity of the foot.

(E) Scoliosis is an abnormal lateral curvature of the spine.

19. Another name for hyperthyroidism is

(A) Graves' disease

(B) goiter

(C) Hashimoto's disease

(D) Paget's disease

(E) Bright's disease

    (A) is correct. Graves' disease is another name for hyperthyroidism.

    (B) A goiter is an enlargement of the thyroid gland.

    (C) Hashimoto's disease is a chronic form of thyroiditis.

    (D) Paget's disease is an inherited disease causing a progressive muscle weakness and atrophy.

    (E) Bright's disease is an inflammatory kidney disease with proteinuria and hematuria.

20. Paget's disease is a/an

(A) deficiency in calcium and vitamin D

(B) metabolic disease of the bone characterized by deformity

(C) autoimmune disorder causing loss of muscle strength and paralysis

(D) inherited disease causing a progressive muscle weakness and deformity

(E) A and B

    (D) is correct. Paget's disease is an inherited disease causing a progressive muscle weakness and atrophy.

21. Another name for Lou Gehrig's disease is

(A) cerebral palsy

(B) Bell's palsy

(C) amyotropic lateral sclerosis

(D) Addison's disease

(E) Bright's disease

    (C) is correct. Lou Gehrig's disease is also called amyotropic lateral sclerosis. Lou Gehrig was a famous baseball player who had the disease.

    (A) Cerebral palsy is a nonprogressive paralysis resulting from a defect or trauma at the time of birth.

    (B) Bell's palsy is a one-sided facial paralysis caused by herpes simplex virus.

    (D) Addison's disease results from a deficiency of adrenocortical hormones that results in skin pigmentation, generalized weakness, and weight loss.

    (E) Bright's disease is an inflammatory degenerative kidney disease.

22. A mitral valve prolapse is a serious condition in which the mitral valve drops back into the

(A) left ventricle during diastole

(B) right ventricle during diastole

(C) right atrium during systole

(D) left atrium during systole

(E) none of the above

(D) is correct. A mitral valve prolapse is a serious condition in which the mitral valve drops back into the left atrium during systole.

23. A lumbar puncture is usually performed at the intervertebral space at the

   (A) 5th level
   (B) 5th or 6th level
   (C) 4th level
   (D) 7th level
   (E) none of the above

   (C) is correct. A lumbar puncture is usually performed at the intervertebral space at the 4th level or space.

24. Narcolepsy is a chronic disorder in which there is an extreme uncontrollable desire to

   (A) yawn
   (B) eat
   (C) sleep
   (D) talk
   (E) urinate

   (C) is correct. Narcolepsy is a disorder in which there is an uncontrollable desire to sleep.

25. A positive Babinski is demonstrated by a great toe that

   (A) extends
   (B) flexes
   (C) turns outward
   (D) turns inward
   (E) none of the above

   (A) is correct. A positive Babinski sign occurs when the great toe extends after the sole of the foot is stimulated.

26. A test developed to establish neurological function and body balance is the

   (A) electromyogram
   (B) positron emission tomography (PET)
   (C) Romberg's sign
   (D) Babinski's sign
   (E) vagotomy

   (C) is correct. Romberg's sign is a test to establish neurological function in which the patient is asked to close his or her eyes and place his or her feet together. The test for balance is positive if the patient sways while the eyes are closed.
   (A) An electromyogram is a written recording of muscle contractions as a result of electrical stimulation.
   (B) Positron emission tomography (PET) is the use of radionuclides to reconstruct brain sections.
   (D) Babinski's sign is a reflex used to determine lesions and abnormalities of the nervous system. In a positive Babinski, the great toe extends instead of flexes when the lateral sole of the foot is stroked.
   (E) A vagotomy is a surgical incision into the vagus nerve.

27. Strabismus is also called

(A) farsightedness
(B) nearsightedness
(C) exophthalmus
(D) lazy eye
(E) glaucoma

(D) is correct. Strabismus is also called lazy eye.

28. The Snellen chart should be hung how many feet from the patient's eye?

(A) 5
(B) 10
(C) 15
(D) 20
(E) 25

(D) is correct. The Snellen chart should be hung 20 feet from the patient's eye.

29. A vision test used to measure refractive error in small children is called

(A) Ishiara test
(B) Snellen test
(C) tonometry
(D) retinoscopy
(E) ophthalmoscopy

(D) is correct. Retinoscopy is a vision test used to measure refractive error in small children.
(A) The Ishiara test is used to test for color vision.
(B) A Snellen test is used to determine sharpness of vision based on a chart of 11 rows of letters set at 20 feet from the patient.
(C) Tonometry is the use of an instrument (tonometer) to measure intraocular pressure to determine the presence of glaucoma.
(E) Ophthalmoscopy is the use of an instrument (ophthalmascope) to examine the internal structure of the eye, including the fundus, macula, optic nerve, and blood vessels.

30. A total loss of hearing is known as

(A) otitis media
(B) presbycusis
(C) anacusis
(D) otosclerosis
(E) cerumen block

(C) is correct. A total loss of hearing is known as anacusis.
(A) Otitis media is a middle ear infection.
(B) Presbycusis is a loss of hearing associated with the aging process.
(D) Otosclerosis is a progressive hearing loss caused by immobility of the stapes bone.
(E) Cerumen block is caused by a build-up of ear wax.

31. When giving an immunization to an infant or child, never administer within

(A) the flu season
(B) 24 hours of a fever
(C) 48 hours of a fever
(D) 24 hours of another immunization
(E) none of the above

(B) is correct. When giving an immunization to an infant or child, never administer within 24 hours of a fever.

32. According to the American Cancer Society, women should examine both breasts

(A) weekly
(B) monthly
(C) bimonthly
(D) quarterly
(E) annually

    (B) is correct. The American Cancer Society recommends that women examine their breasts monthly.

33. A hernia of the bladder that protrudes into the vagina is called a/an

(A) cystoscope
(B) condyloma
(C) colposcopy
(D) cystocele
(E) eclampsia

    (D) is correct. A cystocele is a hernia of the bladder that protrudes into the vagina.

    (A) A cystoscope is a lighted instrument used to visualize the urinary bladder.

    (B) A condyloma is a wartlike skin growth usually found on the genitalia or in the anal area.

    (C) A colposcopy is a visual examination of the cervix and vagina using a colposcope.

    (E) Eclampsia is a condition during the 20th week of pregnancy and the first week of postpartum that results in convulsive seizures and coma.

34. A colposcopy is a/an

(A) examination of the female pelvic cavity using an endoscope
(B) exposing of tissues to high temperatures in order to destroy tissues
(C) visual examination of the bladder and vagina
(D) surgical removal of a core of cervical tissue
(E) examination of the urinary bladder using a lighted instrument

    (C) is correct. Colposcopy is the visual examination of the bladder and vagina.

35. Facilitating the removal of secretions from the bronchi by placing the patient in a position that uses gravity to promote this is known as

(A) intermittent positive pressure breathing
(B) postural drainage
(C) endotracheal intubation
(D) hyperbaric oxygen therapy
(E) none of the above

    (B) is correct. Postural drainage is the removal of secretions from the bronchi by placing the patient in a position that uses gravity to promote this.

    (A) Intermittent positive pressure breathing (IPPB) is a method for assisting the breathing of patients by the use of increased pressure.

(C) Endotracheal intubation is placement of a tube through the mouth to create an airway.

(D) Hyperbaric oxygen therapy is the use of oxygen under great pressure to treat cases of carbon monoxide poisoning, smoke inhalation, and other conditions.

36. The newborn reflex that occurs when the infant turns his or her head in the direction of a stimulus is called the

(A) sucking reflex
(B) rooting reflex
(C) palmar grasp reflex
(D) China doll reflex
(E) Moro reflex

(B) is correct. The rooting reflex is tested by stroking an infant's cheek. The infant with a normal response will turn toward the side that is stroked.

(A) The sucking reflex is an automatic reflex at birth. The infant will suck nipples and other objects placed in his or her mouth.

(C) The palmar grasp reflex occurs when the infant closes his or her hand as the palm is stroked.

(D) The China doll reflex occurs when the infant is pulled into a sitting position. This will cause the infant's eyes to open and shoulders to tense as the infant tries to keep his or her head up.

(E) The Moro reflex occurs when infants become startled. They will normally arch their back, throw back their head, extend their arms, and then quickly close (or flex) into a ball as though they were falling.

37. A test used to assess neonatal status is the

(A) Snellen test
(B) Apgar scale
(C) Moro reflex
(D) sucking reflex
(E) B, C, and D

(B) is correct. The Apgar scale is used immediately after birth, and then 5 minutes later, to assess the status of the newborn. The infant (neonate) is rated in 5 categories (heart rate, respirations, body color, muscle tone, and reflex irritability) on a scale of 1 to 10. In addition, reflexes such as the Moro and sucking reflexes are tested.

CHAPTER 18

ASSISTING WITH MINOR SURGERY

1. Outpatient surgery is generally limited to that which lasts less than

   (A) 15 minutes   (D) 90 minutes
   (B) 30 minutes   (E) 120 minutes
   ✓(C) 60 minutes

   (C)   is correct. Outpatient surgery usually lasts less than 60 minutes. Longer procedures are performed in a surgical center or hospital.

2. Outpatient surgery can be

   (A) an emergency procedure   (D) performed in a surgicenter
   (B) optional surgery   ✓(E) all of the above
   (C) elective surgery

   (E)   is correct.
   (A)   Emergency surgery is required to immediately save a life, such as in the case of hemorrhage, or to prevent further injury or infection.
   (B)   Optional surgery may not be medically necessary, but the patient wishes to have it performed (for example, cosmetic surgery or a vasectomy).
   (C)   Elective surgery is considered medically necessary, but it can be performed when the patient wishes.
   (D)   A surgicenter is a medical facility that performs ambulatory surgery.

3. Any invasive procedure in which the body is entered requires

   (A) oral permission   (D) written and oral permission
   (B) the skin to be sterilized   (E) a board-certified surgeon
   ✓(C) written permission

   (C)   is correct.

4. Another name for surgical asepsis is

   (A) sterile asepsis   (D) surgical sterilization
   (B) medical asepsis   (E) none of the above
   ✓(C) sterile technique

   (C)   is correct. Sterile technique is the same as surgical asepsis.

5. Because the purpose of the surgical scrub clothes is to protect the patient from exposure to pathogens, the scrubs should

   (A) be changed between each patient
   (B) be white only
   (C) be washed separately

✓(D) not be worn home by the medical assistant
(E) all of the above

(D) is correct. The medical assistant should not wear surgical scrubs home.

6. The surgical hand-washing procedure is performed

(A) for 10 minutes using a clean hand brush
(B) for 10 minutes using a sterile hand brush
(C) by scrubbing for 2 minutes after removing all rings and jewelry
✓(D) using a germicidal soap
(E) with a brush and disinfectant

(D) is correct. A germicidal soap is used for the surgical hand-washing procedure. Each hand and wrist is scrubbed with a sterile brush for 5 minutes, moving toward the elbows. After rinsing, the hands are given a second lather of germicidal soap and scrubbed for 3 minutes.

7. A germicidal soap dispenser is preferable to bar soap when doing a surgical scrub primarily because

(A) it produces more lather
(B) it can be sterilized
✓(C) bar soap is frequently a compatible medium for the growth of bacteria
(D) it is less messy
(E) all of the above

(C) is correct. A germicidal soap dispenser does not provide a medium for bacterial growth.

8. When performing a surgical scrub, it is best that the water temperature be

(A) hot for the first scrub, warm for the second
(B) tolerably hot
✓(C) warm
(D) warm for the first scrub, hot for the second
(E) none of the above

(C) is correct. The water temperature should be comfortably warm when performing a surgical scrub.

9. When applying sterile gloves

(A) apply the gloves before setting up the equipment
(B) pick up the first glove under the cuff and pull over the other hand slowly
(C) hold the gloves over the sink while applying them since the sink is considered "clean"
(D) leave the cuffs turned down after applying since the cuff will catch any spilled fluids
✓(E) place the fingers of the gloved hand under the cuff of the second glove, and then apply

(E) is correct. Place the fingers of the gloved hand under the cuff of the second sterile glove, and then apply the second glove. The first sterile glove is applied by using the thumb of the left hand to pick up the first glove by grasping the folded inside edge of the cuff. This glove is pulled onto the right hand using only the thumb and fingers of the left hand. The fingers must not touch the rest of the sterile glove.

10. The rationale for turning surgical gloves inside out while removing them is to

    (A) maintain the sterility of the gloves
✓(B) seal in blood and bodily fluids
    (C) make them easier to remove
    (D) identify them more readily as used and contaminated
    (E) none of the above

        (B) is correct. Turning the gloves inside out during the removal stage seals in the blood and bodily fluids.

11. What is the correct method for shaving a surgical patient during the skin prep?

    (A) dry shave going against the grain
    (B) wet shave going against the grain
✓(C) wet shave going with the grain
    (D) wet shave before preparing the patient's skin
    (E) dry shave after preparing the patient's skin

        (C) is correct. A wet shave going with the grain of the hair is the correct method for shaving a surgical patient during the skin prep.

12. A sterile assistant who passes instruments, among other duties, is called a/an

    (A) surgical assistant
✓(B) scrub assistant
    (C) second "hand"
    (D) operating room assistant
    (E) circulating assistant

        (B) is correct. The scrub assistant has "scrubbed" or performed a surgical hand-washing scrub and wears sterile gown, mask, and gloves. This person passes instruments during the surgical procedure. The person in charge of handing instruments is called a "surgical technologist/technician."

13. Another name for a local anesthetic is

✓(A) conduction
    (B) general
    (C) intravenous
    (D) hypnotic
    (E) none of the above

        (A) is correct. A local anesthetic is also known as a conduction type of anesthesia.
        (B) A general anesthetic is one in which the patient loses consciousness.
        (C) An intravenous (IV) is often used to administer a general anesthetic such as sodium pentothal.
        (D) A hypnotic anesthetic produces sleep when administered in large doses. This is a type of general anesthetic.

14. An example of a local infiltration anesthetic is lidocaine hydrochloride, which is more commonly known as

- **(A)** benzocaine
- **(B)** Novocain
- **(C)** Solarcaine
- ✔**(D)** Xylocaine
- **(E)** none of the above

    (D) is correct. Xylocaine is the local anesthetic lidocaine hydrochloride.

15. An example of a small-gauge suture used for the skin is

- **(A)** stainless steel 0
- ✔**(B)** stainless steel 5-0
- **(C)** chromic gut 2-0
- **(D)** plain gut 3-0
- **(E)** nylon 2-0

    (B) is correct. Stainless steel 5-0 is an example of a small-gauge suture used for the skin.

16. Of the different types of absorbable sutures, which is absorbed the fastest?

- **(A)** plain cat gut
- **(B)** surgical cat gut
- **(C)** chromic cat gut
- **(D)** black silk
- **(E)** none of the above

    (A) is correct. Plain cat gut is absorbed the fastest. It is used in areas where there is rapid healing, such as highly vascular areas of the lips and tongue.

    (B) Surgical cat gut is used on tissues in which there is fast healing, such as the vaginal area.

    (C) Chromic cat gut has a slower absorption rate and can be used to hold tissue together longer, such as for muscle repair.

    (D) Black silk is nonabsorbable suture material.

17. Absorbable suture materials are used

- **(A)** in areas in which they do not have to be removed
- **(B)** when absorption will occur within 5 to 20 days
- **(C)** for internal organs such as the bladder and intestines
- **(D)** for ligating and tying off of blood vessels
- ✔**(E)** all of the above

    (E) is correct.

18. An all-purpose suture, which is considered one of the most dependable types, is

- **(A)** nylon
- ✔**(B)** silk
- **(C)** polyester
- **(D)** steel
- **(E)** cotton

    (B) is correct. Silk, while the most expensive, is also considered the most dependable suture material. Black silk is the most commonly used nonabsorbable suture material.

19. The size, which is gauge or diameter of suture material,

(A) increases in size with the number of zeros
(B) decreases in size with the number of zeros
(C) indicates the amount of scarring that will be present
(D) A and C only
(E) B and C only

      (E)   is correct. The size decreases with the number of zeros. For example, 6-0 (000000) is the smallest and 0 is the thickest. Very fine suture, such as 5-0 and 6-0, leaves little scarring.

20. The smallest suture material is

(A) 0
(B) 2-0
(C) 4-0
(D) 5-0
(E) 6-0

      (E)   is correct. 6-0 is the smallest suture gauge.

21. A swaged needle is one in which

(A) no needle is required
(B) the needle and suture are combined in one length
(C) the needle has a large cutting portion
(D) the surgeon is allowed to go in and out of tissue in a confined space
(E) none of the above

      (B)   is correct. A swaged needle is one in which the needle and suture are combined in one length.

22. Facial sutures, in order to prevent scarring, may be removed after only

(A) 12 to 24 hours
(B) 24 to 48 hours
(C) 48 to 72 hours
(D) 3 to 5 days
(E) they are not removed at all

      (B)   is correct. Facial sutures may be removed after 24 to 48 hours.

23. If instructed to cut suture material once the wound has been closed, cut both ends

(A) $\frac{1}{4}$ to $\frac{1}{2}$ of an inch above the knot
(B) $\frac{1}{8}$ to $\frac{1}{4}$ of an inch above the knot
(C) $\frac{1}{2}$ to $\frac{3}{4}$ of an inch above the knot
(D) $\frac{3}{4}$ to 1 inch above the knot
(E) none of the above

      (B)   is correct. The suture should be cut $\frac{1}{8}$ to $\frac{1}{4}$ of an inch above the knot.

24. An instrument used by an obstetrician to measure an expectant mother's pelvis is the

(A) vaginal speculum
(B) dilator
(C) curette
(D) pelvimeter
(E) none of the above

(D) is correct. A pelvimeter is used to measure the expectant mother's pelvis to determine the size and growth of the baby.

(A) A vaginal speculum is used to visualize the vagina and cervix.

(B) A dilator is used to expand the diameter of a vessel or an opening.

(C) A curette is a spoon-shaped scraping instrument.

25. The portion of the hemostat located near the handle, which protects it from slipping once it is closed, is the

(A) tooth
(B) clamp
(C) ratchet

(D) serrated tip
(E) lock

(C) is correct. The ratchet is the portion of the hemostat located near the handle, which protects it from slipping once it is closed.

26. Hemostats include

(A) mosquito forceps
(B) Pennington forceps
(C) curved forceps

(D) sponge forceps
(E) all of the above

(E) is correct.

27. A hemostat with clawlike teeth at the tip to grasp and hold tissue is called a

(A) thumb forceps
(B) tissue forceps
(C) sterilizer or transfer forceps

(D) needle holder
(E) splinter forceps

(B) is correct. A tissue forceps has clawlike teeth to grasp and hold tissue.

(A) Thumb forceps are tweezer-like forceps that are used to grasp sterile objects, such as dressings and tissue.

(C) Sterilizer or transfer forceps have a long handle and are used to remove materials and objects from sterilizers and containers.

(D) Needle holders are forceps that are used to grasp the needle during a suturing.

(E) Splinter forceps are a type of thumb forceps that have a fine pointed tip to grasp foreign objects imbedded in the skin.

28. A sharply pointed instrument that fits inside a sheath or cannula to act as a guide for the cannula as it moves into an organ, body cavity, or vessel is a/an

(A) probe
(B) obturator
(C) trocar

(D) sound
(E) laryngoscope

(C) is correct. A trocar is a sharply pointed instrument that fits inside a sheath or cannula to act as a guide for the cannula as it moves into an organ, body cavity, or vessel.

(A) A probe is a slender instrument that is used to enter and explore body cavities.

(B) An obturator is an instrument that fits inside a speculum or scope and assists in guiding the speculum or scope into a vessel, organ, or canal.

(D) A sound is a long slender probe.

(E) A laryngoscope is an instrument, containing a light, that is used to examine the larynx.

29. An endoscope is a hollow, cylindrical instrument containing a light source. An endoscope that is used to examine the urinary bladder is called a/an

(A) otoscope
(B) anoscope
(C) proctoscope
(D) cystoscope
(E) sigmoidoscope

(D) is correct. A cystoscope is used to examine the urinary bladder.
(A) An otoscope is used to examine the external and middle ear.
(B) An anoscope is used to examine the superficial rectum (anus).
(C) A proctoscope is used to examine the rectum.
(E) A sigmoidoscope is used to visualize the sigmoid colon.

30. A typical surgical setup consists of

(A) scalpel, blades, trocar, probe, scope
(B) scalpel, blades, hemostat, probe, scope
(C) scalpel, blades, hemostat, scissors, suture, scope
(D) scalpel, blades, hemostat, scissors, suture
(E) scalpel, blades, scissors, suture, speculum

(D) is correct. The typical surgical setup consists of a scalpel and several blades, hemostat(s), scissors, and suture. Other instruments are added as determined by the nature of the procedure.

31. Scalpel blades come in various sizes, depending on the

(A) manufacturer
(B) surgeon's preference
(C) type of tissue and incision
(D) size of the surgeon's hand
(E) whether the patient is an adult or a child

(C) is correct. The most important criteria for selecting the correct scalpel and blade are the type of tissue being operated upon and the type of incision being made.

32. Orthopedic instruments include

(A) drill set
(B) wire cutters
(C) bone clamp
(D) forceps
(E) all of the above

(E) is correct.

33. Surgical scissors used to cut tissue and sutures may be

(A) curved or straight
(B) sharp-sharp
(C) blunt-blunt
(D) sharp-blunt
(E) all of the above

(E) is correct.

34. Bandage scissors have

(A) a sharp-sharp edge
(B) a hook near the tip to facilitate moving under and cutting
(C) a knobby tip to facilitate moving under the bandage
(D) long handles
(E) blades with edges that do not touch

(C) is correct. Bandage scissors have a knobby tip to facilitate placing the edge under a bandage without injuring or cutting the patient's skin.

35. What is the name of the small table used to hold instruments during a surgical procedure?

(A) surgical table
(B) Lister stand
(C) sterile stand
(D) Mayo stand
(E) none of the above

(D) is correct. A Mayo stand is the small table used to hold instruments during a surgical procedure.

36. When transferring sterile solutions to a sterile field

(A) discard the liquid remaining in the bottle
(B) place the cap on a surface with outside edges of the cap facing up
(C) place the cap on a surface with the inside edges of the cap facing up
(D) place the cap on the Mayo stand
(E) pour the liquid by stabilizing the bottle on the edge of the basin

(C) is correct. To avoid contamination of the inside ring of the cap, it is placed on another surface, such as a table, with the inside of the cap facing up.

37. The area that is considered contaminated on a draped Mayo stand is

(A) within a 1-inch border
(B) outside a 1-inch border
(C) within a 2-inch border
(D) outside a 2-inch border
(E) the entire drape is sterile

(B) is correct. The area outside a 1-inch border on the draped Mayo stand is considered contaminated since it is in contact with the nonsterile work surface.

38. Which of the following should NOT touch a sterile field?

(A) sterile instrument container
(B) 4 × 4s
(C) gloved hands
(D) used instruments
(E) transfer forceps

(D) is correct. Used instruments are contaminated and should not touch a sterile work surface. All the other items listed are considered sterile, including the tips of the transfer forceps.

39. The air immediately above a sterile field is considered

  (A) unsterile
  (B) part of the sterile field
  (C) contaminated by droplets in the air
  (D) part of the perimeter of the sterile field
  (E) none of the above

  (B) is correct. The air immediately above the sterile field is considered part of the sterile field. This means that no ungloved hand or unsterile container should be placed over the sterile field.

40. You have an open sore on your hand. What procedure should you follow when preparing to assist the surgeon?

  (A) try to be excused from assisting with the procedure until the sore is completely healed
  (B) if you are not excused from assisting with the procedure, cover the sore with a dressing or bandage and then correctly apply gloves
  (C) if you are not excused from the procedure, apply two sets of sterile gloves
  (D) all of the above are correct
  (E) none of the above is correct

  (D) is correct depending on office policy.

41. When a patient is awakening from a surgical procedure, which of the following complaints needs to be IMMEDIATELY conveyed to the surgeon?

  (A) nausea and vomiting   **(D)** all of the above
  (B) pain   **(E)** none of the above
  (C) bleeding

  (C) is correct. While all of the complaints need to be conveyed to the surgeon, the most immediate need for action is in the case of bleeding.

42. When patients are scheduled to have outpatient surgery, the medical assistant would tell them

  (A) that another person should accompany them
  (B) what food and drink they may take before coming in for the procedure
  (C) that there will be minimal pain
  (D) that the surgeon has performed this procedure many times, and there is no danger to having the procedure
  (E) A and B only

  (E) is correct. Patients should be told about needing someone to accompany them and what food and drink are permissible, but the MA should not make promises about the amount of pain or the outcome of the procedure.

43. The father of a 6-year-old tonsillectomy and adenoidectomy (T & A) postoperative patient has just purchased orange juice through a vending machine and given it to the patient. The father was instructed to give only ice chips to the boy as needed. What does the medical assistant do?

(A) tell the father he may not stay with his son
(B) inform the surgeon
(C) explain that orange juice can cause nausea and vomiting
(D) remain with the boy
(E) B, C, and D only

(E)   is correct.

44. What should be done when trying to obtain a written, surgical informed consent form from a patient who is an immigrant and does not speak or understand English?

(A) contact a relative who can interpret for the patient
(B) use hand signs and pantomime to explain the procedure to the patient
(C) explain the procedure in English since the obligation is to explain the procedure, not to interpret it for the patient
(D) inform the surgeon
(E) A and D only

(E)   is correct. If the patient does not understand the surgical consent form, it is not considered to be an informed consent and is, therefore, illegal.

45. Cryosurgery is surgery done with

(A) heat
(B) freezing temperatures
(C) sufficient anesthesia to cause no pain
(D) chemicals designed to kill cancer cells
(E) laser beams

(B)   is correct. Cryosurgery is performed with freezing temperatures.

46. Small electrocautery units used to perform minor cautery procedures are called

(A) hyfrecators
(B) hemostats
(C) trocars
(D) lasers
(E) cryosurgical units

(A)   is correct. A hyfrecator is a small electrocautery unit.
(B)   Hemostats are applied to blood vessels to hold vessels until they can be sutured.
(C)   A trocar is used to withdraw fluids from cavities.
(D)   A laser is an intense beam of light used in a variety of surgical procedures, including the removal of tumors.
(E)   Cryosurgerical units use extreme cold to control bleeding and treat lesions.

47. A wound in which the outer layers of skin are rubbed away due to scraping is a/an

(A) incision   **(D)** abrasion
(B) laceration   **(E)** none of the above
(C) puncture

    (D)   is correct. An abrasion is a wound in which the outer layers of skin are rubbed away.

    (A)   An incision is a smooth cut resulting from a surgical scalpel or sharp material, such as razor or glass. This may result in excessive bleeding if deep and scarring.

    (B)   A laceration is a wound in which the edges are torn in an irregular shape. This can cause profuse bleeding and scarring.

    (C)   A puncture wound is made by a sharp pointed instrument, such as a bullet, needle, nail, or splinter. External bleeding is usually small, but infection may occur due to penetration with a contaminated object.

48. A patient with a wound should be asked when he or she last received a tetanus shot, and the physician should be notified if it has been more than

(A) 1 year   **(D)** 8 years
(B) 3 years   **(E)** 10 years
(C) 5 years

    (E)   is correct. A tetanus shot is good for 10 years.

49. An EMB consists of

(A) using a curette or suction tool to remove uterine tissue
(B) the tying and cutting of the vas deferens
(C) an incision and drainage (I & D)
(D) an examination of the vagina and cervix, performed using a lighted instrument
(E) none of the above

    (A)   is correct. An endometrial biopsy (EMB) consists of using a curette or suction tool to remove uterine tissue for testing.

    (B)   A vasectomy consists of tying and cutting the vas deferens. This is considered a permanent form of birth control for the male.

    (C)   An incision and drainage (I & D) is performed to relieve the buildup of purulent (pus) material as a result of infection.

    (D)   A colposcopy is an examination of the vagina and cervix, performed using a lighted instrument called a colposcope.

CHAPTER 19

ASSISTING PATIENTS WITH SPECIAL PHYSICAL NEEDS

1. A cerebrovascular accident (CVA) caused by a clot forming in the body and traveling to the brain is called a

   (A) compression
   (B) cerebral hemorrhage
   (C) cerebral thrombosis
   (D) cerebral embolism
   (E) cardioversion

   (D) is correct. A cerebral embolism is a clot that has formed in the body and traveled to the brain.
   (A) A compression relates to an injury caused by pressure exerted against organs or bones (for example, a compression fracture).
   (B) Cerebral hemorrhage is bleeding within the brain, such as from a ruptured blood vessel. This is also referred to as a CVA.
   (C) Cerebral thrombosis is a hardening of vessels within the brain.
   (E) Cardioversion is converting a cardiac arrhythmia (irregular heart action) to a normal sinus rhythm using a cardioverter to give countershocks to the heart.

2. A hemorrhagic lesion within the brain that may result in paralysis and the inability to speak is known as a

   (A) CNA
   (B) CVA
   (C) CPR
   (D) CBC
   (E) DNR

   (B) is correct. A hemorrhagic lesion within the brain that may result in paralysis and the inability to speak is known as a CVA (cerebrovascular accident).
   (A) The initials CNA refer to certified nursing assistant.
   (C) CPR refers to cardiopulmonary resuscitation.
   (D) CBC refers to a complete blood count.
   (E) DNR refers to a do not resuscitate order.

3. A surgical opening into the small intestine for the purpose of allowing waste material to drain is called a/an

   (A) stoma
   (B) colostomy
   (C) iliostomy
   (D) ileostomy
   (E) none of the above

   (D) is correct. An ileostomy is a surgical opening into the small intestine for the purpose of allowing waste material to drain.

(A) A stoma is an opening from the skin.

(B) A colostomy is a surgical opening into the large intestine.

(C) Ilio- is the word root referring to a portion of the hipbone. Ileo- is the word root referring to the small intestine.

4. One of the diseases for which an ostomy might be performed is

(A) chronic diarrhea

(B) Crohn's disease

(C) constipation

(D) irritable bowel syndrome

(E) indigestion

> (B) is correct. One of the surgical treatments for Crohn's disease is an ostomy. Crohn's disease is a form of chronic inflammatory bowel disease affecting the ileum and/or colon. It is also called regional ileitis.

5. A feeding tube is

(A) placed into one of several areas of the digestive system

(B) placed into a vein

(C) intended to have fluids run through as quickly as possible to avoid clotting

(D) used only for cancer patients

(E) is administered through a port in the wrist

> (A) is correct. A feeding tube is placed into the digestive system for the administering of nourishing fluids to patients who are unable to swallow or eat.

6. A patient with a feeding tube can be administered

(A) liquid food supplements only

(B) liquid food supplements and medications

(C) liquid food supplements and water

(D) liquid food supplements, water, and medications

(E) none of the above

> (D) is correct. A patient can receive food supplements, water, and medications through a feeding tube.

7. What symptom should the patient with a feeding tube report to the physician?

(A) vomiting

(B) nausea

(C) diarrhea

(D) cramping

(E) all of the above

> (E) is correct.

8. Patients who are receiving a single-dose medication intravenously on a regular basis may have a small needle with a port inserted into their wrist, which is called a

(A) clamp

(B) drip chamber

(C) heparin lock

(D) piggy-back

(E) none of the above

(C)   is correct. A heparin lock consists of a small needle with a port, containing heparin to prevent blood clotting, that is inserted into the patient's wrist. Medication can then be instilled into the port without having to insert a needle into the patient for each dose.

9. Which of the following is a dangerous condition for a patient with a cast?

(A)   cast becomes wet
(B)   limb itches
(C)   limb becomes swollen
(D)   cast becomes dirty
(E)   none of the above

(C)   is correct. A swollen limb within a cast can be dangerous since circulation may become compromised.

10. The main advantage of casts made out of fiberglass material over conventional plaster is that they are

(A)   lighter in weight
(B)   so easy to apply that a medical assistant can do it
(C)   less expensive
(D)   available in different colors
(E)   all of the above

(A)   is correct. The main advantage to a fiberglass cast is that it is lighter in weight than the conventional plaster cast.

11. During the drying process of a cast application, a patient may complain or express anxiety about

(A)   how long the cast will remain in place
(B)   the removal of the cast
(C)   a sensation of warmth, even heat
(D)   the appearance of the cast
(E)   none of the above

(C)   is correct. It is normal for the patient to experience a mild sensation of warmth as the cast material is drying on the limb.

12. When assisting patients who have a terminal disease, the best method is to

(A)   encourage them by telling them they look wonderful and will get better
(B)   avoid them
(C)   don't allow them to dwell on the depressing subject of death
(D)   allow them to talk about it
(E)   none of the above

(D)   is correct. Allow the dying person to talk about his or her concerns.

13. The handicap that is considered to be the most difficult for a patient to deal with is

(A)   blindness
(B)   deafness
(C)   loss of speech
(D)   clubfoot
(E)   speech impediment

(B) is correct. Deafness is said to be the most difficult of all handicaps since the person can become isolated from what is happening around him or her.

14. In addition to profound memory loss, an Alzheimer's patient, particularly in later stages of the disease, exhibits

(A) constipation
(B) weight gain
(C) hearing loss
(D) agitation
(E) meticulous concern for appearance

(D) is correct. Agitation is a frequent effect of Alzheimer's disease.

15. A painful, infectious viral disease that attacks the nerve endings is

(A) scabies
(B) verruca
(C) tinea
(D) herpes zoster
(E) herpes simplex

(D) is correct. Herpes zoster is a painful, infectious viral disease that attacks the nerve endings. It is also called shingles.
(A) Scabies is a contagious skin disease caused by an egg-laying mite that causes intense itching.
(B) Verruca is a benign neoplasm (tumor), which has a rough surface that is removed by chemicals and/or laser therapy. It is also called warts.
(C) Tinea is a fungal skin disease resulting in itching, scaling lesions.
(E) Herpes simplex is an infectious disease caused by herpes simplex virus 1 and characterized by thin vesicles that tend to recur in the same area, such as the lips or conjunctiva.

16. Another term meaning tumor is

(A) wart
(B) nodule
(C) papule
(D) nevus
(E) neoplasm

(E) is correct. A neoplasm is a tumor.
(A) A wart is also called verruca.
(B) A nodule is a solid, raised group of cells.
(C) A papule a small, solid, raised spot on the surface of the skin.
(D) A nevus is a pigmented (colored) skin blemish. This is also called a birthmark or mole.

17. A change that results in thick, white patches on the mucous membranes of the tongue and inside cheek is called

(A) lipoma
(B) leukoplakia
(C) keratosis
(D) hemangioma
(E) Kaposi's sarcoma

(B) is correct. Leukoplakia is a change in the mucous membranes of the tongue and inside cheek resulting in thick, white patches.
(A) A lipoma is a fatty tumor that generally does not metastasize.

(C) Keratosis is an overgrowth and thickening of cells in the epithelium located in the epidermis of the skin.

(D) A hemangioma is a benign tumor of dilated blood vessels.

(E) Kaposi's sarcoma is a form of skin cancer frequently seen in acquired immune deficiency syndrome (AIDS) patients.

18. Intermittent attacks of pallor or cyanosis of the fingers and toes associated with the cold or emotional distress is a condition known as

(A) thrombophlebitis
(B) varicose veins
(C) Reynaud's phenomenon
(D) aortic insufficiency
(E) angina pectoris

(C) is correct. Reynaud's phenomenon is a condition in which there are intermittent attacks of pallor or cyanosis of the fingers and toes associated with the cold or emotional distress.

(A) Thrombophlebitis is inflammation and clotting of blood within a vein.

(B) Varicose veins are swollen and distended veins, usually in the legs, resulting from pressure, such as occurs during a pregnancy.

(D) Aortic insufficiency is a failure of the aortic valve in the heart to close completely, which results in leaking and inefficient heart action.

(E) Angina pectoris is a condition in which there is severe pain with constriction around the heart. It is caused by a deficiency of oxygen to the heart muscle.

19. A surgical procedure of altering the structure of a vessel by dilating the vessel using a balloon inside the vessel is called an

(A) artery graft
(B) angioplasty
(C) angiography
(D) aneurysmectomy
(E) artificial pacemaker

(B) is correct. An angioplasty is a surgical procedure in which the blood vessel is altered by dilating it with a balloon.

(A) An artery graft is a piece of blood vessel that is transplanted from a part of the body to the aorta to repair a defect.

(C) Angiography is an x-ray taken after the injection of an opaque material into a blood vessel.

(D) An aneurysmectomy is the surgical removal of the sac of an aneurysm, which is an abnormal dilation of a blood vessel.

(E) An artificial pacemaker is an electrical device that substitutes for the natural pacemaker of the heart.

20. A disease resulting from a deficiency in adrenocortical hormones in which there is an increased pigmentation of the skin, generalized weakness, and weight loss is

(A) Cushing's syndrome
(B) dwarfism
(C) Graves' disease
(D) Addison's disease
(E) myasthenia gravis

(D) is correct. Addison's disease is the result of a deficiency in adrenocortical hormones that causes an increased pigmentation of the skin, generalized weakness, and weight loss.

(A) Cushing's syndrome is a set of symptoms that results from hypersecretion of the adrenal cortex. This may be the result of a tumor of the adrenal gland.

(B) Dwarfism is a condition of being abnormally small. It may be the result of a hereditary condition or an endocrine dysfunction.

(C) Graves' disease results from an overactivity of the thyroid gland and can result in a crisis situation.

(E) Myasthenia gravis is a condition in which there is great muscular weakness and progressive fatigue. There may be difficulty in chewing or swallowing. Drooping eyelids may be present.

21. A condition resulting from a hypofunction of the thyroid gland, which can include symptoms of anemia, slowed speech, enlarged tongue and facial features, edematous skin, drowsiness, and mental apathy, is called

(A) von Recklinghausen's disease
(B) thyrotoxicosis
(C) myxedema
(D) myasthenia gravis
(E) ketoacidosis

(C) is correct. Myxedema is a condition of hypofunction of the thyroid gland.

(A) von Recklinghausen's disease is caused by excessive production of parathyroid hormone, which results in degeneration of the bones.

(B) Thyrotoxicosis is a condition that results from overproduction of the thyroid gland. Symptoms include a rapid heart action, enlarged thyroid gland, exophthalmos, and weight loss.

(D) Myasthenia gravis is a condition in which there is great muscular weakness and progressive fatigue. There may be difficulty in chewing or swallowing. Drooping eyelids may be present.

(E) Ketoacidosis is acidosis due to an excess of ketone bodies (waste products), which can result in death for the diabetic patient if not reversed.

22. A disorder caused by the inadequate secretion of the antidiuretic hormone (ADH) by the posterior lobe of the pituitary gland is called

(A) diabetes insipidus (DI)
(B) diabetes mellitus (DM)
(C) acromegaly
(D) hyperkalemia
(E) hypercalcemia

(A) is correct. Diabetes insipidus (DI) is caused by an inadequate secretion of the antidiuretic hormone (ADH) by the posterior lobe of the pituitary gland.

(B) Diabetes mellitus (DM) is a chronic disorder of carbohydrate metabolism, which results in hyperglycemia and glycosuria (sugar in the blood).

(C) Acromegaly is a chronic disease of middle-aged persons, which results in an elongation and enlargement of the bones of the head and extremities.

(D) Hyperkalemia is an excessive amount of potassium in the blood.

(E) Hypercalcemia is an excessive amount of calcium in the blood.

23. A test used to measure the concentration of thyroxin (T4) circulating in the bloodstream is

(A) PBI
(B) RAIU
(C) RIA
(D) GTT
(E) none of the above

(A) is correct. The protein-bound iodine (PBI) test is used to measure the concentration of thyroxin (T4) circulating in the bloodstream. The iodine becomes bound to the protein in the blood and can be measured. This test is useful in establishing thyroid function.

(B) Radioactive iodine uptake (RAIU) is a test in which radioactive iodine is taken orally (PO) or intravenously (IV), and the amount that is eventually taken into the thyroid gland (the uptake) is measured to assist in determining thyroid function.

(C) The radioimmunoassay (RIA) test is used to measure the levels of hormones in the plasma of the blood.

(D) The glucose tolerance test (GTT) is used to determine the blood sugar level.

24. A condition in which the intestine slips or telescopes into another section of the intestine just below it is called

(A) reflux esophagitis
(B) ileitis
(C) inguinal hernia
(D) intussusception
(E) diverticulosis

(D) is correct. Intussusception occurs when the intestine slips or telescopes into another section of the intestine. This is more common in children.

(A) Reflux esophagitis occurs when acid from the stomach backs up into the esophagus, causing inflammation and pain.

(B) Ileitis is an inflammation of the ileum of the small intestine.

(C) An inguinal hernia is an outpouching of intestines into the inguinal region of the body.

(E) Diverticulosis is an inflammation of a diverticulum or sac in the intestinal tract, especially in the colon.

25. Bad or offensive breath, which is often a sign of disease, is called

(A) gastroenteritis
(B) halitosis
(C) gastritis
(D) dyspepsia
(E) cirrhosis

(B) is correct. Halitosis is bad or offensive breath, which may be a sign of disease within the body.

(A) Gastroenteritis is an inflammation of the stomach and small intestine.

(C) Gastritis is an inflammation of the stomach, which can result in pain, tenderness, nausea, and vomiting.

(D) Dyspepsia is another term for indigestion.

(E) Cirrhosis is a chronic disease of the liver.

26. Inflammation of the gallbladder is called

(A) cholelithiasis
(B) cholelithotripsy
(C) cholecystitis

(D) cholecystolith
(E) choledochal

    (C)   is correct. Cholecystitis is an inflammation of the gallbladder.
    (A)   Cholelithiasis is the formation or presence of stones or calculi in the gallbladder or common bile duct.
    (B)   Cholelithotripsy is the crushing of a gallstone in the common bile duct.
    (D)   Cholecystolith is a stone or calculus in the gallbladder.
    (E)   Choledochal means pertaining to the bile duct.

27. The return of fluids from the stomach into the mouth is

(A) emesis
(B) vomit
(C) regurgitation

(D) A and B only
(E) A, B, and C

    (E)   is correct. Emesis, vomit, and regurgitation are all terms that refer to the return of fluids from the stomach into the mouth.

28. A malignant growth found in the shaft of the long bones that spreads through the periosteum is called

(A) myeloma
(B) Kaposi's sarcoma
(C) fibrosarcoma

(D) Ewing's sarcoma
(E) thymoma

    (D)   is correct. Ewing's sarcoma is a malignant (cancerous) growth found in the shaft of the long bones that spreads through the periosteum.
    (A)   A myeloma is a malignant (cancerous) tumor originating in plasma cells in the bone.
    (B)   Kaposi's sarcoma is a type of skin cancer that is prevalent in AIDS patients.
    (C)   A fibrosarcoma is a tumor that contains connective tissue that occurs in bone marrow. It is found most frequently in the femur, humerus, and jawbone.
    (E)   A thymoma is a malignant tumor of the thymus gland.

29. A complex of symptoms that appears in the early stages of AIDS, which includes weight loss, fatigue, skin rash, and anorexia, is called

(A) ELISA
(B) Western blot
(C) ARC

(D) HIV
(E) TIA

    (C)   is correct. AIDS-related complex (ARC) is a complex of symptoms that appears in the early stage of AIDS.
    (A)   ELISA refers to the enzyme-linked immunoabsorbent assay test, which is used to test blood for an antibody to the AIDS virus. There may be a false-positive; then the Western blot would be used to verify the results.
    (B)   The Western blot test is used to back up the ELISA blood test to detect the presence of the antibody to HIV (AIDS virus) in the blood.
    (D)   HIV refers to human immunodeficiency virus.

(E) Transient ischemic attack (TIA) is a temporary interference with blood supply to the brain, causing neurological symptoms such as dizziness, numbness, and hemiparesis.

30. Paralysis of one-half of the body is known as

(A) quadriplegia
(B) paraplegia
(C) hemiplegia
(D) all of the above
(E) none of the above

(C) is correct. Hemiplegia is a paralysis on one-half (hemi) of the body.
(A) Quadriplegia refers to paralysis of all four extremities.
(B) Paraplegia refers to paralysis of both legs.

31. Abnormal lateral curvature of the spine is

(A) lordosis
(B) scoliosis
(C) kyphosis
(D) rickets
(E) spinal stenosis

(B) is correct. Scoliosis is an abnormal lateral curvature of the spine.
(A) Lordosis is an abnormal increase in the forward curvature of the lumbar spine. This is also known as swayback.
(C) Kyphosis is an abnormal increase in the outward curvature of the thoracic spine. This is also known as hunchback or humpback.
(D) Rickets is a condition caused by a deficiency in calcium and vitamin D in early childhood that results in bone deformities, especially bowed legs.
(E) Spinal stenosis is a narrowing of the spinal canal, causing pressure on the cord and nerves.

32. The measurement of bone density using an instrument for the purpose of detecting osteoporosis is called

(A) photon absorptiometry
(B) MRI
(C) myelography
(D) menisectomy
(E) muscle biopsy

(A) is correct. Photon absorptiometry is the measurement of bone density using an instrument for the purpose of detecting osteoporosis.
(B) Magnetic resonance imaging (MRI) uses radio-frequency radiation as its source of energy. The technique is useful for visualizing the large blood vessels, heart, brain, and soft tissues.
(C) Myelography is the study of the spinal column after injecting opaque contrast medium.
(D) Menisectomy is the surgical removal of the knee cartilage (meniscus).
(E) A muscle biopsy is the removal of muscle tissue for pathological examination.

33. A one-sided facial paralysis caused by the herpes simplex virus is

(A) autism
(B) aphasia
(C) anorexia nervosa
(D) Bell's palsy
(E) Huntington's chorea

(D) is correct. Bell's palsy is a one-sided facial paralysis caused by the herpes simplex virus.

(A) Autism is a form of mental introversion in which the patient, usually a child, shows no interest in anything or anyone except himself or herself.

(B) Aphasia is a loss of the ability to speak.

(C) Anorexia nervosa is a loss of appetite, which generally occurs in females between the ages of 12 and 21, due to a fear of obesity.

(E) Huntington's chorea is a disease of the central nervous system that results in progressive dementia, with bizarre involuntary movements of parts of the body.

34. A swelling or mass of blood that is confined to a specific area, such as in the brain, is

(A) glioma
(B) hydrocephalus
(C) chorea
(D) coma
(E) hematoma

(E) is correct. A hematoma is a swelling or mass of blood that is confined to a specific area.

(A) A glioma is a sarcoma (cancerous tumor) of neurological origin.

(B) Hydrocephalus is an accumulation of cerebrospinal fluid within the ventricles of the brain, causing pressure on the brain and an enlarged head.

(C) Chorea is an involuntary nervous disorder that results in muscular twitching of the limbs or facial muscles.

(D) A coma is an abnormal deep sleep or stupor resulting from an illness or injury.

35. A degenerative, inflammatory disease of the central nervous system (CNS) in which there is extreme weakness and numbness is known as

(A) Reye's syndrome
(B) multiple sclerosis
(C) Parkinson's disease
(D) spina bifida
(E) tic douloureux

(B) is correct. Multiple sclerosis is a degenerative, inflammatory disease of the CNS in which there is extreme weakness and numbness.

(A) Reye's syndrome is a combination of symptoms that generally occurs in children under 15 years of age 1 week after they have had a viral infection.

(C) Parkinson's disease is a chronic progressive disorder of the nervous system, with fine tremors, muscular weakness, rigidity, and a shuffling gait.

(D) Spina bifida is a congenital defect in the walls of the spinal cord in which the laminae of the vertebra do not meet or close.

(E) Tic douloureux is a painful condition in which the trigeminal nerve is affected by pressure or degeneration.

36. The application of a mild electrical stimulation to skin electrodes placed over a painful area, causing interference with the transmission of the painful stimuli, is called

(A) TENS
(B) PET
(C) MRI

(D) TIA
(E) CAT

    (A) is correct. Transcutaneous electrical nerve stimulation (TENS) is the application of a mild electrical stimulation to skin electrodes placed over a painful area, causing interference with the transmission of the painful stimuli.

    (B) Positron emission tomography (PET) is the use of positive radionuclides to reconstruct brain sections. Measurement can be taken of oxygen and glucose uptake, cerebral blood flow and blood volume.

    (C) Magnetic resonance imaging (MRI) uses radio-frequency radiation as its source of energy. It is used to visualize the blood vessels, heart, brain, and soft tissues.

    (D) Transient ischemic attack (TIA) is a temporary interference with blood supply to the brain, causing neurological symptoms.

    (E) Computerized axial tomography (CAT) is the use of computer-assisted x-rays to detect tumors and fractures.

37. Which test is used to detect defects or abnormal blood supply in the brain?

(A) PET
(B) MRI
(C) CAT

(D) A and B only
(E) A, B, and C

    (E) is correct. The PET, MRI, and CAT are all used to detect defects or abnormal blood supply in the brain.

38. A condition of the eye in which there is an increase in intraocular pressure is

(A) strabismus
(B) nystagmus
(C) trachoma

(D) glaucoma
(E) cataract

    (D) is correct. Glaucoma is a condition of the eye in which there is an increase in intraocular pressure. This can result in blindness if untreated.

    (A) Strabismus is an eye muscle weakness resulting in the eyes looking in different directions at the same time.

    (B) Nystagmus is a jerky-appearing, involuntary eye movement.

    (C) Trachoma is a chronic infectious disease of the conjunctiva and cornea caused by bacteria. This occurs most commonly in people living in hot, dry climates. Untreated, it may lead to blindness when the scarring invades the cornea.

    (E) A cataract is diminished vision resulting from the lens of the eye becoming opaque or cloudy.

39. A test for ear function in which the physician measures the movement of the tympanic membrane is the

(A) Rinne tuning fork test
(B) Weber tuning fork test
(C) tympanometry
(D) audiometric test
(E) A and B only

(C) is correct. Tympanometry is a test for ear function in which the physician measures the movement of the tympanic membrane.

(A) and (B) The Rinne and Weber tuning fork tests are performed by a physician holding the tuning fork, an instrument that produces a constant pitch when it is struck, against or near the bones on the side of the head. These tests assess both nerve and bone conduction of sound.

(D) The audiometric test is a test of hearing ability by determining the lowest and highest intensities and frequencies that a person can distinguish.

40. An emergency obstetrical condition in which the placenta tears away from the uterine wall before the 20th week of pregnancy, which requires immediate delivery of the baby, is

(A) breech presentation
(B) placenta previa
(C) abruptio placenta
(D) prolapsed uterus
(E) PID

(C) is correct. Abruptio placenta is an emergency obstetrical condition in which the placenta tears away from the uterine wall before the 20th week of pregnancy.

(A) A breech presentation is the position of the fetus within the uterus in which the buttocks or feet are presented first for delivery, rather than the head of the baby.

(B) Placenta previa occurs when the placenta has become attached to the lower portion of the uterus and, in turn, blocks the birth canal.

(D) A prolapsed uterus is a fallen uterus that can cause the cervix to protrude through the vaginal opening.

(E) Pelvic inflammatory disease (PID) is any inflammation of the female reproductive organs, generally bacterial in nature.

41. A puncturing of the amniotic sac using a needle and syringe for the purpose of withdrawing amniotic fluid for testing is

(A) Doppler
(B) culdoscopy
(C) D&C
(D) cauterization
(E) amniocentesis

(E) is correct. Amniocentesis is the puncturing of the amniotic sac using a needle and syringe for the purpose of withdrawing amniotic fluid for testing.

(A) A Doppler ultrasound uses an instrument (Doppler) placed externally over the uterus to detect the presence of fibroid tumors or to outline the shape of the fetus.

(B) Culdoscopy is an examination of the female pelvic cavity using an endoscope.

(C) A dilatation and curettage (D&C) is a surgical procedure in which the opening of the cervix is dilated and the uterus is scraped or suctioned of its lining or tissue.

(D) Cauterization is the destruction of tissue using an electric current, a caustic product, a hot iron, or freezing.

42. The surgical removal of the prostate gland by inserting a device through the urethra and removing prostate tissue is

(A) vasectomy

(B) TUR

(C) orchidopexy

(D) castration

(E) cauterization

(B) is correct. A transurethral resection (TUR) is the surgical removal of the prostate gland by inserting a device through the urethra and removing the prostate gland.

(A) A vasectomy is the removal of a segment or all of the vas deferens to prevent sperm from leaving the male body.

(C) An orchidopexy is the surgical fixation to move undescended testes into the scrotum, and attaching them to prevent retraction.

(D) Castration is the excision of the testicles in the male or the ovaries in the female.

(E) Cauterization is the destruction of tissue with an electric current, a caustic agent, a hot iron, or freezing.

43. A disorder that produces moderate to severe mental retardation and multiple defects is

(A) Duchenne's muscular dystrophy

(B) Down syndrome

(C) cystic fibrosis

(D) Cooley's anemia

(E) Tay-Sachs disease

(B) is correct. Down syndrome is a disorder that produces moderate to severe mental retardation and multiple defects.

(A) Duchenne's muscular dystrophy is a muscular disorder in which there is progressive wasting away of various muscles, including leg, pelvic, and shoulder muscles.

(C) Cystic fibrosis is a disorder of the exocrine glands, which causes these glands to produce abnormally thick secretions of mucus.

(D) Cooley's anemia is a rare form of anemia, or a reduction of red blood cells, which is found in some people of Mediterranean origin.

(E) Tay-Sachs disease is a disorder caused by a deficiency of an enzyme, which can result in mental and physical retardation and blindness. It is transferred by a recessive gene and is most commonly found in families of Eastern European Jewish descent.

44. A congenital disorder that results in a defect in the walls of the spinal column, causing the membranes of the spinal cord to push through to the outside, is

(A) sickle cell anemia

(B) Tay-Sachs disease

(C) retinitis pigmentosa

(D) Huntington's chorea

(E) spina bifida

(E) is correct. Spina bifida is a congenital disorder that results in a defect in the walls of the spinal column, causing the membranes of the spinal cord to push through to the outside.

(A) Sickle cell anemia is a severe, chronic, incurable disorder that results in anemia and that causes joint pain, chronic weakness, and infections. This disease occurs more commonly in people of Mediterranean and African heritage.

(B) Tay-Sachs disease is a disorder caused by a deficiency of an enzyme, which can result in mental and physical retardation and blindness. It is transferred by a recessive gene and is most commonly found in families of Eastern European Jewish descent.

(C) Retinitis pigmentosa is a chronic progressive disease that begins in early childhood and is characterized by degeneration of the retina.

(D) Huntington's chorea is a rare condition characterized by bizarre involuntary movements, called chorea.

45. A condition in which the lung tissue collapses is

(A) atelectasis
(B) asthma
(C) emphysema
(D) hyaline membrane disease
(E) COPD

(A) is correct. Atelectasis is a condition in which the lung tissue collapses, which prevents the respiratory exchange of oxygen and carbon dioxide.

(B) Asthma is a disease caused by various conditions, such as allergens, resulting in constriction of the bronchial airways and labored respirations.

(C) Emphysema is a pulmonary condition that can occur as a result of long-term heavy smoking.

(D) Hyaline membrane disease is a condition seen in premature infants whose lungs have not had time to develop. The lungs are not able to expand fully, and a membrane (hyaline membrane) forms, which causes extreme difficulty in breathing and may result in death.

(E) Chronic obstructive pulmonary disease (COPD) is a chronic, progressive, and usually irreversible condition in which the lungs have a diminished capacity for inspiration (inhalation) and expiration (exhalation).

Laboratory Specimens and Specimen Collection

CHAPTER 20

URINALYSIS

1. The presence of blood in the urine is known as

   (A) anuria
   (B) oliguria
   (C) glycosuria

   (D) hematuria
   (E) dysuria

   (D) is correct. Hematuria is the presence of blood in the urine.
   (A) Anuria refers to the complete suppression of urine formed by the kidneys and a complete lack of urine excretion.
   (B) Oliguria refers to a reduction of urine, or a scant amount.
   (C) Glycosuria refers to the presence of sugar in the urine. This is commonly found in persons with diabetes mellitus.
   (E) Dysuria refers to painful urination.

2. The presence of sugar in the urine is known as

   (A) albuminuria
   (B) glycosuria
   (C) polyuria

   (D) nocturia
   (E) dysuria

   (B) is correct. Glycosuria refers to the presence of sugar in the urine.
   (A) Albuminuria is the presence of serum albumin in the urine.
   (C) Polyuria refers to an excessive amount of urine. This is commonly present in the disease diabetes insipidus.
   (D) Nocturia refers to the need to urinate during the night.
   (E) Dysuria refers to painful urination.

3. Glycosuria, an abnormal condition, is the presence of what in the urine?

   (A) red blood cells
   (B) white blood cells
   (C) bacteria

   (D) sugar
   (E) parasites

   (D) is correct. Glycosuria is the presence of sugar in the urine.

4. The presence of which of the following in urine may signal the onset of liver disease?

   (A) nitrites
   (B) ketones
   (C) erythrocytes

   (D) leukocytes
   (E) bilirubin

   (E) is correct. Bilirubin in the urine may signal the onset of liver disease.

5. An infection, such as a urinary tract infection, that is acquired while in the hospital is called

(A) tertiary infection

(B) *E. coli*

(C) nosocomial infection

(D) none of the above

(E) all of the above

(C) is correct. A hospital-acquired infection is referred to as a nosocomial infection.

6. When handling a patient's urine, a medical assistant must follow the universal handling of fluid precautions, meaning

(A) gloves and a lab coat must be worn

(B) aseptic procedures must be followed

(C) gloves, lab coat, and goggles must be worn

(D) A and B

(E) A, B, and C

(E) is correct. Gloves, lab coat, and goggles must be worn while handling a urine specimen since there is danger of spilling and fluid splashing.

7. A foul urine odor can be described as

(A) aromatic

(B) fruity

(C) turbid

(D) fetid

(E) sediment

(D) is correct. A fetid odor is a foul odor.

(A) Normal urine has an aromatic odor.

(B) A fruity odor might be present in disease conditions such as uncontrolled diabetes.

(C) Turbid refers to the appearance of urine. Turbid means the same as cloudy.

(E) Sediment is the substance that settles to the bottom of a specimen.

8. The normal color of urine is

(A) turbid

(B) orange

(C) fetid

(D) straw

(E) clear

(D) is correct. The normal color of urine is a straw color.

(A) Turbid refers to a cloudy appearance.

(B) Orange-colored urine may be present in a very concentrated specimen.

(C) Fetid refers to odor.

(E) Clear refers to clarity or lack of cloudiness in urine.

9. A greenish-brown urine may be indicative of

(A) diabetes

(B) infection

(C) hepatitis

(D) hematuria

(E) none of the above

(C) is correct. Greenish-brown urine may be present in a person suffering from a liver disorder such as hepatitis.

10. Sediment in urine, both organized and unorganized, includes

   (A) casts, cells, and crystals
   (B) casts, cells, bacteria, parasites, yeast, and fungi
   (C) casts, cells, bacteria, parasites, yeast, fungi, and spermatozoa
   (D) casts, cells, bacteria, parasites, yeast, fungi, spermatozoa, and crystals
   (E) casts, cells, bacteria, parasites, yeast, fungi, spermatozoa, crystals, and amorphous material

   (E)   is correct.

11. Which of the following statements is TRUE?

   (A) cells are visualized microscopically under low power
   (B) casts are visualized microscopically under high power
   (C) crystals are visualized microscopically under low power
   (D) the findings are charted after averaging what has been seen in 10 fields
   (E) the findings are charted after averaging what has been seen in five fields

   (D)   is correct. Microscopic findings are charted after averaging what has been seen in 10 fields.

12. The normal specific gravity of urine, which measures the ability of the kidneys to concentrate urine, ranges from

   (A) 1.000 to 1.005   **(D)** 1.010 to 1.030
   (B) 1.005 to 1.010   **(E)** 1.010 to 1.014
   (C) 1.010 to 1.020

   (D)   is correct. The normal specific gravity of urine ranges from 1.010 to 1.030.

13. Specific gravity is the weight of a substance in relation to the weight of that same amount of

   (A) urine   **(D)** ordinary tap water
   (B) blood   **(E)** none of the above
   (C) distilled water

   (C)   is correct. Specific gravity (SG) is the weight of a substance, such as urine, in relation to the weight of that same amount of distilled water. Water is used as the standard and has a specific gravity of 1.000.

14. A urinometer or refractometer is used with urine to measure

   (A) pH   **(D)** specific gravity
   (B) red and white blood cells   **(E)** hemoglobin
   (C) glucose

   (D)   is correct. A urinometer or refractometer is used to measure the specific gravity of urine.
   (A)   A chemical analysis, such as used with reagent strips or dipsticks, is used to determine the pH of urine.
   (B)   A hemacytometer is used to aid in determining the number of red and white blood cells in a specimen.

(C) Glucose is detected in the urine using a glucometer.

(E) Hemoglobin in the blood is measured manually using a hemoglobinometer or an automated blood analyzer.

15. If the specific gravity falls below the normal range, it could indicate that

(A) the kidney's ability to dilute or concentrate the urine is not functioning properly

(B) there is a kidney disease

(C) the patient may be on a salt-restriction diet

(D) the disease of diabetes insipidus may be present

(E) all of the above

(E) is correct.

16. The pH of a solution is measured on a scale from 0 to

(A) 5   **(D)** 12

(B) 7   **(E)** 14

(C) 10

(E) is correct. The pH of a solution can range from 0 to 14, with 7 as the midpoint between an acid versus a base (alkalinity).

17. On a pH scale, the point of 14 measures

(A) the lowest level of acidity   **(D)** the lowest level of alkalinity

(B) the highest level of acidity   **(E)** none of the above

(C) the highest level of alkalinity

(C) is correct. The pH measurement of 14 is the highest level of alkalinity.

18. On a pH scale, the point 0 measures

(A) the lowest level of acidity   **(D)** the lowest level of alkalinity

(B) the highest level of acidity   **(E)** none of the above

(C) the highest level of alkalinity

(B) is correct. On a pH scale, 0 measures the highest level of acidity.

19. Chemical dipsticks for urine testing are used to measure all of the following EXCEPT

(A) specific gravity and pH

(B) protein, glucose, and ketones

(C) casts, bacteria, parasites, yeast, and fungi

(D) occult blood and leukocytes

(E) bilirubin and nitrite

(C) is correct. A microscopic examination must be used to identify and measure casts, bacteria, parasites, yeast, and fungi in the urine.

20. Normal kidneys can produce urine ranging from a pH of

(A) 3 to 6
(B) 4.5 to 8
(C) 3.5 to 6
(D) 5.0 to 8.5
(E) 8.5 to 14

(B) is correct. Normal kidneys can produce urine ranging from 4.5 to 8 in pH.

21. Urine voided by patients on a normal diet is slightly acidic at around

(A) 2
(B) 4
(C) 6
(D) 8
(E) 10

(C) is correct. Urine voided by patients on a normal diet is slightly acidic at around 6.

22. A pH lower than 7 might be present in

(A) urinary tract infections
(B) metabolic or respiratory acidosis
(C) diets high in fruits and vegetables
(D) all of the above
(E) none of the above

(D) is correct.

23. A pH higher than 7 is common in

(A) fever
(B) high-protein diets
(C) when taking large amounts of vitamin C
(D) all of the above
(E) none of the above

(D) is correct.

24. Which of the following statements is TRUE?

(A) urine voided by healthy patients on a normal diet is slightly alkaline
(B) urine voided by healthy patients on a normal diet is slightly acidic
(C) a pH lower than 7.0 is common if a patient is consuming large amounts of vitamin C
(D) a pH greater than 7.0 is common in the presence of a UTI
(E) all of the above

(B) is correct. Urine voided by healthy patients on a normal diet is slightly acidic.

25. UTI refers to

(A) unaccounted for infection
(B) urinary trace infection
(C) urinary tract infection
(D) upper tract infection
(E) none of the above

(C) is correct. UTI refers to a urinary tract infection.

26. When instructing a patient how to collect a routine urine specimen, the patient should be told to fill the container

(A) ½ full

(B) ¾ full

(C) ⅔ full

(D) completely

(E) it doesn't matter

    (C) is correct. The patient should be instructed to fill the container ⅔ full to avoid spillage.

27. Collected urine specimens should be examined within

(A) 15 minutes

(B) 30 to 60 minutes

(C) 60 to 90 minutes

(D) 1 to 2 hours

(E) 1 to 2 days

    (B) is correct. Collected urine specimens should be examined within 30 to 60 minutes.

28. Which of the following statements regarding the collection of a routine (random) urine sample is FALSE?

(A) it is collected in a nonsterile container

(B) it should remain at room temperature at all times prior to testing

(C) it can be collected anytime during the day

(D) at least 10 mL of urine should be collected

(E) the container should be labeled with the date and the patient's name

    (B) is correct. Urine should be refrigerated if it cannot be tested within 30 minutes.

29. A routine urinalysis is divided into three categories: physical characteristics, chemical examination, and the

(A) appearance

(B) specific gravity

(C) microscopic analysis

(D) glucose

(E) ketones

    (C) is correct. A microscopic analysis is the third category of a routine urinalysis.

    (A) Appearance is a part of the physical examination.

    (B) Specific gravity is part of the chemical examination.

    (D) Glucose is part of the chemical analysis.

    (E) Ketones are part of the chemical analysis.

30. One of the by-products found in urine when hemoglobin breaks down, which is generally not found in urine, is

(A) nitrite

(B) glucose

(C) ketone bodies

(D) bilirubin

(E) none of the above

    (D) is correct. Bilirubin is a by-product found in the urine, which occurs when hemoglobin breaks down.

31. Ketone bodies will be present in the urine with the improper metabolism of

(A) sugars
(B) fat
(C) protein

(D) carbohydrates
(E) all of the above

(B) is correct. Ketone bodies may be present in the urine with the improper metabolism of fats.

32. Ketones may be found in the urine in

(A) poorly controlled diabetes
(B) dehydration
(C) starvation
(D) ingestion of large amounts of aspirin
(E) all of the above

(E) is correct.

33. Generally, a positive indicator of a urinary tract infection is the presence of

(A) nitrites
(B) bilirubin
(C) urobilinogen

(D) ketones
(E) glucose

(A) is correct. The presence of nitrites in the urine may be an indication of a urinary tract infection.

34. When protein forms in the kidney tubules and appears in the urine, it is called

(A) bacteria
(B) casts
(C) crystals

(D) cells
(E) contamination

(B) is correct. When protein forms in the kidney tubules and appears in the urine, it is called casts.

35. When performing a microscopic examination of urine, which of the following would be the first indication of an abnormal finding per high-power field (hpf)?

(A) 0 red blood cells
(B) 1–2 red blood cells
(C) 3–4 red blood cells

(D) 5–6 red blood cells
(E) none of the above

(C) is correct. More than two red blood cells per high-power field (hpf) is considered abnormal. Therefore, three or four red blood cells is abnormal.

36. Urine should be centrifuged for how many minutes in preparation for a microscopic examination?

(A) 1 minute
(B) 2 minutes
(C) 3 minutes

(D) 5 minutes
(E) 10 minutes

(D) is correct. Urine should be centrifuged for 5 minutes in preparation for a microscopic examination.

37. Another term for urination is

(A) voiding
(B) micturition
(C) passing water

(D) A and B only
(E) A, B, and C

(E) is correct. Voiding and micturition are used by medically trained personnel. Some patients may use the phrase "passing water" to indicate urination.

38. If a urine collection is to be collected 2 hours after eating a meal, this is called a

(A) preprandial specimen
(B) 2-hour timed specimen
(C) 2-hour postprandial specimen

(D) catheterized specimen
(E) none of the above

(C) is correct. A urine specimen collected 2 hours after consuming a meal is called a 2-hour postprandial specimen.

39. When a patient is unable to control the flow of urine, he or she is said to be

(A) retaining urine
(B) circumcised
(C) catheterized

(D) incontinent
(E) none of the above

(D) is correct. Incontinent means to be unable to control the flow of urine.
(A) When a patient is unable to void, and retains urine as a result, he or she may need to be catheterized by inserting a sterile tube into the bladder to draw off urine.
(B) Circumcision refers to the surgical removal of the foreskin covering the head of the penis in the male.
(C) Catheterization refers to the insertion of a sterile tube into the bladder for the purpose of drawing off sterile urine, either for testing or to relieve retention.

40. The normal quantity of urine for an adult during a 24-hour period will average

(A) 1 pint
(B) 2 pints
(C) 3 pints

(D) ½ gallon
(E) 1 gallon

(E) is correct.

41. Glucose will "spill" into the urine when the blood glucose level exceeds

(A) 120 to140 mg/100 mL
(B) 140 to 160 mg/100 mL
(C) 160 to 180 mg/100 mL

(D) 180 to 200 mg/100 mL
(E) 200 mg/100 mL

(C) is correct.

42. Collecting a urine sample in midstream is called a

(A) catheterized specimen
(B) 2-hour postprandial specimen
(C) clean-catch specimen

(D) first-morning specimen
(E) none of the above

(C) is correct. Collecting a urine sample in midstream is called a clean-catch specimen.

43. The abbreviation KUB refers to

(A) ketones, urobilinogen, and blood
(B) kidneys
(C) ureters
(D) bladder
(E) B, C, and D

(E) is correct. KUB refers to kidneys, ureters, and bladder.

44. Normal bacteria that are found in the intestinal tract and that are the most common cause of lower-tract urinary infections, due to improper hygiene after bowel movements, are

(A) ketones
(B) nitrites
(C) *E. coli*
(D) electrolytes
(E) phimosis

(C) is correct. *Escherichia coli (E. coli)* are normal bacteria that are found in the intestinal tract and are the most common cause of lower-tract urinary infections due to improper hygiene.

45. Insulin-dependent diabetes mellitus is

(A) due to a lack of insulin
(B) Type I
(C) Type IA and Type IB
(D) Type II
(E) A, B, and C only

(E) is correct. Diabetes mellitus is due to a lack of insulin in the body. It has a sudden onset. Type I is insulin-dependent diabetes mellitus (IDDM). Type IA develops during the childhood and young adult years. Type IB develops in the adult.
(D) Type II is non-insulin dependent diabetes mellitus (NIDDM). This type has a slower onset than IDDM.

46. The signs and symptoms of IDDM include

(A) ketonuria and glycosuria
(B) hyperglycemia and polyuria
(C) weight gain
(D) weight loss
(E) A, B, and D

(E) is correct. Ketonuria (ketones excreted in the urine), glycosuria (glucose excreted in the urine), hyperglycemia (elevated blood glucose levels), polyuria (excessive urination) and weight loss are all symptoms of diabetes mellitus Type I.

47. Diabetic coma, which occurs when there is a lack of insulin and the body breaks down too much of its fat supply for energy needs, has the following signs and symptoms

   (A) diaphoresis, shock with pale, clammy skin, and disorientation
   (B) ketonuria, ketoacidosis, drowsiness, with skin that is hot and dry
   (C) deep labored breathing
   (D) A and C
   (E) B and C

   (E)   is correct. The signs of diabetic coma include ketonuria (ketone bodies in the urine), ketoacidosis (lowered pH resulting in a fruity breath odor), drowsiness, dry and hot skin, and deep, labored breathing.

   (A)   Diaphoresis, shock with pale, clammy skin, and disorientation are signs of an insulin reaction or insulin shock.

CHAPTER 21

MICROBIOLOGY

1. Histology is the study of

    (A) cells
    (B) disease and its origins
    (C) the color and shape of microorganisms
    (D) tissue microscopically
    (E) microorganisms

    (D) is correct. Histology is the microscopic study of tissue.
    (A) The science that deals with the formation, function, and structure of cells is called cytology.
    (B) The study of disease and its origins is called pathology.
    (C) The study of the color and shape of microorganisms is known as morphology.
    (E) Microbiology is the scientific study of microorganisms.

2. Disease-producing organisms are known as

    (A) microorganisms   **(D)** cultures
    (B) pathogens   **(E)** a streak culture
    (C) agglutinates

    (B) is correct. Pathogens are disease-producing organisms.
    (A) Microorganisms are organisms that are visible only by using a microscope. They may or may not be disease-producing.
    (C) Agglutinates refer to the clumping of cells.
    (D) Cultures refer to the propagation of microorganisms or of living tissue cells in special media that are conducive to their growth, such as broth or agar.
    (E) A streak culture is performed by spreading of the bacteria across a culture plate by drawing a wire containing the inoculum across the surface of the medium.

3. Microorganisms that are able to live only in the presence of oxygen are

    (A) anaerobes   **(D)** bacteria
    (B) aerobes   **(E)** none of the above
    (C) microbes

    (B) is correct. Aerobes are microorganisms that are able to live only in the presence of oxygen.
    (A) Anaerobes are microorganisms able to survive without oxygen.
    (C) Microbes are small organisms, including bacteria, protozoa, algae, fungi, and defined viruses.
    (D) Bacteria are single-celled microorganisms that lack a true nucleus.

4. An organism that is capable of living is said to be

(A) anaerobic
(B) aerobic
(C) serological
(D) viable
(E) none of the above

(D) is correct. Viable means capable of living.
(A) Anaerobic refers to microorganisms that are capable of living without oxygen.
(B) Aerobic refers to microorganisms that are able to live only in the presence of oxygen.
(C) Serological refers to the study of serum.

5. The majority of microbes present in and around the human body are nonpathogenic and are called

(A) gram-negative
(B) aseptic
(C) antiseptic
(D) normal flora
(E) none of the above

(D) is correct. Normal flora are the majority of microbes present in and around the human body. These are nonpathogenic.
(A) Gram-negative bacteria retain only the safranine color of pink after staining.
(B) Aseptic means that a specimen or individual is free of septic and/or infectious matter.
(C) Antiseptic is an agent or material that is capable of preventing the growth of pathogenic microorganisms.

6. Which of the following statements is TRUE about laboratory safety?

(A) if you cannot see blood, it isn't present
(B) caustic material is best stored at eye level
(C) always have a pencil ready to use by placing it behind your ear
(D) remove PPE when leaving the lab area
(E) wear PPE outside the lab to protect street clothing

(D) is correct. Personal protective equipment (PPE) should be removed before leaving the lab area.
(A) Always assume that blood is present, even if it is not visible, and take appropriate precautions.
(B) Caustic materials, such as acids and other fluids, should be stored below eye level to avoid accidental spillage into the eyes.
(C) Avoid any hand contact with the mouth, nose, ears, or eyes while in the lab. The hands are easily contaminated.
(E) Personal protective equipment, such as lab coats, should not be worn outside of the lab. They are used to protect street clothing from contamination.

7. What federal regulation provides guidelines for quality assurance and control, record keeping, and personnel qualifications in the clinical laboratory?

   (A) OSHA   (D) CLIA
   (B) CDC   (E) FDA
   (C) POL

   (D) is correct. The Clinical Laboratory Improvement Act (CLIA) is the federal regulation for quality assurance and control, record keeping, and personnel qualifications in the clinical laboratory.

   (A) OSHA refers to the Occupational Safety and Health Administration, which provides guidelines for employee safety in the workplace.

   (B) The CDC refers to the Centers for Disease Control in Atlanta, Georgia. This agency provides guidelines and research related to health and infectious disease issues.

   (C) POL refers to physician office laboratories, which are the smaller clinical laboratories that are found in many physicians' offices.

   (E) FDA refers to the Food and Drug Administration, which regulates controlled substances and drug testing.

8. CLIA has established three categories of testing. These include

   (A) high-complexity tests   (D) home tests
   (B) moderate-complexity tests   (E) A, B, and C only
   (C) waiver tests

   (E) is correct.

9. A waiver test as established by CLIA

   (A) makes up about 75 percent of all laboratory tests
   (B) is a highly complex test that must be performed by pathologists and/or physicians in a specific field of medical science
   (C) is a simple, stable test that requires a minimum of judgment and interpretation
   (D) A and B only
   (E) none of the above

   (C) is correct. The waiver test category, established by CLIA, is a simple, stable test that requires a minimum of judgment and interpretation, such as a visual color comparison for a pregnancy test.

   (A) Moderate-complexity tests make up approximately 75 percent of lab tests.

   (B) High-complexity tests require the skills of pathologists or other medical specialists to perform them.

10. Material taken for a throat culture can include which area(s)?

    (A) back of tongue
    (B) teeth
    (C) throat
    (D) mucous membranes on inside of cheek
    (E) all the of above

    (C) is correct. Only material taken from the throat should be used for a throat culture.

11. Material for a sputum specimen is collected from what area?

(A) nose
(B) mouth
(C) throat
(D) lungs and bronchial tubes
(E) pharynx

> (D) is correct. A sputum specimen should be collected from the lungs and bronchial tubes. Spitting into the sputum container is to be avoided since this specimen will contain saliva.

12. A self-contained, disposable plastic tube, containing a sterile swab, used for specimen collection in the office is known as a

(A) gelatin culture
(B) Gram stain
(C) culture
(D) culturette
(E) none of the above

> (D) is correct. A culturette is a self-contained, disposable plastic tube, containing a sterile swab, that is used for specimen collection in the office.
>
> (A) Gelatin culture is a type of media used to grow microorganisms in the laboratory.
>
> (B) A Gram stain is applied to specimens to determine if the organism is gram-negative (pink stain retained) or gram-positive (violet stain).
>
> (C) A culture is the propagation of living tissue cells in special media that are conducive to their growth.

13. When using a culturette system to collect a throat culture, the tongue should be depressed and the

(A) patient asked to hold his or her breath
(B) patient asked to close his or her eyes so as not to flinch
(C) swab rolled firmly across the back of the patient's throat
(D) swab dabbed at the back of the throat so as not to gag the patient
(E) none of the above

> (C) is correct. The swab should be firmly rolled across the back of the throat when obtaining a throat culture.

14. A microorganism, serum, or toxic substance that is introduced by inoculation is called the

(A) aerobe
(B) anaerobe
(C) swab
(D) inoculum
(E) inoculate

> (D) is correct. An inoculum is a microorganism, serum, or toxic substance that is introduced into growth material, such as agar, or into the human body for inoculation.
>
> (A) An aerobe is a microorganism that is capable of living only in the presence of oxygen.
>
> (B) An anaerobe is a microorganism that is able to survive without oxygen, such as the deadly botulism.

(C) A swab is a cotton or gauze on the end of a slender stick used for cleansing, applying remedies, or obtaining tissue or secretions for bacteriologic examination.

(E) To inoculate means to inject or transfer a microorganism, serum, or toxic material into the body, onto culture medium, or onto a slide.

15. A sputum specimen may be ordered by the physician to isolate and diagnose

    (A) tuberculosis
    (B) *Haemophilis*
    (C) streptococcal pneumonia

    (D) B and C only
    (E) A, B, and C

    (E) is correct.

16. What type of culture requires the use of a concave depression on the slide?

    (A) smear culture
    (B) hanging drop culture
    (C) wet mount culture

    (D) gelatin culture
    (E) streak culture

    (B) is correct. The hanging drop culture requires the use of a concave depression on the slide.

    (A) A smear culture is performed by spreading bacteria on a surface, such as a microscope slide or a culture medium.

    (C) A wet mount culture is performed by inoculating a dry slide by rolling a swab containing the specimen across the surface of the slide. A coverslip is then placed over the specimen, and the entire specimen is immediately observed under the microscope.

    (D) A gelatin culture is performed using gelatin as the media.

    (E) A streak culture is performed by spreading of bacteria by drawing a wire containing the inoculum across the surface of the medium. This is called "streaking a plate."

17. Broth, gelatin, and agar are examples of

    (A) cultures
    (B) media
    (C) inoculate

    (D) specimens
    (E) none of the above

    (B) is correct. Media for growing microorganisms in the laboratory include broth, gelatin, and agar.

    (A) Cultures are the propagation of microorganisms or of living tissue cells in special media that are conducive to their growth, and/or the process by which organisms are grown on media and identified.

    (C) Inoculate refers to the injection of an antigen, antiserum, or antitoxin into an individual.

    (D) Specimens refer to a part of a thing that is intended to show the kind and quality of the whole, such as a specimen of urine.

18. When preparing a smear, holding the slide and passing it over a flame

(A) inoculates the slide
(B) sterilizes the specimen
(C) fixes the smear to the slide
(D) kills the bacteria on the slide
(E) allows the technician to see the microorganisms

 (C) is correct. Passing a slide with a smear over a flame fixes the smear to the slide.

19. A culture is allowed to grow in an incubator at 37 degrees Celsius for how long?

(A) 2 hours
(B) 24 hours
(C) 48 hours
(D) 72 hours
(E) B, C, and D are all correct

 (E) is correct. Depending on the test ordered by the physician, the incubation period may be 24, 48, or 72 hours.

20. A secondary culture is

(A) taken from another site on the patient
(B) obtained by selecting an isolated colony from the initial agar plate and placing it onto another media plate
(C) taken if the first one is lost
(D) not to be used
(E) none of the above

 (B) is correct. A secondary culture is obtained by selecting an isolated colony from the initial agar plate and placing it onto another media plate.

21. Gram-negative bacteria, when stained, retain the

(A) blue color
(B) pink color
(C) violet color
(D) green/blue color
(E) none of the above

 (B) is correct. Gram-negative bacteria retain the pink color when stained.
 (C) Gram-positive bacteria take on a violet color in the gram-staining process.

22. The method of detecting which antibiotics will be effective in killing a particular bacteria is known as

(A) smear fixation
(B) gram staining
(C) sensitivity testing
(D) agglutination
(E) incubation

 (C) is correct. Sensitivity testing is a method of detecting which antibiotics will be effective in killing a particular bacteria.
 (A) Smear fixation is holding or fastening a bacterial specimen to a slide with heat or other fixative.
 (B) Gram staining refers to preparing a slide for a Gram stain to differentiate a gram-positive organism from a gram-negative organism.

(D)   Agglutination refers to clumping of cells.
(E)   Incubation is the period of culture development or the time it takes from placing an inoculated agar plate in an incubator or "oven" to when the microorganisms start to grow.

23. What should you look for when identifying bacteria?

(A)   shape, such as cocci, bacilli, spirilla
(B)   distribution, such as clusters and chains
(C)   structural features, such as spores
(D)   staining characteristics
(E)   all of the above

(E)   is correct.

24. What invention by van Leeuwenhoek in 1680 allowed microbes to be observed for the very first time?

(A)   Gram stain
(B)   telescope
(C)   stethoscope
(D)   microscope
(E)   none of the above

(D)   is correct. van Leeuwenhoek, the founder of microbiology, was one of the first to use the microscope to examine "tiny little beasties." Zacharias Janssen, an eyeglass maker in Holland, invented the first microscope.

25. What position should the microscope stage be in when beginning to use the microscope?

(A)   up position
(B)   first have the slide placed on the stage and then raise the stage up
(C)   down position with 100x objective directly over the slide
(D)   down position
(E)   none of the above

(D)   is correct. The stage should be in the down position to avoid breaking the glass slide.

26. Microscopic slides are placed on what portion of the microscope?

(A)   substage
(B)   stage
(C)   diaphragm
(D)   revolving nosepiece
(E)   rheostat

(B)   is correct. The microscopic slide is placed on the stage of the microscope.
(A)   The substage condenser is a lens system used to increase light for a sharper image.
(C)   The diaphragm is an adjustable aperture, like a camera shutter, that controls the amount of light.
(D)   The revolving nosepiece holds objectives and rotates for selection.
(E)   The rheostat regulates the intensity of light.

27. A substage condenser on a microscope is a

   (A) control for vertical and horizontal movement of the slide
   (B) part of the microscope that holds the illuminator
   (C) lens system used to concentrate and direct light for a sharper image
   (D) small knob atop a larger knob that adjusts the stage up and down
   (E) directional light source

      (C) is correct. The substage condenser is a lens system used to concentrate and direct light for a sharper image.
      (A) The mechanical stage adjustment is the control for vertical and horizontal slide movement.
      (B) The base of the microscope holds the illuminator.
      (D) The coarse/fine adjustment knob is a small knob atop a large knob that adjusts the stage up and down.
      (E) The body tube is the directional light source.

28. The movable device that holds a slide on a microscope is known as a/an

   (A) stage   **(D)** body tube
   (B) mechanical stage adjustment   **(E)** diaphragm
   (C) objective

      (B) is correct. The mechanical stage adjustment holds a slide on a microscope and is the adjustment for horizontal and vertical movement.
      (A) The stage is the platform the slide sets on.
      (C) The objective is the magnification level, such as 10x, 40x, or 100x.
      (D) The body tube is the directional light source.
      (E) The diaphragm is the adjustable aperture, like a camera shutter, that controls light for sharper focus.

29. When working with the microscope, which of the following is correct?

   (A) lower stage after removing slide
   (B) carry the microscope with one hand, using only the arm of the microscope
   (C) 10x setting is used for oil immersion
   (D) 40x setting is used for a high-power, dry specimen
   (E) all of the above

      (D) is correct. The objective setting 40x is used for a high-power, dry specimen.

30. The oculars, objectives, and microscope stage should be cleaned using

   (A) water and a soft cloth   **(D)** lens paper and cleaner
   (B) glass cleaner   **(E)** all of the above
   (C) soap and water

      (D) is correct. Only lens paper and cleaner should be used to clean the parts of the microscope. Other cleaners may cause abrasive damage.

31. The oil immersion power of the microscope, like that used to perform a differential blood test, is

    (A) 10x
    (B) 40x
    (C) 70x

    (D) 100x
    (E) 200x

        (D) is correct. The objective setting 100x is the oil immersion power.

32. All of the following should be included on a lab slip EXCEPT

    (A) date specimen is obtained
    (B) time specimen is obtained
    (C) time specimen is sent to lab

    (D) physician's name
    (E) patient's name

        (C) is correct.

33. Quality control (QC) in the physician's office laboratory (POL) includes

    (A) running control samples for each test performed
    (B) reagent management
    (C) instrument calibration
    (D) patient preparation and specimen collection procedures
    (E) all of the above

        (E) is correct.

CHAPTER 22

HEMATOLOGY

1. A physician who specializes in the study of blood is a/an

   (A) oncologist
   (B) pathologist
   ✓**(C)** hematologist
   (D) urologist
   (E) neurologist

    (C) is correct. A hematologist specializes in the study of blood.
    (A) An oncologist specializes in the study of cancer.
    (B) A pathologist specializes in diagnosing the abnormal changes in tissues that are removed during a surgical operation and in postmortem examinations.
    (D) A urologist specializes in disorders and diseases of the bladder and urinary tract.
    (E) A neurologist treats the nonsurgical patient who has a disorder or disease of the nervous system.

2. The largest cellular component of the blood consists of

   ✓**(A)** erythrocytes
   (B) leukocytes
   (C) platelets
   (D) lymphocytes
   (E) phagocytes

    (A) is correct. Erythrocytes, or red blood cells (RBCs), are the largest cellular component of the blood. RBCs contain hemoglobin, the iron-carrying component of the blood.
    (B) The second largest component of the blood is leukocytes, or white blood cells (WBCs).
    (C) Platelets, or thrombocytes, are the smallest of all the formed elements in the blood and are one-half the size of an erythrocyte. Platelets have no hemoglobin and are critical in the blood-clotting process.
    (D) Lymphocytes are white blood cells that provide protection for the body through an immunity activity.
    (E) Phagocytes are neutrophils, or WBCs, a component of the blood that has the ability to ingest and destroy bacteria.

3. The protein component of the blood that contains antibodies, which help to resist infection, is

   (A) hemoglobin
   ✓**(B)** gamma globulin
   (C) fibrinogen
   (D) plasma
   (E) platelets

    (B) is correct. Gamma globulin is the protein component of the blood that contains antibodies, which help to resist infection.

(A) Hemoglobin is the component of red blood cells (erythrocytes) responsible for carrying oxygen in the bloodstream.

(C) Fibrinogen is a blood protein that is essential for clotting to take place.

(D) Plasma is the fluid portion of the blood and contains the fibrinogen.

(E) Platelets are the cells that are responsible for the coagulation of blood.

4. The component of the blood that assists in the clotting process is

(A) fibrinogen   **(D)** prothrombin

(B) plasma   ✓**(E)** all of the above

(C) platelets

(E) is correct.

5. A type of white blood cell with a clear cytoplasm is a/an

(A) erythrocyte   **(D)** platelet

✓**(B)** agranulocyte   **(E)** thrombocyte

(C) granulocyte

(B) is correct. An agranulocyte is a white blood cell (leukocyte) with a clear cytoplasm.

(A) An erythrocyte is a mature red blood cell.

(C) A granulocyte is a polymorphonuclear leukocyte (WCB). There are three types of granulocytes: neutrophils, eosinophils, and basophils.

(D) A platelet is a blood cell responsible for the coagulation of blood.

(E) Thrombocyte is another term for a platelet.

6. Another term for platelet is

(A) erythrocyte   ✓**(D)** thrombocyte

(B) leukocyte   **(E)** reticulocyte

(C) neutrophil

✓(D) is correct. Thrombocyte is another term for platelet, the cell responsible for coagulation (clotting) of the blood.

(A) An erythrocyte is a mature red blood cell (RBC).

(B) A leukocyte is a white blood cell (WBC).

(C) A neutrophil is a type of granulocyte (WBC).

(E) A reticulocyte is an immature red blood cell (RBC).

7. The largest WBC in the blood is the

✓**(A)** monocyte   **(D)** neutrophil

(B) basophil   **(E)** eosinophil

(C) segmented neutrophil

(A) is correct. The monocyte is the largest WBC in the blood.

(B) The basophil, a granulocytic leukocyte (WBC), releases histamine and heparin to damaged tissue.

(C) A neutrophil and (D) a segmented neutrophil are important for the phagocytosis process. Neutrophils are the most numerous of all granulocytic white blood cells.

(E) An eosinophil increases during an allergic reaction and acts to destroy parasites. It is a type of granulocytic leukocyte (WBC).

8. The normal percentage of neutrophils in the body is

   (A) 1 to 4 percent
   (B) 5 to 10 percent
   (C) 20 to 35 percent
   (D) 50 to 70 percent
   (E) none of the above

   (D) is correct. The normal percentage of neutrophils in the blood is 50 to 70 percent.

9. Proteins that defend the body against infection are

   (A) antigens
   (B) anticoagulants
   ✓**(C)** antibodies
   (D) buffy coat
   (E) platelets

   (C) is correct. Antibodies are proteins that defend the body against infection.
   (A) Antigens are foreign substances that stimulate the production of antibodies.
   (B) Anticoagulants are substances that prevent blood from clotting (such as EDTA and heparin).
   (D) A buffy coat is the white-colored layer that forms between packed blood cells and the plasma after centrifuging a whole blood sample. It is composed of white blood cells (WBCs) and platelets.
   (E) Platelets are blood cells that aid in the blood-clotting process.

10. A complete blood count (CBC) includes all of the following EXCEPT

   (A) white blood cell (WBC) count
   (B) red blood cell (RBC) count
   (C) hemoglobin and hematocrit
   (D) white blood cell differential (diff)
   ✓**(E)** all of the above

   (E) is correct.

11. A test to measure the time it takes for blood to coagulate is the

   (A) hemoglobin test (Hb, Hgb)
   (B) CBC
   ✓**(C)** bleeding time
   (D) ESR
   (E) differential (diff)

   (C) is correct. A bleeding time test measures the amount of time for the blood to coagulate.
   (A) A hemoglobin test measures the amount of oxygen-carrying hemoglobin present in a blood sample.
   (B) A CBC is a complete blood count.
   (D) ESR stands for erythrocyte sedimentation rate. This is a blood test to determine the rate at which mature red blood cells settle out of the blood after the addition of an anticoagulant. It can be an indicator of an inflammatory disease.
   (E) A differential (diff) blood count determines the number of each variety of leukocytes or white blood cells (WBCs).

12. The white-colored layer that forms between the packed red blood cells and the plasma after centrifuging a sample of whole blood is known as

(A) plasma
(B) serum
(C) hemoglobin

(D) buffy coat
(E) electrolytes

✓(D) is correct. The buffy coat is the layer that forms between the packed red blood cells and the plasma after centrifuging. It is composed of white blood cells and platelets.

(A) Plasma is the fluid portion of the blood, which comprises 55 percent of the total blood volume, and contains fibrinogen.

(B) Serum is the clear, sticky fluid that remains after the blood has clotted. It contains no fibrin.

(C) Hemoglobin is the component of red blood cells responsible for carrying oxygen.

(E) Electrolytes are ionized salts in the blood, such as sodium (NA), potassium (K), and chloride (Cl).

13. The process in which white blood cells ingest and digest foreign material is called

✓(A) phagocytosis
(B) erythroblastosis
(C) leukocytes

(D) hemolysis
(E) hematopoiesis

(A) is correct. Phagocytosis is the process in which white blood cells (WBCs) ingest and digest foreign material in the body.

(B) Erythroblastosis is a condition in which there are excessive numbers of erythroblasts in the blood. Erythroblasts are immature red blood cells.

(C) Leukocytes are white blood cells (WBCs).

(D) Hemolysis refers to the destruction of blood cells.

(E) Hematopoiesis refers to the formation of blood cells.

14. The average adult blood volume is

(A) 4.0 to 5.0 liters
(B) 4.5 to 5.0 liters
✓(C) 5.5 to 6.0 liters

(D) 6.5 to 7.0 liters
(E) 7.5 to 8 liters

(C) is correct. The average adult blood volume is 5.5 to 6.0 liters.

15. Serum is the

(A) clear, straw-colored liquid portion of the blood
(B) process of withdrawing blood from a vein
(C) destruction of blood cells
✓(D) liquid portion of blood containing no fibrin
(E) collection of blood underneath the skin

(D) is correct. Serum is the liquid portion of blood containing no fibrin.

(A) Plasma is the clear, straw-colored liquid portion of the blood.

(B) Venipuncture is the process of withdrawing blood from a vein.

(C) Hemolysis is the destruction of blood cells.

(E) A hematoma is a collection of blood underneath the skin.

16. Plasma is approximately what percent of the total blood volume?

(A) 50 percent   (D) 65 percent
(B) 55 percent   (E) 70 percent
(C) 60 percent

✓(B)   is correct. Plasma is approximately 55 percent of the total blood volume.

17. Which is an immature red blood cell containing a nucleus?

(A) platelet   ✓(D) reticulocyte
(B) leukocyte   (E) phagocyte
(C) erythrocyte

(D)   is correct. A reticulocyte is an immature red blood cell containing a nucleus.
(A)   A platelet is a cell that aids in the blood-clotting process.
(B)   A leukocyte is another term for a white blood cell (WBC).
(C)   An erythrocyte is a red blood cell (RBC).
(E)   A phagocyte is a white blood cell (WBC), which ingests and digests foreign material.

18. The red color of blood comes from

(A) serum   ✓(D) hemoglobin
(B) plasma   (E) platelets
(C) leukocytes

(D)   is correct. The red color of blood comes from hemoglobin.

19. The normal adult female hemoglobin is

(A) 6 to 8 g/dl   (D) 14 to 18 g/dl
(B) 8 to 12 g/dl   (E) none of the above
✓(C) 12 to 16 g/dl

(C)   is correct. The normal adult female hemoglobin is 12 to 16 g/dl.
(D)   The normal adult male hemoglobin is 14 to 18 g/dl.

20. Jerome White's hemoglobin is 12 g/dl. This is

(A) within a normal range   (D) normal
(B) high   (E) none of the above
✓(C) low

(C)   is correct. The normal range for a male's hemoglobin is from 14 to 18 g/dl.

21. All of the following are examples of white blood cells EXCEPT

(A) neutrophil   (D) basophil
(B) lymphocyte   (E) eosinophil
✓(C) reticulocyte

(C)   is correct. A reticulocyte is an immature red blood cell containing a nucleus.

22. A white blood cell count above 11,000 may indicate a/an

(A) clotting disorder
(B) viral infection
✓(C) bacterial infection
(D) anemia
(E) none of the above

(C) is correct. A white blood cell count above 11,000 may indicate a bacterial infection.

23. Which type of blood collection tube contains a clot activator and a gel that permanently separates the serum from the clot after centrifugation?

(A) green top
(B) purple top
(C) red top
✓(D) marbled top
(E) gray top

(D) is correct. The marbled (red and gray/black) top tube is also called a serum separator tube (SST). It contains a gel that will permanently separate the serum from the clot after centrifugation. It also contains a clot activator.

(A) The green top tube contains heparin. This tube is used if whole blood or plasma is needed.

(B) The purple/lavender top tube contains ethylenediaminetetraacetic acid (EDTA), which is used if whole blood or plasma is needed. This tube is commonly used for a CBC or a glycosylated hemoglobin.

(C) The red top tube contains no anticoagulant. Blood will clot in this tube after centrifugation. A red top tube is used for serum chemistry testing.

(E) A gray top tube, containing potassium oxalate, is used if whole blood or plasma is needed for testing. This tube is commonly used for a glucose tolerance test (GTT).

24. When drawing blood for a PT and/or a PTT, which type of blood collection tube should be used?

(A) green top
(B) purple top
(C) red top
✓(D) light blue top
(E) gray top

(D) is correct. A light blue top tube contains sodium citrate. This tube is used if whole blood or plasma is needed, and it is commonly used for a PT (prothrombin time) or PTT (partial thromboplastin time).

(A) The green top tube contains heparin. This tube is used if whole blood or plasma is needed.

(B) A purple/lavender top tube contains ethylenediaminetetraacetic acid (EDTA), which is used if whole blood or plasma is needed. This tube is commonly used for a CBC or a glycosylated hemoglobin.

(C) The red top tube contains no anticoagulant. Blood will clot in this tube after centrifugation. A red top tube is used for serum chemistry testing.

(E) A gray top tube, containing potassium oxalate, is used if whole blood or plasma is needed for testing. This tube is commonly used for a glucose tolerance test (GTT).

25. In phlebotomy, a red top tube is commonly used for

    (A) serum separation
    ✓**(B)** serum chemistry testing
    (C) prothrombin time
    (D) complete blood counts
    (E) none of the above

        (B) is correct. The red top tube, which contains no anticoagulant, is commonly used for serum chemistry testing.

26. An example of an anticoagulant is

    (A) sodium
    (B) potassium
    ✓**(C)** heparin
    (D) chloride
    (E) none of the above

        (C) is correct. Heparin is an example of an anticoagulant. Sodium (A), potassium (B), and chloride (D) are electrolytes.

27. The most commonly used anticoagulant for blood tests is

    ✓**(A)** EDTA
    (B) sodium citrate
    (C) potassium citrate
    (D) potassium oxylate
    (E) heparin

        (A) is correct. EDTA is a commonly used anticoagulant for a CBC or a glycosylated hemoglobin test.

28. Capillary punctures are best performed

    (A) on the ring finger
    (B) for an infant, on the plantar surface of the heel
    (C) using the patient's nondominant hand
    (D) A and C only
    ✓**(E)** all of the above

        (E) is correct.

29. As soon as a venipuncture has been completed, ask patients

    (A) if the procedure hurt them
    (B) what their name is
    (C) to bend their arm over the venipuncture site
    ✓**(D)** to apply steady pressure on the venipuncture site with a cotton ball or gauze
    (E) all of the above

        (D) is correct. Have the patient apply steady pressure over the venipuncture site using a cotton ball or gauze square.

30. A hemacytometer is a special glass-chambered slide used to

    (A) store a blood sample
    ✓**(B)** count red and white blood cells under a microscope
    (C) perform an erythrocyte sedimentation rate (ESR)
    (D) perform autohemotherapy
    (E) perform a hematocrit

(B) is correct. A hemacytometer is used to count the numbers of red and white blood cells.

(A) Blood samples are stored in collection tubes and stored under refrigeration if not used or tested immediately.

(C) Wintrobe and Westergren tests are used for an erythrocyte sedimentation rate (ESR).

(D) Autohemotherapy is the treatment of using a person's own blood in a transfusion by withdrawing and injecting the blood intramuscularly.

(E) A hematocrit is a blood test to measure the volume of erythrocytes in a given volume of blood.

31. A test to determine the rate at which RBCs settle at the bottom of a tube is called a/an

(A) hematocrit   **(D)** differential
✓**(B)** ESR   **(E)** CBC
(C) hemoglobin

(B) is correct. An erythrocyte sedimentation rate (ESR) is a test to determine the rate at which RBCs settle at the bottom of a tube.

(A) A hematocrit blood test is a measurement of red blood cells (erythrocytes) within the total volume of blood.

(C) A hemoglobin (Hb, Hgb) test tests for the component of packed red blood cells that are responsible for carrying oxygen.

(D) A differential blood count is used to determine the number of each variety of leukocytes.

(E) A CBC is a complete blood count, which consists of a red blood cell (RBC) count, white blood cell (WBC) count, hemoglobin (Hg), hematocrit (Hct), and white blood cell differential.

32. A low hematocrit count might indicate

(A) dehydration   **(D)** polycythemia
(B) anemia   ✓**(E)** B and C only
(C) hemorrhage

(E) is correct. A low hematocrit would be present in conditions such as anemia and hemorrhage.

(A) Dehydration may result in an elevated hematocrit.

(D) Polycythemia means a condition of excessive red blood cells.

33. A low hemoglobin (Hb, Hgb) may be present in

(A) cases of severe burns   **(D)** leukemia
✓**(B)** iron-deficiency anemia   **(E)** none of the above
(C) polycythemia vera

(B) is correct. Hemoglobin, the iron-containing pigment of red blood cells that carries oxygen from the lungs to the tissue, is decreased in the disorder of iron-deficiency anemia.

(A) There may be an elevated hemoglobin in cases of severe burns.

(C) Polycythemia vera causes the production of too many red blood cells.

(D) Leukemia, a disease characterized by an excess of white blood cells, may result in severe anemia.

34. A normal ESR in an adult is

    (A) 0–5 mm/hr.   **(D)** 20–30 mm/hr.
    (B) 5–10 mm/hr.   **(E)** 40–60 mm/hr.
   ✓**(C)** 0–20 mm/hr.

        (B̶) is correct. A normal ESR in an adult is 0–20 mm/hr.

35. Which of the following blood tests does NOT require fasting?

    (A) glucose tolerance   **(D)** triglyceride level
    (B) FBS   **(E)** total cholesterol
   ✓**(C)** CBC

        (C) is correct. A complete blood count (CBC) does not require fasting beforehand.

36. A disorder in which there is an overabundance of erythrocytes is

    (A) anemia   **(D)** polycythemia
    (B) leukemia   **(E)** none of the above
    (C) agranulocytosis

     ✓(D) Polycythemia is a disorder of the blood in which there is an overabundance of erythrocytes.
     (A) Anemia is a reduction in the number of red blood cells (RBCs).
     (B) Leukemia is a disease characterized by a great excess of white blood cells.
     (C) Agranulocytosis is a condition in which there is a reduction of granular leukocytes in the blood. This results in destructive ulcerative lesions in the throat (leukopenia).

37. A collection of blood below the surface of the skin is called a

    (A) hemolysis   **(D)** hematuria
  ✓**(B)** hematoma   **(E)** hematology
    (C) hematemesis

     (B) is correct. A hematoma is a collection of blood below the surface of the skin. This is commonly called a bruise.
     (A) Hemolysis is the destruction of red blood cells (RBCs).
     (C) Hematemesis is the vomiting of blood.
     (D) Hematuria is the presence of blood in the urine.
     (E) Hematology is the study of blood.

38. What process occurs if a person with Rh^- blood receives a transfusion of Rh^+ blood?

  ✓**(A)** agglutination   **(D)** purpura
    (B) anemia   **(E)** hemophilia
    (C) polycythemia

     (A) is correct. Anti-Rh agglutination will occur. Agglutination is an antigen-antibody reaction in which a solid antigen clumps together with a soluble antibody. Any transfusion after the first one can have serious results.

(B) Anemia is a reduction in the number of red blood cells (RBCs), which results in less oxygen reaching the tissues.

(C) Polycythemia is a condition in which there are too many red blood cells (RBCs).

(D) Purpura is a condition in which there are multiple small hemorrhages under the skin, in the mucous membranes, and within tissues and organs.

(E) Hemophilia is a hereditary blood disease in which there is a prolonged blood-clotting time.

39. A pregnant woman who is Rh⁻ may become sensitized by an Rh⁺ fetus. In pregnancies after the first pregnancy, the maternal antibodies may cross the placenta and destroy fetal cells resulting in what condition?

(A) tetralogy of Fallot   (D) all of the above
(B) patent ductus arteriosus   (E) none of the above
✓(C) erythroblastosis fetalis

(C) is correct. Erythroblastosis fetalis is a potentially fatal condition in the newborn, which develops anytime after the first pregnancy whenever a mother is Rh⁻ and a fetus is Rh⁺. It is also called hemolytic disease of the newborn.

(A) Tetralogy of Fallot is a congenital defect in the newborn resulting in a combination of four symptoms (tetralogy): pulmonary stenosis, septal defect, abnormal blood supply to the aorta, and hypertrophy of the right ventricle.

(B) Patent ductus arteriosus is the congenital presence of a connection between the pulmonary artery and the aorta in the newborn that remains after birth. This condition is normal in the fetus.

40. A blood test for mononucleosis that tests for the nonspecific heterophile antibody is

(A) prothrombin time   ✓(D) Monospot
(B) ESR   (E) differential
(C) WBC

(D) is correct. The Monospot is a blood test for mononucleosis that tests for the nonspecific heterophile antibody.

(A) A prothrombin time (pro time) test determines the coagulation rate of the blood. Prothrombin is the component of blood that interacts with calcium salts to form thrombin, a coagulation factor.

(B) ESR refers to erythrocyte sedimentation rate, which is a blood test to determine the rate at which mature red blood cells settle out of the blood after the addition of an anticoagulant.

(C) A white blood cell (WBC) count measures the number of leukocytes in a volume of blood.

(E) A differential blood count determines the number of each variety of leukocyte.

CHAPTER 23

PHARMACOLOGY AND MEDICATION ADMINISTRATION

1. The prevention of disease is

   (A) contraindicated
   (B) habituation
   (C) idiosyncrasy

   (D) prophylaxis
   (E) toxicity

   (D) is correct.
   (A) Contraindicated is a condition in which a specific drug should not be used.
   (B) Habituation is the development of an emotional dependence on a drug, due to repeated use.
   (C) Idiosyncrasy is an unusual or abnormal response to a drug or food by an individual.
   (E) Toxicity is the extent or degree to which a substance is poisonous.

2. A condition in which the use of a drug should NOT be used is

   (A) contraindicated
   (B) habituation
   (C) idiosyncrasy

   (D) prophylaxis
   (E) toxicity

   (A) is correct. Pregnancy, high blood pressure, kidney disease, and other diseases may prevent an individual from being allowed to use certain drugs.
   (B) Habituation is the development of an emotional dependence on a drug, due to repeated use.
   (C) Idiosyncrasy is an unusual or abnormal response to a drug or food.
   (D) Prophylaxis is the prevention of disease.
   (E) Toxicity is the extent or degree to which a substance is poisonous.

3. A response to a drug other than the effect desired is

   (A) addiction
   (B) side effects
   (C) toxicity

   (D) placebo
   (E) habituation

   (B) is correct.
   (A) Addiction is an acquired physical and psychological dependence on a drug.
   (C) Toxicity is the extent or degree to which a substance is poisonous.
   (D) Placebo is an inactive, harmless substance used to satisfy a patient's desire for medication.
   (E) Habituation is the development of an emotional dependence on a drug, due to repeated use.

4. A drug tolerance is

 (A) an acquired physical and psychological dependence on a drug
 (B) the ability of a drug to be effective against a wide range of microorganisms
 (C) to weaken the strength of a substance by the addition of something else
 (D) the development of an emotional dependence on a drug, due to repeated use
 (E) a decrease in susceptibility to a drug after the continued use of the drug

 (E) is correct.

5. The official federal agency with responsibility for the regulation of food, drugs, cosmetics, and medical devices is the

 (A) BNDD
 (B) FDA
 (C) PDR
 (D) USP-NF
 (E) DEA

 (B) is correct.
 (A) BNDD is the Bureau of Narcotics and Dangerous Drugs, which enforces drug control.
 (C) PDR is the *Physician's Desk Reference*, a book used as a quick reference on drugs.
 (D) USP-NF is the *United States Pharmacopeia-National Formulary*, a drug book listing all the official drugs that are authorized for use in the United States.
 (E) DEA is the Drug Enforcement Agency, which controls the use of narcotics.

6. The proprietary name of a drug is also known as the

 (A) trade name
 (B) brand name
 (C) generic name
 (D) A & B
 (E) A & C

 (D) is correct. The trade name or brand name is the commercial name that is patented by the pharmaceutical company that manufactures the drug.
 (C) The generic name is the common name by which a drug or product is known (for example, aspirin).

7. An OTC drug is

 (A) a drug that can only be ordered by a physician
 (B) accessible without a prescription
 (C) controlled due to a potential for addiction
 (D) labeled: Caution: Federal law prohibits dispensing without a prescription
 (E) a drug that must be administered directly by a physician

 (B) is correct.

8. Which schedule for controlled substances has a high potential for addiction and abuse?

 (A) Schedule I
 (B) Schedule II
 (C) Schedule III
 (D) Schedule IV
 (E) Schedule V

(B)   is correct.
(A)   Schedule I has the highest potential for addiction and abuse.
(C)   Schedule III has a moderate to low potential for addiction.
(D)   Schedule IV has a lower potential for addiction and abuse than Schedule III.
(E)   Schedule V has the lowest potential for addiction and abuse.

9. The drug classification that relieves pain without the loss of consciousness is

(A) adrenergic
(B) analgesic
(C) anesthetic
(D) antibiotic
(E) antiseptic

(B)   is correct.
(A)   Adrenergic increases the rate and strength of the heart muscle.
(C)   Anesthetic produces a lack of feeling, which may be of local or general effect.
(D)   Antibiotic destroys or prohibits the growth of microorganisms.
(E)   Antiseptic prevents the growth of microorganisms.

10. The drug classification that controls nausea and vomiting is

(A) antacid
(B) antidote
(C) anti-emetic
(D) antipruritics
(E) antipyretic

(C)   is correct.
(A)   Antacid neutralizes acid in the stomach.
(B)   Antidote counteracts the effects of poisons.
(D)   Antipruritic relieves itching.
(E)   Antipyretic reduces fever.

11. The drug classification that controls itching is

(A) antacid
(B) antidote
(C) anti-emetic
(D) antipruritic
(E) antipyretic

(D)   is correct.

12. The drug classification that lowers blood sugar is

(A) antihistamine
(B) antihypertensive
(C) diuretic
(D) hemostatic
(E) hypoglycemic

(E)   is correct.
(A)   Antihistamine counteracts histamine and controls allergic reactions.
(B)   Antihypertensive controls high blood pressure.
(C)   Diuretic increases the excretion of urine, which promotes the loss of water and salt from the body.
(D)   Hemostatic controls bleeding.

13. The drug classification that controls or relieves coughing is

(A) antibiotic
(B) antitussive
(C) bronchodilator
(D) decongestant
(E) expectorant

    (B) is correct.
    (A) Antibiotic destroys or prohibits the growth of microorganisms.
    (C) Bronchodilator dilates or opens the bronchi to improve breathing.
    (D) Decongestant reduces nasal congestion and swelling.
    (E) Expectorant assists in the removal of secretions from the bronchopulmonary membranes.

14. Anesthetics

(A) increase peripheral circulation and decrease blood pressure and vasodilation
(B) produce relaxation without causing sleep
(C) produce sleep
(D) produce a lack of feeling, which may be of local or general effect
(E) are used to reduce mental anxiety and tensions

    (D) is correct.
    (A) Adrenergic blocking agents increase peripheral circulation and decrease blood pressure and vasodilation.
    (B) Sedatives produce relaxation without causing sleep.
    (C) Hypnotics produce sleep.
    (E) Tranquilizers are used to reduce mental anxiety and tensions.

15. Mydriatics

(A) dilate the pupils
(B) strengthen the heart muscle
(C) control bleeding
(D) stimulate bowel movements
(E) are given to promote resistance to infectious diseases

    (A) is correct.
    (B) Cardiogenics strengthen the heart muscle.
    (C) Hemostatics control bleeding.
    (D) Purgatives stimulate bowel movements.
    (E) Vaccines are given to promote resistance to infectious diseases.

16. Acetaminophen is the generic name for

(A) aspirin
(B) Advil
(C) Tylenol
(D) Demerol
(E) Valium

    (C) is correct.
    (A) Acetylsalicylic acid is aspirin.
    (B) Ibuprofen is Advil.
    (D) Meperidine is Demerol.
    (E) Diazepam is Valium.

17. Darvon is classified as a/an

(A) analgesic   (D) anesthetic
(B) anti-anxiety   (E) antipyretic
(C) antibiotic

    (A)   is correct. Darvon, an analgesic, relieves pain.
    (B)   An anti-anxiety drug relieves or reduces anxiety.
    (C)   An antibiotic destroys or prohibits the growth of microorganisms.
    (D)   An anesthetic drug produces a lack of feeling.
    (E)   An antipyretic drug reduces fever.

18. Xanax is classified as a/an

(A) antibiotic   (D) stimulant
(B) anti-anxiety   (E) tranquilizer
(C) psychedelic

    (E)   is correct. Xanax is used as a tranquilizer to reduce mental tensions.
    (A)   An antibiotic destroys or prohibits the growth of microorganisms.
    (B)   An anti-anxiety drug relieves or reduces anxiety and muscle tension.
    (C)   A psychedelic drug can produce visual hallucinations.
    (D)   A stimulant acts to speed up the heart and respiratory system.

19. Lanoxin is classified as a/an

(A) antibiotic   (D) antitussive
(B) diuretic   (E) laxative
(C) cardiogenic

    (C)   is correct. Lanoxin, a cardiogenic, strengthens the heart.
    (A)   An antibiotic destroys or prohibits the growth of microorganisms.
    (B)   A diuretic drug increases the excretion of urine.
    (D)   An antitussive drug controls or relieves coughing.
    (E)   A laxative is used to promote normal bowel function.

20. Premarin is classified as a/an

(A) antibiotic   (D) antihypertensive
(B) decongestant   (E) estrogen
(C) expectorant

    (E)   is correct. Premarin is a replacement for estrogen.
    (A)   An antibiotic destroys or prohibits the growth of microorganisms.
    (B)   A decongestant reduces nasal congestion and swelling.
    (C)   An expectorant assists in the removal of secretions from pulmonary membranes.
    (D)   An antihypertensive drug prevents or controls high blood pressure.

21. Tenormin is classified as a/an

(A) antibiotic   (D) diuretic
(B) beta-blocker   (E) antidiabetic
(C) antihistamine

(B) is correct. Tenormin is a beta-blocker that reduces blood pressure, which works for the good of the heart.

22. Dyazide is classified as a/an

    (A) antibiotic
    (B) antihypertensive
    (C) antihistamine
    (D) diuretic
    (E) emetic

    (D) is correct. Dyazide, a diuretic, causes an increased production of urine.

23. Dilantin is classified as a/an

    (A) emetic
    (B) bronchodilator
    (C) diuretic
    (D) analgesic
    (E) anticonvulsant

    (E) is correct. Dilantin, an anticonvulsant, helps to reduce or control seizure activity in the epileptic.
    (A) An emetic induces vomiting.
    (B) A bronchodilator opens or dilates the bronchi.
    (C) A diuretic increases the excretion of urine.
    (D) An analgesic relieves pain.

24. Micronase is classified as a/an

    (A) antibiotic
    (B) decongestant
    (C) oral hypoglycemic agent
    (D) antihypertensive
    (E) antacid

    (C) is correct. Micronase, an oral hypoglycemic, works to reduce blood sugar and is given orally.

25. Coumadin is classified as a/an

    (A) anticoagulant
    (B) antibiotic
    (C) expectorant
    (D) antihypertensive
    (E) antitussive

    (A) is correct. Coumadin, an anticoagulant, delays or prevents blood from clotting. Patients taking Coumadin must have their blood monitored frequently to make sure that the blood isn't too thick or too thin. Aspirin is contraindicated when using Coumadin since aspirin is a blood thinner in itself.

26. Prozac is classified as a/an

    (A) tranquilizer
    (B) sedative
    (C) hypnotic
    (D) anesthetic
    (E) antidepressant

    (E) is correct. Prozac, an antidepressant, elevates the mood of a depressed individual.

27. Theo-Dur is classified as a

(A) bronchodilator
(B) beta-blocker
(C) tranquilizer
(D) diuretic
(E) vasoconstrictor

(A) is correct. Theo-Dur, a bronchodilator, opens the bronchi to make breathing easier.

28. Vasotec is classified as a/an

(A) antidiarrheal
(B) antihypertensive
(C) vasodilator
(D) vasoconstrictor
(E) vitamin

(B) is correct. Vasotec, an antihypertensive, lowers blood pressure.

29. Synthroid is classified as a/an

(A) antibiotic
(B) cardiogenic
(C) analgesic
(D) hormone
(E) anti-inflammatory

(D) is correct. Synthroid is used either to replace the hormone lacking in hypothyroidism or if the thyroid has been removed surgically.

30. Motrin is classified as a/an

(A) analgesic
(B) anti-inflammatory
(C) antacid
(D) decongestant
(E) anti-emetic

(B) is correct. Motrin, an anti-inflammatory, is prescribed for inflammatory conditions of the musculoskeletal system.

31. An injection under the skin and fat layers is

(A) intradermal
(B) subcutaneous
(C) intramuscular
(D) intravenous
(E) intracavity

(B) is correct. A subcutaneous injection is administered under the skin and fat layers.
(A) An intradermal injection is administered within the top layer of the skin.
(C) An intramuscular injection is given into a muscle.
(D) An intravenous injection is administered into a vein.

32. An injection into the veins is

(A) intradermal
(B) subcutaneous
(C) intramuscular
(D) intravenous
(E) intracavity

(D) is correct. Medical assistants are not permitted to administer intravenous medications.

33. The method commonly used in skin testing for allergies and tuberculosis is

(A) intradermal
(B) subcutaneous
(C) intramuscular
(D) intravenous
(E) intracavity

    (A)   is correct. The intradermal method is a very shallow injection, just within the top layer of skin.

34. Rx is Latin for

(A) take thou
(B) mark
(C) taken by mouth
(D) name
(E) prescription

    (A)   is correct. Rx is taken from the Latin term *recipe*, which means "take thou."

35. Which one is NOT a part of a prescription?

(A) patient's name and address
(B) name of drug
(C) method of taking drug
(D) instructions for taking drug
(E) the FDA number

    (E)   is correct. The DEA number is usually listed on a prescription in the event the drug is a narcotic. FDA is the Food and Drug Administration, a federal agency that regulates food, drugs, cosmetics, and medical devices.

36. Which is NOT one of the "six rights" of medication administration?

(A) right patient
(B) right medication
(C) right physician
(D) right dosage
(E) right route

    (C)   is correct. The "six rights" are right patient, right medication, right dosage, right route, right time, and right documentation.

37. Bid is an abbreviation for

(A) once a day
(B) twice a day
(C) three times a day
(D) four times a day
(E) every day

    (B)   is correct. Bid means to give the medication twice a day.

38. OD is an abbreviation for

(A) overdose
(B) right ear
(C) after meals
(D) once daily
(E) right eye

    (E)   is correct. OD is right eye, OS is left eye, and OU is both eyes.

39. PRN is an abbreviation for

(A) stat

(B) before meals

(C) as needed

(D) after meals

(E) evening

    (C)   is correct. PRN means that the medication is only given when the patient needs it.

40. The abbreviation for "hours of sleep" is

(A) PO

(B) H

(C) ss

(D) hs

(E) s

    (D)   is correct. hs means hours of sleep.

    (A)   PO means after meals.

    (B)   H means hour.

    (C)   ss means one-half.

    (E)   s means without.

41. Which weight or measure is NOT in the metric system?

(A) mL

(B) cc

(C) gm

(D) L

(E) gr

    (E)   is correct. The grain (gr) is an apothecary measurement.

42. To change grams to milligrams, the decimal point is moved how many spaces?

(A) 2 spaces to the left

(B) 3 spaces to the left

(C) 3 spaces to the right

(D) 2 spaces to the right

(E) none of the above

    (C)   is correct. To convert grams to milligrams, multiply by 1,000, or move the decimal three places to the right. Example: 15 grams = 15,000 milligrams.

43. To change grams to kilograms, the decimal point is moved how many spaces?

(A) 2 spaces to the left

(B) 3 spaces to the left

(C) 3 spaces to the right

(D) 2 spaces to the right

(E) none of the above

    (B)   is correct. To change grams to kilograms, divide grams by 1,000, or move the decimal point 3 spaces to the left. Example: 150 grams = 0.15 kilogram.

44. The equivalent metric measurement of the apothecary measurement of 1 dram is

(A) 15 mL

(B) 30 cc

(C) 1 m

(D) 4 mL

(E) 1 ounce

    (D)   is correct. 1dr (dram) = 4 mL (milliliter).

45. The equivalent metric measurement of the apothecary measurement of 1 fl. oz. is

(A) 5 mL
(B) 10 mL
(C) 15 mL

(D) 30 mL
(E) 50 mL

(D) is correct. 1 fl. oz. (fluid ounce) = 30 mL (milliliter).

46. The equivalent metric measurement of the apothecary measurement of 1 oz. is

(A) 5 cc
(B) 10 cc
(C) 15 cc

(D) 30 cc
(E) 50 cc

(D) is correct. 1 cc (cubic centimeter) = 1 mL (milliliter). Therefore 1 ounce (oz.) is equal to 30 cc or 30 mL.

47. The common household measurement of 1 T is equal to how many milliliters?

(A) 1 mL
(B) 5 mL
(C) 10 mL

(D) 15 mL
(E) 30 mL

(D) is correct. 1 T (tablespoon) = 15 mL (milliliter).

48. The common household measurement of 1 t is equal to how many milliliters?

(A) 1 mL
(B) 5 mL
(C) 10 mL

(D) 15 mL
(E) 30 mL

(B) is correct. 1 t (teaspoon) = 5 mL (milliliter).

49. The common household measurement of 15 gtts is equal to the apothecary measurement of

(A) 1 m
(B) 5 m
(C) 10 m

(D) 15 m
(E) 30 m

(D) is correct. 1 gtt (drop) = 1 m (minim). Therefore 15 drops = 15 minims.

50. The household measurement of 1 t is equal to the apothecary measurement of

(A) 1 fl. dr
(B) 2 fl. dr
(C) 3 fl. dr

(D) 4 fl. dr
(E) 5 fl. dr

(A) is correct. 1 t (teaspoon) = 1 fl. dr (fluid dram).

51. Which pediatric dosage calculation is based on the child's age (if over 1 year)?

(A) Clark's rule
(B) Fried's law
(C) Young's rule

(D) West's nomogram
(E) none of the above

(C) is correct. To use Young's rule, divide the child's age in years by the same number plus 12. Multiply this number by the adult dose to determine the correct pediatric dose.

52. Which pediatric dosage calculation is based on the child's weight?

   (A) Clark's rule   **(D)** West's nomogram
   (B) Fried's law   **(E)** none of the above
   (C) Young's rule

   (A) is correct. Clark's rule divides the weight of the child by 150 pounds and multiplies this number by the adult dose to arrive at the pediatric dosage.

53. To take medication by injection is to take medication

   (A) orally   **(D)** by inhalation
   (B) sublingually   **(E)** parenterally
   (C) topically

   (E) is correct. Parenteral medication is administered by injection.
   (A) Orally is by mouth.
   (B) Sublingually is under the tongue.
   (C) Topically is applied on the outside of the body on the skin.
   (D) By inhalation is by breathing in the medication.

54. When administering oral or sublingual medication

   (A) assemble all equipment using aseptic technique
   (B) use the "three befores" and select the correct medication
   (C) pour the medication into the bottle cap instead of the hand
   (D) A and C
   (E) A, B, and C

   (E) is correct.

55. Which one of the following is NOT a parenteral route to administer medication?

   (A) intradermal   **(D)** elixir
   (B) intramuscular   **(E)** Z-track
   (C) subcutaneous

   (D) is correct. Elixir is given orally.

56. The $3/8$-inch needle length is used in a/an

   (A) intradermal injection   **(D)** intravenous injection
   (B) subcutaneous injection   **(E)** Z-track injection
   (C) intramuscular injection

   (A) is correct.
   (B) Subcutaneous injection uses a $1/2$-inch or $5/8$-inch needle.
   (C) Intramuscular injection uses a 1- to 3-inch needle.
   (D) Intravenous injections are not given by medical assistants.
   (E) Z-track is a deep intramuscular injection and ranges from $1 1/2$ to 3 inches.

57. The most common gauge(s) for subcutaneous injections is/are

(A) 27–28
(B) 25–26
(C) 20–23
(D) 27
(E) 23

    (B) is correct.

58. Infants' immunizations are usually injected into the

(A) deltoid muscle
(B) gluteus medius muscle
(C) vastus lateralis muscle
(D) bicep muscle
(E) tricep muscle

    (C) is correct. The vastus lateralis muscle is used in infants because their gluteus medius muscle is not well developed yet.

59. The angle at which subcutaneous injections are administered is

(A) 10–15 degrees
(B) 25 degrees
(C) 30 degrees
(D) 45 degrees
(E) 90 degrees

    (D) is correct. Subcutaneous injections are administered at a 45-degree angle, except for insulin and heparin, which are given at a 90-degree angle.

60. Immunizations scheduled for a child 4 to 5 months of age are

(A) HBV 1, DPT 1, oral polio 1
(B) DPT 2, oral polio 2, HIB 2
(C) DPT 1, oral polio 1, HBV 2, HIB 1
(D) DPT 1, oral polio 2, HBV 2
(E) DPT 2, oral polio 2, MMR

    (B) is correct.

61. Immunizations scheduled for a child 1 year of age are

(A) TB test, rubeola
(B) DPT 3, HBV 3
(C) DPT booster, oral polio booster
(D) DPT 3, MMR
(E) MMR, TB test

    (E) is correct. Immunizations for a 1-year-old child are mumps, measles, and rubella (MMR), and a TB test.

62. Gauge 20–23, length 1–3 inches is the needle size for

(A) intradermal injections
(B) subcutaneous injections
(C) intramuscular injections
(D) insulin injections
(E) tuberculin skin tests

    (C) is correct.
    (A) Intradermal injections use 27–28, $3/8$-inch needles.
    (B) Subcutaneous injections use 25–26, $1/2$- or $5/8$-inch needles.
    (D) Insulin injections are given subcutaneously.
    (E) Tuberculin skin tests are done intradermally.

63. The intradermal injection is administered at what degree of angle?

(A) 5-degree angle
(B) 15-degree angle
(C) 20-degree angle
(D) 45-degree angle
(E) 90-degree angle

(B) is correct.

64. Intradermal injections are given for

(A) influenza prevention
(B) iron-replacement therapy
(C) insulin therapy
(D) tuberculin skin testing
(E) pain management

(D) is correct. The Mantoux tuberculin test is administered intradermally.

65. Which site is used in administering intradermal injections?

(A) lateral thigh
(B) deltoid
(C) stomach
(D) upper arm
(E) forearm

(E) is correct. The inner center aspect of the forearm, as well as the upper chest and upper back, is an intradermal injection site.

66. When administering an intradermal injection, a visible sign of proper technique is a

(A) slight allergic reaction
(B) small wheal
(C) needlestick mark
(D) small cyst
(E) discoloration of the site

(B) is correct. Intradermal injections enter only the top level of skin where the substance injected leaves a wheal or bubble on the skin.

67. Which site can be used for subcutaneous injections?

(A) deltoid
(B) forearm
(C) upper chest
(D) buttocks
(E) abdomen

(E) is correct. Subcutaneous injections are administered in the abdomen, upper outer arm, anterior thigh, and subscapular portion of the back.

68. Which site can be used for intramuscular injections?

(A) upper chest
(B) abdomen
(C) vastus lateralis
(D) forearm
(E) subscapular portion of back

(C) is correct. Intramuscular injections can be given in the deltoid, vastus lateralis, and the gluteus medius muscles.

69. The muscle site most commonly used for administering tetanus boosters in adults is

(A) quadriceps
(B) vastus lateralis
(C) deltoid
(D) gluteus medius
(E) biceps

    (C)   is correct.

70. The muscle site that is considered the safest for an intramuscular injection is

(A) vastus lateralis
(B) deltoid
(C) gluteus medius
(D) quadriceps
(E) gluteus maximus

    (A)   is correct. The vastus lateralis muscle has fewer major blood vessels located in it and is considered safest.

71. When administering intramuscular injections in the dorsogluteal muscle, there must be care not to damage the

(A) femur
(B) spinal cord
(C) sciatic nerve
(D) iliac crest
(E) pelvic girdle

    (C)   is correct. To avoid the sciatic nerve, draw an imaginary line from the greater trochanter of the femur to the posterior superior iliac spine, and inject above and lateral to the imaginary line.

72. The agency that issues universal precautions pertaining to the handling of body fluids is the

(A) DEA
(B) OSHA
(C) FDA
(D) AAMA
(E) AMA

    (B)   is correct. OSHA is the Occupational Safety and Health Administration.
    (A)   DEA is the Drug Enforcement Agency.
    (C)   FDA is the Food and Drug Administration.
    (D)   AAMA is the American Association of Medical Assistants.
    (E)   AMA is the American Medical Association.

73. Epinephrine for allergic reactions is administered

(A) SC (subcutaneous)
(B) IM (intramuscular)
(C) IV (intravenous)
(D) Z-track (deep intramuscular)
(E) ID (intradermal)

    (A)   is correct.

74. A small sealed glass tube that contains medication is called a/an

(A) single-dose vial
(B) multidose vial
(C) ampule
(D) prefilled cartridge
(E) none of the above

    (C)   is correct.

75. To remove all of the medication from the neck of an ampule

  (A) gently shake the ampule
  (B) gently roll the ampule
  (C) tip the ampule upside down
  (D) gently tap the neck of the ampule on the counter
  (E) snap your thumb and middle finger gently against the tip of the ampule

  (E) is correct. Tapping the ampule in this manner rids the neck of the medication. Do not use your bare fingers to break the neck of the ampule to remove the medication.

76. A formula that is frequently used in dosage calculations is

  (A) $D/Q \times H$
  (B) $D/H \times Q$
  (C) $H/Q \times D$
  (D) $Q/D \times H$
  (E) $Q/H \times D$

  (B) is correct. $D/H \times Q$ means desired strength divided by the strength on hand, multiplied by the quantity per cc of the on-hand strength. This equals the quantity to be given for the desired strength.

77. The physician has ordered 50 mg of Demerol to be administered. Demerol on hand is 25 mg/cc. How much should be given?

  (A) 0.5 cc
  (B) 1 cc
  (C) 1.5 cc
  (D) 2 cc
  (E) 2.5 cc

  (D) is correct. 50 mg divided by 25 mg multiplied by 1 cc equals 2 cc.
      $50/25 = 2 \times 1\ cc = 2\ cc$

78. The physician has ordered 5 mg of Compazine to be administered. Compazine on hand is 10 mg/cc. How much should be given?

  (A) 0.5 cc
  (B) 1 cc
  (C) 2 cc
  (D) 2.5 cc
  (E) 3 cc

  (A) is correct. 5 mg divided by 10 mg multiplied by 1 cc equals 0.5 cc.
      $5/10 = 0.5 \times 1\ cc = 0.5\ cc$

79. The physician has ordered 1,000 mg of Keflin to be administered. Keflin on hand is 1 g/2 cc. How much should be given?

  (A) 0.5 cc
  (B) 1 cc
  (C) 2 cc
  (D) 2.5 cc
  (E) 3 cc

  (C) is correct. 1,000 mg equals 1 g multiplied by 2 cc equals 2 cc.
      $1,000\ mg = 1\ g;\ 1/1 = 1 \times 2\ cc = 2\ cc$

80. The physician has ordered 250 mg of penicillin to be administered. Penicillin on hand is 0.25 g/5 cc. How much should be given?

(A) 1 cc   (D) 4 cc

(B) 2 cc   (E) 5 cc

(C) 3 cc

    (E) is correct. 250 mg divided by 250 mg multiplied by 5 cc equals 5 cc.
0.25 g = 250 mg; 250/250 = 1 $\times$ 5 cc = 5 cc

CHAPTER 24

PATIENT EDUCATION AND NUTRITION

1. The most effective combination of teaching methods for the older adult is

   (A) lecture, printed materials, and models
   (B) lecture, return demonstration, and programmed instruction
   (C) role play, group teaching, and return demonstration
   (D) video, test of knowledge, and group teaching
   (E) all of the above

   > (A) is correct. The most effective combination of teaching methods for older adults is lecture, printed materials to refresh their memory, and models for demonstration of the concepts.

2. When writing instructional booklets to teach diabetics nutritional planning, which statement is TRUE?

   (A) use of medical terminology is fine as long as detailed definitions are given
   (B) sprinkle material with medical abbreviations so the patient will know this is medical education
   (C) combine several ideas into one grouping in order to save space
   (D) avoid the use of too many examples
   (E) none of the above are true

   > (E) is correct.

3. Patients who must learn new skills are best taught using

   (A) group teaching
   (B) demonstration
   (C) programmed instruction
   (D) simulations
   (E) role play

   > (B) is correct. The demonstration method of teaching is appropriate for patients who must learn a new skill, such as giving their own insulin injections.
   >
   > (A) Group teaching brings together patients who have common learning needs.
   >
   > (C) Programmed instructions are printed instructions that force the learner to understand one concept before going on to the next.
   >
   > (D) Simulations create a pretend scenario for learning purposes.
   >
   > (E) Role playing is using a short play or scenario in which the learner participates in "playing out" the story.

4. Building learning on what has been learned rather than creating a new set of knowledge is known as

(A) role playing
(B) group teaching
(C) simulation
(D) past experience
(E) programmed instruction

    (D) is correct. Building learning on what has already been learned is known as past experience.

    (A) Role playing is using a short play or scenario in which the learner participates in "playing out" the story.

    (B) Group teaching brings together patients who have common learning needs.

    (C) Simulations create a pretend scenario for learning purposes.

    (E) Programmed instructions are printed instructions that force the learner to understand one concept before going on to the next.

5. One of the disadvantages of programmed instruction is that it

(A) requires learner decision making
(B) may exclude significant facts
(C) may be impersonal and boring
(D) is limited to a small group
(E) may be threatening

    (C) is correct. Programmed instruction may be impersonal and boring if it is not well constructed.

6. The advantage of a printed handout is that it

(A) gives visual reinforcement
(B) involves the patient in the learning process
(C) offers direct application of the skill
(D) shows proportions and relationships
(E) all of the above

    (A) is correct. Printed materials offer a visual reinforcement for the learner of material that has been presented by the medical assistant.

7. Which of the following statements is TRUE?

(A) the intellectual capacity of the older adult diminishes with age
(B) long-term memory is often decreased in the older adult
(C) short-term memory is often increased in the older adult
(D) older adults frequently take longer to process new material
(E) none of the above are true

    (D) is correct. The older adult may take longer to process new material. However, intellectual capacity does not necessarily diminish with age.

8. In regard to using medical abbreviations in patient teaching

(A) use only the ones that pertain to the current medical condition
(B) do NOT use abbreviations with the patient
(C) use only very common ones
(D) use them all since the patient should understand the physician's vocabulary
(E) quiz the patient to be sure he or she understands

(B) is correct. It is better not to use medical abbreviations at all with patients.

9. Which situation is a potential legal dilemma for the CMA?

(A) the patient asks for information regarding an alternative treatment for breast cancer

(B) the patient asks for a list of the foods that her baby, who has diarrhea, can eat

(C) the patient is discharged after day surgery for a hernia repair with only an instructional pamphlet

(D) the patient states that he or she won't follow instructions, so none are given

(E) all of the above

(E) is correct.

10. The process by which food is broken down mechanically and chemically in the alimentary canal is called

(A) regurgitation   (D) hydrogenation
(B) ingestion   (E) obesity
(C) digestion

(C) is correct. Digestion is the process by which food is broken down mechanically and chemically in the alimentary canal.

(A) Regurgitation is the process of food that has entered the stomach coming back up into the mouth. This is also called vomiting.

(B) Ingestion occurs when food or drink is taken orally.

(D) Hydrogenation is a process of changing an unsaturated fat to a solid saturated fat by the addition of hydrogen.

(E) Obesity is an abnormal amount of fat on the body of an individual who is 20 percent over the average weight for his or her age, sex, and/or height.

11. A person is considered obese when the individual is what percent over the average weight for his or her age, sex, and/or height?

(A) 10 percent   (D) 25 percent
(B) 15 percent   (E) 30 percent
(C) 20 percent

(C) is correct. A person is considered obese when that individual is 20 percent over the average weight for his or her age, sex, and height.

12. The average adult stomach holds approximately

(A) ½ quart   (D) 2 quarts
(B) 1 quart   (E) 5 quarts
(C) 1½ quarts

(C) is correct. The average adult stomach holds approximately 1½ quarts.

13. Approximately 25 percent of all the energy released by nutrients is used by the body to carry on its normal functions. The rest becomes

(A) heat
(B) fat
(C) sugar
(D) muscle
(E) bone

(A) is correct. The remaining 75 percent of energy released by nutrients becomes heat.

14. The six classifications of nutrients are carbohydrates, protein, fat, water, vitamins, and

(A) sugars
(B) antioxidants
(C) insulin
(D) minerals
(E) fructose

(D) is correct. Minerals are one of the six classifications of nutrients.

15. The recommended daily number of glasses of water is

(A) 2 to 4
(B) 4 to 6
(C) 6 to 8
(D) 8 to 10
(E) 10 to 12

(C) is correct. Six to eight glasses of water is the recommended daily amount.

16. An example of a simple sugar is

(A) sucrose
(B) fructose
(C) lactose
(D) maltose
(E) milk sugar

(B) is correct. Fructose is an example of a simple sugar.

17. An example of a complex carbohydrate is

(A) pasta
(B) potatoes
(C) broccoli
(D) grapefruit
(E) all of the above

(E) is correct.

18. The nutrient "building blocks" of the body, which form the base of each living cell, are

(A) minerals
(B) carbohydrates
(C) fats
(D) vitamins
(E) proteins

(E) is correct. Proteins are the "building blocks" of the body, which form the base of each living cell.

19. An example of a water-soluble vitamin is

(A) vitamin A
(B) vitamin B
(C) vitamin D
(D) vitamin E
(E) vitamin K

    (B) is correct. Vitamin B is an example of a water-soluble vitamin. Fat-soluble vitamins are vitamins A, D, E, and K.

20. What are the food sources for the water-soluble vitamin Niacin?

(A) egg yolks, legumes, and meat
(B) enriched cereals, tuna, peanuts, liver, and poultry
(C) beef, milk, and shellfish
(D) milk, yeast, wheat germ, almonds, and egg white
(E) eggs, pork, yeast-enriched cereals, and nuts

    (B) is correct. Enriched cereals, tuna, peanuts, liver, and poultry are good sources of Niacin.
    (A) Egg yolks, legumes, and meat are good sources of biotin.
    (C) Beef, milk, and shellfish are sources of vitamin B_{12}.
    (D) Milk, yeast, wheat germ, almonds, and egg white are sources of vitamin B_2.
    (E) Eggs, pork, yeast-enriched cereals, and nuts are sources of vitamin B_1.

21. The disease scurvy was found to be caused by a deficiency in vitamin

(A) A
(B) B
(C) C
(D) D
(E) E

    (C) is correct. Scurvy was found to be caused by a deficiency in vitamin C.

22. The disease rickets, which produced bowed legs in young babies and children, is caused by a deficiency of vitamin

(A) A
(B) B
(C) C
(D) D
(E) K

    (D) is correct. Rickets is caused by a deficiency of vitamin D.

23. According to the food pyramid issued by the U.S. Department of Agriculture, the number of servings of vegetables per day should be

(A) 1–2
(B) 2–3
(C) 3–5
(D) 6–11
(E) none of the above

    (C) is correct. The average American diet should contain 3 to 5 servings of vegetables per day.

24. According to the food pyramid, the number of servings of bread, cereal, rice, and pasta is

(A) 1–2　　　　　　　　　　　　(D) 5–6
(B) 2–3　　　　　　　　　　　　(E) 6–11
(C) 3–5

　　　(E) is correct. The average American diet should contain 6 to 11 servings of bread, cereal, rice, and pasta per day.

25. Fat contains how many calories of energy per gram?

(A) 2　　　　　　　　　　　　　(D) 7
(B) 4　　　　　　　　　　　　　(E) 9
(C) 5

　　　(E) is correct. Fat contains 9 calories of energy per gram. Both proteins and carbohydrates contain 4 calories of energy per gram.

26. A good source of vitamin B_1 is

(A) milk　　　　　　　　　　　　(D) molasses
(B) yeast-enriched cereals　　　　(E) pork
(C) bananas

　　　(B) is correct. Yeast-enriched cereals are a good source of vitamin B_1.

27. Calcium and phosphorus absorption is facilitated by vitamin

(A) A　　　　　　　　　　　　　(D) D
(B) B　　　　　　　　　　　　　(E) E
(C) C

　　　(D) is correct. Vitamin D facilitates the absorption of calcium and phosphorus.

28. The recommended percentage of foods from proteins in the daily diet is

(A) 5 percent　　　　　　　　　(D) 30 percent
(B) 8 percent　　　　　　　　　(E) 50 percent
(C) 12 percent

　　　(C) is correct. The recommended percentage of foods from proteins in the daily diet is 12 percent.

29. A BRAT diet has been ordered for Emily Krenz, who is 2 years old. What foods will be included on that diet?

(A) baby cereal　　　　　　　　(D) bananas and rice
(B) milk　　　　　　　　　　　　(E) vegetables
(C) strained meat

　　　(D) is correct. The BRAT diet includes Bananas, Rice, Applesauce, and Toast.

30. Another name for a high-fiber diet is

(A) BRAT
(B) low residue
(C) high residue
(D) bland
(E) soft

(C) is correct. A high-residue diet is the same as a high-fiber diet.

31. When restricting food on a 1,200-calorie diet that is being adapted for a diabetic patient using food exchange lists, what needs to be remembered?

(A) the food pyramid
(B) the amount of exercise the patient has
(C) 1,200 calories may be too restrictive for a diabetic patient
(D) vitamins A, B, C, D, E, K
(E) all of the above

(E) is correct.

32. An example of a complex carbohydrate is

(A) jelly
(B) table sugar
(C) orange
(D) syrup
(E) honey

(C) is correct. An orange is an example of a complex carbohydrate. All the other examples are simple carbohydrates (simple sugars).

33. Which of the following statements about cholesterol is TRUE?

(A) all cholesterol is bad
(B) good cholesterol is low-density lipoprotein (LDL)
(C) there is no evidence that high cholesterol is linked to disease
(D) cholesterol is an essential element normally found in the body
(E) the information "cholesterol 0 mg," found on a food label, means that there is no fat present

(D) is correct. Cholesterol is an essential element normally found in the body.

34. The lipoprotein that is classified as a "bad cholesterol" is the same as

(A) HDL
(B) LDL
(C) total cholesterol
(D) saturated fat
(E) none of the above

(B) is correct. Lipoprotein, or "bad cholesterol," is the same as LDL.

CHAPTER 25

ELECTROCARDIOGRAPHY, RADIOLOGY, AND PHYSICAL THERAPY

1. The heart is located

   (A) on the right side of the chest
   (B) entirely on the left side of the chest
   (C) behind the scapula
   (D) between the lungs
   (E) just to the right of the liver

   (D) is correct. The heart is located between the lungs and slightly to the left side of the body.

2. The serous inner membrane lining of the heart is the

   (A) myocardium
   (B) endocardium
   (C) pericardium
   (D) pacemaker
   (E) cardiac cycle

   (B) is correct. The endocardium is the serous inner membrane lining of the heart.
   (A) The myocardium is the muscular middle layer of the heart.
   (C) The pericardium is the double-walled sac surrounding the heart.
   (D) The pacemaker is the portion of cardiac electrical tissue that establishes the beat. This is also known as the sinoatrial (SA) node.
   (E) The cardiac cycle is one heartbeat, designed arbitrarily as P, Q, R, S, and T. It consists of contraction and relaxation of both atria and ventricles. It is one pulse.

3. The primary purpose of the heart valves is to

   (A) force blood through the chambers of the heart
   (B) prevent blood from rushing through the heart too fast
   (C) separate the chambers of the heart
   (D) prevent the backward flow of blood
   (E) none of the above

   (D) is correct. The primary purpose of the heart valves is to prevent the backward flow of blood.

4. When listening to the heart with a stethoscope, the sound heard is actually the

   (A) epicardium
   (B) the closing of the heart valves
   (C) pacemaker
   (D) myocardium
   (E) pericardium

(B)   is correct. The sound heard through the stethoscope is actually the closing of the heart valves.

(A)   The epicardium is the outer layer of the heart.

(C)   The pacemaker of the heart is located in the sinoatrial node and is silent.

(D)   The myocardium of the heart is the muscular middle layer of the heart.

(E)   The pericardium of the heart is the double-walled sac surrounding the heart.

5. The SA node, located in the right atrium of the heart, is known as the

   (A)   sensor
   (B)   electrode
   (C)   sinoatrial node
   (D)   pacemaker of the heart
   (E)   C and D

   (E)   is correct. The sinoatrial (SA) node is known as the pacemaker of the heart.

   (A)   A sensor is a device that detects electrical charges, also called an electrode.

   (B)   An electrode and sensor are the same.

6. The SA node is located in or on the

   (A)   right atrium
   (B)   right ventricle
   (C)   apex
   (D)   valve between right atrium and right ventricle
   (E)   septum between atria

   (A)   is correct. The SA node is located in or on the right atrium.

7. The "little spark" that begins or starts the heartbeat originates in the

   (A)   Purkinje fibers
   (B)   vagus nerve
   (C)   SA node
   (D)   AV node
   (E)   artificial pacemaker

   (C)   is correct. The SA node produces the "little spark" that begins or starts the heartbeat and sets its pace. The SA node has a rate between 60 and 80 impulses per minute.

   (A)   The Purkinje fibers extend from the right and left bundle branches of the heart to the ventricular walls and cause the ventricles to contract.

   (B)   The vagus nerve is the 10th cranial nerve. It affects the actions of the heart, pharynx, larynx, lungs, bronchi, esophagus, stomach, small intestines, and gallbladder.

   (D)   The atrioventricular (AV) node is a cardiac muscle located in the lower right atrial septum.

   (E)   An artificial pacemaker is one that is surgically implanted into a patient's chest, which will automatically control the rate of the heart.

8. The correct order of stimulation in the electrical conduction system of the heart is

(A) bundle of HIS, AV node, SA node, bundle branches, Purkinje network
(B) AV node, SA node, bundle of HIS, bundle branches, Purkinje network
(C) SA node, AV node, bundle of HIS, bundle branches, Purkinje network
(D) Purkinje network, Purkinje fibers, SA node, AV node
(E) bundle of HIS, SA node, AV node, bundle branches, Purkinje network

(C) is correct. The order of stimulation in the electrical conduction of the heart originates in the SA node and moves through the AV node, bundle of HIS, bundle branches, and Purkinje network.

9. The portion of the EKG that relates to ventricular depolarization is the

(A) P wave
(B) QRS complex
(C) T wave
(D) U wave
(E) P-R interval

(B) is correct. The QRS complex is the portion of the EKG that relates to ventricular depolarization.

(A) The P wave is the first upward deflection and represents atrial depolarization (contraction).

(C) The T wave represents the electrical repolarization (recovery), which gives the cells time to recharge in preparation for ventricular depolarization (contraction).

(D) The U wave, when present, is a small upward deflection, which occurs after the T wave.

(E) The P-R interval occurs at the beginning of the P wave and ends at the onset of the QRS wave. It represents the conduction of the electrical impulse through the atria from the SA node to the AV node.

10. The contraction and relaxation of both atria and ventricles equal

(A) one cardiac cycle
(B) two cardiac cycles
(C) three cardiac cycles
(D) four cardiac cycles
(E) none of the above

(A) is correct. One cardiac cycle consists of the contraction and relaxation of both atria and ventricles.

11. The electrical state of the heart in which the cardiac cells are in a state of resting is

(A) depolarization
(B) polarization
(C) negatively charged
(D) A and C
(E) B and C

(E) is correct. During the state of polarization, the cardiac cells are in a state of rest and are negatively charged.

12. When the cardiac cells are discharging a positively charged electrical impulse, which creates a contraction, they are said to be in a state of

(A) repolarization   **(D)** rest
(B) depolarization   **(E)** none of the above
(C) polarization

       (B)   is correct. The cardiac cells are in a state of depolarization when they are discharging a positive electrical impulse and in a state of contraction.
       (A)   Repolarization or recovery occurs when cardiac cells are transformed from a state of depolarization (active) to a state of polarization (rest).
       (C)   Polarization occurs when the cardiac cells are negatively charged and in a state of rest.

13. What wave on an EKG reflects the repolarization of the ventricles?

(A) P wave   **(D)** U wave
(B) QRS wave   **(E)** none of the above
(C) T wave

       (C)   is correct. The T wave reflects the repolarization of the ventricles.
       (A)   The P wave reflects the electrical impulse coming from the atria.
       (B)   The QRS wave represents the electrical impulse as it passes through the ventricles.
       (D)   The U wave, when present, is the small upward deflection that follows a T wave.

14. An electrocardiogram is a

(A) recording of the mechanical action of the heart
(B) recording of the voltage with respect to time
(C) technique for making recordings of heart activity
(D) machine used to make cardiac tracings
(E) recording of the size of the heart

       (B)   is correct. An electrocardiogram is a recording of the voltage with respect to time.

15. An electrocardiogram is also referred to as an

(A) ECG   **(D)** A and B only
(B) EKG   **(E)** A, B, and C
(C) EEG

       (D)   is correct. The abbreviations ECG and EKG both mean electrocardiogram.
       (C)   EEG stands for electroencephalogram, which is a study of the electrical impulses of the brain.

16. Another name for an electrode is a/an

(A) lead   **(D)** channel
(B) tracing   **(E)** artifact
(C) sensor

(C) is correct. An electrode is also called a sensor.

(A) A lead is an electrical connection to the body to receive data from a specific combination of sensors.

(B) A tracing is a recording of data.

(D) On an EKG machine capable of receiving more than one signal at once, a channel is the pathway for one signal.

(E) An artifact is a deflection caused by electrical activity other than from the heart. This is an irregular and erratic marking.

17. Normally, a complete ECG/EKG consists of how many sensors and how many leads?

(A) 8, 10   (D) 12, 10
(B) 10, 10   (E) 10, 12
(C) 6, 12

(E) is correct. A complete ECG/EKG consists of 10 sensors and 12 leads.

18. The type of EKG sensors that appear to be small suction cups are called

(A) styluses   (D) leads
(B) electrolytes   (E) none of the above
(C) Welch electrodes

(C) is correct. The small suction cup sensors are known as Welch electrodes.

(A) A stylus is the penlike apparatus on an EKG machine that records the electrical impulses onto the EKG paper.

(B) Electrolytes are the gel materials applied to the skin to enhance contact between the skin and the sensor.

(D) Leads are the electrical connections to the body to receive data from a combination of sensors.

19. The only cardiac sensor that is NOT actually used in the recording of an EKG is the

(A) LL   (D) LA
(B) RL   (E) all of the above are used
(C) RA

(B) is correct. The right leg (RL) is used to ground the system. The left arm (LA), right arm (RA), and left leg (LL) are all used in recording the EKG.

20. A lead is

(A) one negative pole   (D) all of the above
(B) one positive pole   (E) none of the above
(C) one ground

(D) is correct. A lead consists of one negative pole, one positive pole, and a ground (the right leg).

21. Remembering all of the EKG leads and sensors can be facilitated by visualizing the

   (A) Einthoven's triangle
   (B) chambers of the heart
   (C) polarization and repolarization of the heart
   (D) alphabet
   (E) none of the above

        (A) is correct. Einthoven's triangle is a method for picturing where the leads should be placed.

22. The landmarks for the chest leads for an EKG are the sternum, both clavicles, the left axilla, and the

   (A) right axilla
   (B) supracostal space
   (C) fourth intercostal space
   (D) third intercostal space
   (E) second intercostal space

        (C) is correct. The fourth intercostal space is used as a landmark for the chest leads.

23. The time markers printed on all EKG paper are referred to as

   (A) 1-second markers
   (B) 2-second markers
   (C) 3-second markers
   (D) 4-second markers
   (E) 5-second markers

        (C) is correct. The time markers on the EKG paper are referred to as 3-second markers. They are found at the top of single-channel paper and between channels in multichannel paper.

24. The small squares on EKG paper are

   (A) 1 mm square and represent 0.0 mv of voltage
   (B) 1 mm square and represent 0.1 mv of voltage
   (C) 5 mm square and represent 0.5 mv of voltage
   (D) 5 mm square and represent 0.1 mv of voltage
   (E) none of the above

        (B) is correct. The small squares on EKG paper are 1 mm square and represent 0.1 mv of voltage.

25. To use the EKG to estimate heart rate, you would

   (A) use the "six-second method"
   (B) begin at one 3-second marker and go to the right for 2 additional markers
   (C) count the number of QRS complexes between the first and third markers and add a zero
   (D) all of the above
   (E) none of the above

        (D) is correct. The "six-second method" can be used to estimate the heart rate by beginning at one 3-second marker and moving to the right for 2 additional markers (6 seconds). Then count the number of QRS complexes between the first and third markers and add a zero to get the heart rate.

26. A normal P wave is how many squares/blocks on the EKG paper?

(A) 2.5
(B) 3
(C) 3–5
(D) can be all of the above
(E) none of the above

    (B) is correct. A normal P wave is 3 squares or blocks on the EKG paper.
    (A) The duration of the QRS complex is normally 2.5 squares wide.
    (C) The PR interval is normally 3 to 5 small blocks wide.

27. The paper on an EKG machine, as part of an international standard, moves at the rate of

(A) 10 mm per second
(B) 15 mm per second
(C) 20 mm per second
(D) 25 mm per second
(E) 30 mm per second

    (D) is correct. The paper on an EKG machine moves at the rate of 25 mm per second.

28. When performing an EKG, if the baseline begins to drift to such a degree that it exceeds the parameters of the graph

(A) stop the procedure, standardize, and begin again
(B) reduce the sensitivity from 1 to ½
(C) decrease the speed with which the paper moves through the machine
(D) all of the above
(E) none of the above

    (B) is correct. If the baseline begins to drift to such a degree that it exceeds the parameters of the graph, reduce the sensitivity from 1 to ½.

29. A deflection on an EKG tracing caused by electrical activity other than from the heart is known as a/an

(A) isoelectric line
(B) wave
(C) segment
(D) artifact
(E) interval

    (D) is correct. An artifact is a deflection on an EKG tracing caused by electrical activity other than from the heart.
    (A) The isoelectric line, or baseline, is the point on an EKG line in which there is no electrical charge or activity. This is a flat line on the EKG recording.
    (B) A wave, or deflection, is any upward or downward deviation from zero or the isoelectric (baseline) line.
    (C) A segment on an EKG tracing is the time from the end of one phase to the beginning of another phase. This is the distance between selected wave marks but not including them.
    (E) An interval is the time between the beginning of one phase and the beginning of the next phase.

30. The degree of variation from zero, up or down, in recording the electrical output of the heart is known as the

(A) isoelectric line
(B) baseline
(C) deflection

(D) amplitude
(E) none of the above

 (C) is correct. The degree of variation from zero, up or down, in recording the electrical output of the heart is known as the deflection.

31. During an EKG, a tense muscle or a muscular contraction may produce an artifact called a/an

(A) erratic stylus defect
(B) somatic tremor
(C) AC interference

(D) baseline shift
(E) none of the above

 (B) is correct. A somatic tremor artifact is produced by a tense muscle or muscular contraction during the process of taking an EKG.

32. An artifact in leads 1, 2, and AVR would cause you to recheck the sensors attached to which body part?

(A) chest
(B) left arm
(C) left leg

(D) right arm
(E) right leg

 (D) is correct.

33. A standard limb lead monitors voltage from

(A) any limb sensor
(B) any two limb sensors
(C) the chest sensor

(D) two of the following: RA, LL, RL
(E) two of the following: RA, LA, LL

 (E) is correct. A standard limb lead monitors voltage from two of the following: RA, LA, LL.

34. Lead V1 of the precordial chest leads is placed at the

(A) fourth intercostal space just to the left of the sternum
(B) fourth intercostal space just to the right of the sternum
(C) line midway between leads V2 and V4
(D) left midaxillary line at the same level as V4
(E) left midclavicular line in the fifth intercostal space

 (B) is correct. Lead V1 is placed at the fourth intercostal space just to the right of the sternum.
 (A) Lead V2 is placed at the fourth intercostal space just to the left of the sternum.
 (C) Lead V3 is placed at the line midway between leads V2 and V4.
 (D) Lead V6 is placed at the left midaxillary line at the same level as lead V4.
 (E) Lead V4 is placed at the left midclavicular line in the fifth intercostal space.

35. Lead I of the limb leads measures electrical activity from the

(A) left arm to left leg (LA to LL)
(B) right arm to left leg (RA to LL)
(C) right arm to left arm (RA to LA)
(D) augmented vector right side
(E) augmented vector left side

    (C)   is correct. Lead I of the limb leads measures electrical activity from the right arm to the left arm (RA to LA).

    (A)   Lead III of the limb leads measures electrical activity from the left arm to the left leg (LA to LL).

    (B)   Lead II of the limb leads measures electrical activity from the right arm to the left leg (RA to LL).

    (D)   The augmented vector for the right side is indicated by aVR.

    (E)   The augmented vector for the left side is indicated by aVL.

36. The marking codes used on the older models of EKG machines indicate lead III as

(A) .
(B) ..
(C) ...
(D) ---
(E) -.

    (C)   is correct. Three dots (...) mark lead III on the EKG paper.

    (A)   One dot (.) indicates lead I.

    (B)   Two dots (..) indicate lead II.

    (D)   Three dashes (---) indicate AVF lead.

    (E)   A dash and dot (-.) indicate V1 lead.

37. When performing an EKG on a patient with a right lower leg cast, the leg sensors are

(A) on the left leg
(B) on both upper legs
(C) on both upper arms
(D) on the bottom of the feet
(E) eliminated

    (B)   is correct. The leg sensors are placed on both upper legs when performing an EKG on a patient with a right lower leg cast.

38. A majority of patients who have had a heart attack have an EKG tracing that exhibits

(A) PACs
(B) PVCs
(C) a PAT
(D) a ventricular fibrillation
(E) AV heart block

    (B)   is correct. Premature ventricular contractions (PVCs) appear in the heart tracings of a majority of patients who have had a heart attack.

    (A)   Premature atrial contractions (PACs) occur when an early P wave appears before expected, usually from a source outside the sinus node.

    (C)   A paroxysmal atrial tachycardia (PAT) is a common arrhythmia, seen in young adults with normal hearts. There are no visible P waves. The atrial rate is between 140 and 250/minute.

    (D)   Ventricular fibrillation appears on the EKG tracing as irregular and rounded waves in which the contractions are uncoordinated. Death may occur in as little as 4 minutes with ventricular fibrillation.

(E) An AV heart block occurs when the node is diseased and does not conduct the impulse well. There are three types: first-degree, second-degree, and third-degree heart blocks.

39. An elevated T wave may be present on a patient's EKG when the patient

(A) is suffering an acute myocardial infarction
(B) is suffering from ischemia
(C) is taking digitalis
(D) has enlarged ventricles
(E) has an elevated serum potassium

(E) is correct. An elevated T wave may be present if the patient has an elevated serum potassium blood level.
(A) An acute myocardial infarction may be apparent on an EKG with an ST elevation.
(B) Ischemia may be evidenced by a flat, inverted T wave on the EKG.
(C) The drug digitalis may cause an ST depression on the EKG tracing.
(D) Enlarged ventricles may be indicated by a tall R wave on the EKG.

40. One of the dangers of performing a stress test in the medical office is the risk of a

(A) tachycardia   (D) all of the above
(B) bradycardia   (E) none of the above
(C) heart attack

(C) is correct. One of the dangers of performing a stress test in the medical office is the risk of the patient suffering a heart attack. This is the reason that emergency equipment and a physician should always be in the medical office when a stress test is administered.

41. A device used to record cardiac activity while the patient is ambulatory for at least 24 hours is called a/an

(A) ECG   (D) Holter monitor
(B) portable EKG   (E) none of the above
(C) cardiac stress monitor

(D) is correct. A Holter monitor is a device used to record cardiac activity while the patient is ambulatory for at least 24 hours.

42. The test performed to evaluate lung volume and capacity in a patient is called a

(A) spirometry procedure   (D) total lung capacity
(B) pulmonary function test   (E) none of the above
(C) pulmonary volume test

(B) is correct. A pulmonary function test is performed to evaluate lung volume and capacity in a patient.

43. A COPD patient may use what instrument to monitor his or her breathing at home?

(A) oximeter
(B) spirometer
(C) peak flowmeter
(D) pressurized oxygen meter
(E) none of the above

> (C) is correct. A peak flowmeter is used by the patient to monitor his or her breathing at home.

44. Which of the following procedures, relating to x-rays, are NOT performed by medical assistants?

(A) instruct the patient
(B) handle x-ray film
(C) position the patient
(D) interpret x-ray film
(E) prepare the patient

> (D) is correct. The MA does not interpret x-ray film. Only a physician can interpret x-rays. In some states, only licensed personnel are permitted to assist with radiological procedures.

45. Secondary radiation is

(A) emitted by the direct x-ray beam
(B) scattered from the patient being x-rayed
(C) emitted through the radiology walls
(D) the second beam of x-ray coming from equipment
(E) none of the above

> (B) is correct. Secondary radiation is scattered from the patient being x-rayed.

46. An example of contrast medium is

(A) lidocaine
(B) epinephrine
(C) sodium chloride
(D) barium oxylate
(E) barium sulfate

> (E) is correct. Barium sulfate is a contrast medium that is used for radiological procedures, such as the upper and lower gastrointestinal (GI) series.

47. If a patient notices a white stool after having a lower GI, what advice can be given?

(A) drink plenty of fluids
(B) eat a large meal
(C) take an antacid product
(D) take a laxative
(E) only a physician can give medical advice

> (E) is correct. Only a physician can give medical advice.

48. A radiological procedure that does not require a contrast medium is a/an

(A) IVP
(B) mammogram
(C) LGI
(D) UGI
(E) cholecystogram

> (B) is correct. A mammogram is a radiological procedure that does not require a contrast medium.

49. A patient is scheduled for an IV pyelogram. This is an examination of the

(A) gallbladder
(B) small intestine
(C) kidneys, ureters, and bladder
(D) colon
(E) pyloric sphincter of the stomach

> (C) is correct. An IV pyelogram is an x-ray examination of the kidneys, ureters, and bladder after the intravenous injection of a dye.

50. A symptom the patient should NOT expect after having radiation treatments is

(A) hair loss
(B) nausea
(C) diarrhea
(D) hemorrhage
(E) irritated throat

> (D) is correct. The patient should not experience hemorrhage after receiving radiation therapy. The other symptoms mentioned in the question may be present to some extent.

51. NPO means

(A) nothing by mouth except water
(B) nothing by mouth after the procedure
(C) only clear fluids
(D) nothing by mouth
(E) nothing by mouth except medications

> (D) is correct. NPO means nothing by mouth (including food, water, and medications).

52. The electrical activity of a muscle is recorded using which test?

(A) somatosensory evoked potential (SEP)
(B) electromyography (EMG)
(C) evoked potential studies (EPS)
(D) brain stem auditory evoked response (BAER)
(E) none of the above

> (B) is correct. The electrical activity of a muscle is recorded using an electromyography (EMG) test.

53. The process that provides a medicinal or healthful effect is called

(A) suppuration
(B) erythema
(C) therapeutic
(D) contraindicated
(E) supination

(C) is correct. A therapeutic process provides a medicinal or healthful effect.
(A) Suppuration is the formation of pus.
(B) Erythema is redness of the skin.
(D) Contraindicated means a thing is not recommended.
(E) Supination means to turn the palm or hand anteriorly.

54. When applying hot compresses, the correct temperature is

(A) 90°F
(B) 105°F
(C) 115°F
(D) 120°F
(E) 125°F

(B) is correct. The correct temperature when applying a hot compress is 105°F.

55. Moist heat application includes which of the following?

(A) hypothermia blanket
(B) aquamatic K-pad
(C) warm-water bottle
(D) heat lamp
(E) sitz bath

(E) is correct. A sitz bath is a combination of warm and moist heat. The other examples are only warm, not moist, heat.

56. Movement that bends a body part backward is

(A) inversion
(B) supination
(C) pronation
(D) dorsiflexion
(E) rotation

(D) is correct. Dorsiflexion is a movement that bends a body part backward.

57. Range-of-motion exercises performed without assistance from another person are

(A) AROM
(B) PROM
(C) active resistive
(D) A and B
(E) none of the above

(A) is correct. Active range-of-motion (AROM) exercises are performed without assistance from another person.
(B) Passive range-of-motion (PROM) exercises require a therapist to put the patient's joints through a full range of motion without assistance from the patient.
(C) Active resistive exercises are performed when the patient applies movement while another person applies resistance.

58. The crutch-walking gait used when a patient is able to bear weight on both legs is

(A) two-point
(B) three-point
(C) four-point
(D) swing-to
(E) swing-through

(C) is correct. The four-point gait is used when the patient is able to bear weight on both legs. To use this gait, the patient moves the right crutch forward, then the left foot, then the left crutch, and then the right foot.

(A) The two-point gait is used in one of two ways. Both crutches can be put ahead, and then the body is moved through with one foot. A second type of two-point gait occurs when a crutch and the opposite foot are moved forward at the same time.

(B) The three-point gait is used when one leg is stronger than the other or when there is no weight bearing on one leg. The crutches are moved forward, and the weaker leg is brought through the crutches.

(D) The swing-to gait occurs when the patient moves the crutches forward and then swings the legs up to the same point.

(E) To use a swing-through gait, the patient moves the crutches forward and then swings the legs past the crutches.

59. The safest type of crutch gait for a person to use is the

(A) one-point gait
(B) two-point gait
(C) three-point gait
(D) four-point gait
(E) swing-through

(D) is correct. The four-point gait is the safest and most stable gait.

60. The type of exercise program that would be prescribed to strengthen the cardio-vascular system is

(A) isotonic
(B) cardiopulmonary
(C) aerobic
(D) isometric
(E) none of the above

(C) is correct. Aerobic exercise is used to strengthen the cardiovascular system.

61. Ultrasound would be effective treating all EXCEPT

(A) tendons
(B) ligaments
(C) soft tissue
(D) bone
(E) none of the above

(D) is correct. Ultrasound is not used to treat bone.

CHAPTER 26

EMERGENCY SERVICES

1. The EMS includes

   (A) you as the first responder
   (B) the hospital ED
   (C) ambulance paramedics
   (D) all of the above
   (E) none of the above

   > (A) is correct. The medical assistant who places an emergency call to 911 is considered the first responder in the emergency medical system (EMS).

2. Your overall impression about the appearance of a patient in shock is

   (A) not affected by your medical experience
   (B) not an important consideration
   (C) an important finding
   (D) irrelevant
   (E) none of the above

   > (C) is correct. Your general overall impression of a patient in shock is extremely important. The patient's skin may be cold to the touch with a pale, almost white appearance. There may be dizziness and diaphoresis (excessive sweating).

3. The best single question to ask patients before you ask them anything else is

   (A) what happened
   (B) why they came into the physician's office
   (C) their name
   (D) which doctor they want to see
   (E) none of the above

   > (C) is correct. If you have the name of the patient, then medical records can be obtained, which may assist in the diagnosis and treatment of this patient.

4. The first thing you need to do when you discover that a patient has arrested is

   (A) call for help
   (B) check the airway
   (C) contact EMS
   (D) drag the person somewhere where you have some room to work
   (E) get the crash cart and charge the defibrillator paddles

   > (A) is correct. Immediately call for some help. Then begin to administer CPR by checking the airway first.

5. Heatstroke is usually defined by a number of signs, in addition to

    (A) a temperature of 104°F
    (B) a rectal temperature of 105°F
    (C) any central temperature over 100°F
    (D) high blood pressure
    (E) none of the above

        (B) is correct. A person suffering from heatstroke should have a rectal temperature taken. A rectal body temperature over 105°F is one of the indications of heatstroke.

6. A patient in a diabetic coma, if administered sugar,

    (A) will have no response to the sugar
    (B) will get worse
    (C) will respond immediately
    (D) would not be given insulin
    (E) none of the above

        (A) is correct. A patient in a diabetic coma will have no response to the sugar. He or she should be given insulin.

7. A patient suffering from an insulin reaction, if administered sugar,

    (A) will have no response to the sugar
    (B) will get worse
    (C) will respond immediately
    (D) would be given insulin
    (E) none of the above

        (C) is correct. Patients suffering an insulin reaction will respond immediately to sugar. They have too much insulin in their system and need to have a dose of sugar or a sugary liquid to offset the insulin. They should not be given insulin.

8. Patients who have suffered a major amputation are very likely to

    (A) be in a state of shock
    (B) suffer from a critical loss of blood
    (C) have other injuries that may be overshadowed at first glance
    (D) be taken somewhere besides a doctor's office for treatment
    (E) all of the above

        (E) is correct.

9. The patient who has been bitten by a rattlesnake

    (A) will have immediate pain and swelling
    (B) does not need to go to the hospital if he or she receives antivenin
    (C) can be treated with coral snake antivenin if rattlesnake venin is unavailable
    (D) has a better chance for recovery if he or she is very young
    (E) needs to have the venom sucked out of his or her wounds

        (A) is correct. There will be immediate pain and swelling with a rattlesnake bite. The patient needs to receive antivenin specific for a rattlesnake bite. He or she should be seen in a hospital even if he or she has received antivenin. The young are especially susceptible to death from poisonous snakebites. The venom should not be sucked out of the wound.

10. Sunburn is

    (A) not really a burn
    (B) most often a first-degree burn
    (C) most often a second-degree burn
    (D) usually safe to treat with cool water and an ointment or cream
    (E) B and D

        (E) is correct. Sunburn is generally a first-degree burn, which responds well to cool water and a cream.

11. Burns are classified in two ways, by depth and

    (A) length   **(D)** type
    (B) breadth   **(E)** none of the above
    (C) surface area

        (C) is correct. Burns are classified by depth and surface area.

12. A burn that results in reddening, a swelling of the epidermis and outer dermis, and a few blisters is said to be a

    (A) first-degree burn   **(D)** all of the above
    (B) second-degree burn   **(E)** none of the above
    (C) third-degree burn

        (B) is correct. A second-degree burn results in reddening, swelling of the epidermis and outer dermis, and blisters.
        (A) A first-degree burn causes reddening and swelling of the epidermis.
        (C) A third-degree burn results in charring of all layers of the skin and at least some deeper structures.

13. To check the responsiveness level of a patient in an emergency, say firmly

    (A) "Are you all right?"
    (B) "Can you hear me?"
    (C) "Shake your head if you can hear me."
    (D) "Can you feel this needlestick?"
    (E) none of the above

        (A) is correct. Say firmly, "Are you all right?" to check the level of consciousness of an emergency patient.

14. When performing CPR on an infant, use

    (A) one hand
    (B) two hands clasped, but with a lighter touch than on the adult
    (C) two fingers from each hand
    (D) two fingers
    (E) none of the above

(D) is correct. Only two fingers should be used to administer CPR to an infant.

15. A person who is suffering cardiac arrest should be administered chest compressions at a rate of

    (A) 12 times a minute
    (B) 15 times a minutes
    (C) 50 to 70 times a minute
    (D) 80 to 100 times a minute
    (E) this person should not receive chest compressions at all

        (D) is correct. Chest compressions should be administered at the rate of 80 to 100 times a minute.

16. When performing CPR on an adult with another medical assistant, use the compressions:breaths ratio of

    (A) 10:1   (D) 15:1
    (B) 5:1   (E) 20:1
    (C) 15:2

        (B) is correct. The ratio of 5 compressions to 1 breath is the correct ratio when performing two-person CPR.

17. When performing one-person CPR on an adult, the compression:breath ratio is

    (A) 10:1   (D) 15:1
    (B) 5:1   (E) 20:1
    (C) 15:2

        (C) is correct. The ratio of 15 compressions to two breaths is the correct ratio when performing one-person CPR.

18. The first thing you should do if conscious patients appear to be choking is

    (A) stand behind them, encircle their abdomen with both arms, and squeeze them
    (B) help them to lie down so they do not fall
    (C) ask them if they are choking
    (D) look down their throat
    (E) none of the above

        (C) is correct. Ask if they are choking. If they can answer you, they are still able to breathe in some air and may be able to cough up the obstruction by themselves. If there is a complete obstruction, then begin the Heimlich maneuver.

19. If a patient is choking and unconscious, place the patient on his or her back on the floor and

    (A) deliver upward chest thrusts
    (B) ventilate, using an airway
    (C) raise the patient's head until the paramedics arrive
    (D) try to administer water in an attempt to arouse the patient
    (E) none of the above

(A) is correct. If a patient is choking and unconscious, place the patient on his or her back on the floor and deliver upward chest thrusts.

20. Another name for the inability to breathe is

(A) syncope   (D) gag reflex

(B) seizure   (E) aspiration

(C) asphyxia

    (C) is correct. Asphyxia is suffocation or the inability to breathe.

    (A) Syncope is a sudden loss of consciousness. This is also called fainting.

    (B) A seizure is the same as a convulsion.

    (D) The gag reflex is a closure of the glottis and constriction of its associated musculature in response to stimulation of the posterior pharynx by an object or substance in that area.

    (E) Aspiration refers to a substance being sucked into an object, such as into the lungs.

21. Closure of the glottis is known as

(A) asphyxia   (D) swallowing

(B) syncope   (E) none of the above

(C) the gag reflex

    (C) is correct. The gag reflex is closure of the glottis.

22. The xiphoid process is the

(A) death of myocardial tissue

(B) relaxation and contraction of heart muscle

(C) membrane that covers the shaft of long bone

(D) piece of cartilage that forms the lowermost tip of the sternum

(E) none of the above

    (D) is correct. The xiphoid process is the piece of cartilage that forms the lowermost tip of the sternum.

    (A) Death of myocardial tissue can occur in a myocardial infarction (heart attack).

    (B) The relaxation and contraction of heart muscle forms the cardiac cycle.

    (C) The membrane that covers the shaft of long bone is the periosteum.

23. A crash cart in a medical office contains everything EXCEPT

(A) emergency medications   (D) heart/lung machine

(B) intubation equipment   (E) all of the above are included

(C) monitor/defibrillator

    (D) is correct. A heart/lung machine is not normally found in a physician's office on a crash cart.

24. A patient presenting with chest pain should be positioned on the examination table with his or her chest and head elevated to an angle of

(A) 10 degrees   (D) 60 degrees

(B) 15 degrees   (E) 90 degrees

(C) 45 degrees

(C) is correct. The patient should be placed in a semi-Fowler's position with the head elevated 45 degrees. This facilitates breathing for the patient.

25. In an emergency situation, a medical assistant needs to be aware that oxygen is always delivered at a relatively high flow rate, such as

(A) 4 liters per minute
(B) 6 liters per minute
(C) 8 liters per minute
(D) 10 liters per minute
(E) 20 liters per minute

(D) is correct. Paramedics will generally deliver oxygen at a high flow rate, such as 10 liters per minute.

26. Patients experiencing an allergic reaction, in addition to other symptoms, may experience a systolic blood pressure below

(A) 40
(B) 60
(C) 80
(D) 100
(E) 150

(D) is correct. The patient suffering an allergic reaction may have a systolic blood pressure reading below 100.

27. People who are bleeding internally (into their digestive system) tend to have firm, oversized abdomens due to the

(A) accumulation of fluid
(B) whole blood that accumulates
(C) presence of gas as a by-product of digested blood
(D) body's reaction to the bleeding
(E) none of the above

(C) is correct. The presence of gas as a by-product of digested blood can cause a patient with internal bleeding to have a firm, distended abdomen.

28. Another name for a mild stroke is

(A) CVA
(B) transient ischemic attack
(C) infarction
(D) syncope
(E) aneurysm

(B) is correct. A transient ischemic attack (TIA) is a name for a small or mild stroke.
(A) A cerebrovascular accident (CVA) is the term for a major stroke or blood clot in the brain.
(C) An infarction is a blood clot causing a heart attack.
(D) Syncope is fainting.
(E) An aneurysm is a weakening or outpouching in the wall of an artery.

29. Perhaps the most important thing a medical assistant can do to assist a patient who is having convulsions is to

(A) prevent the patient from biting his or her tongue
(B) administer oxygen

(C) restrain the patient to prevent injury during the convulsion
(D) guard against any injury such as falling
(E) all of the above

(D) is correct. Guard the patient against injury by assisting them into a flat position.

30. When a diabetic patient takes the prescribed amount of insulin but strays from his or her diet, causing a decrease in blood sugar, it could cause a

(A) diabetic coma
(B) diabetic crisis
(C) crisis known as insulin shock
(D) hyperglycemic reaction
(E) none of the above

(C) is correct. Insulin shock may result when a diabetic patient strays from his or her diet, even though the prescribed amount of insulin is taken.

31. Insulin-dependent diabetes mellitus is

(A) due to a lack of insulin
(B) Type I
(C) Type IA and Type IB
(D) Type II
(E) A, B, and C only

(E) is correct. Diabetes mellitus is due to a lack of insulin in the body. It has a sudden onset. Type I is insulin-dependent diabetes mellitus (IDDM). Type IA develops during the childhood and young adult years. Type IB develops in the adult.
(D) Type II is non-insulin-dependent diabetes mellitus (NIDDM). This type has a slower onset than IDDM.

32. The signs and symptoms of IDDM include

(A) ketonuria and glycosuria
(B) hyperglycemia and polyuria
(C) weight gain
(D) weight loss
(E) A, B, and D

(E) is correct. Ketonuria (ketones excreted in the urine), glycosuria (glucose excreted in the urine), hyperglycemia (elevated blood glucose levels), polyuria (excessive urination), and weight loss are all symptoms of diabetes mellitus Type I (IDDM).

33. Diabetic coma, which occurs when there is a lack of insulin and the body breaks down too much of its fat supply for energy needs, has which of the following signs and symptoms?

(A) diaphoresis, shock, pale, clammy skin that is hot and dry
(B) ketonuria, ketoacidosis, drowsiness, skin that is hot and dry
(C) deep labored breathing
(D) A and C
(E) B and C

(E) is correct. The signs of diabetic coma include ketonuria (ketone bodies in the urine), ketoacidosis (lowered pH resulting in a fruity breath odor), drowsiness, dry and hot skin, and deep labored breathing.
(A) Diaphoresis, shock with pale, clammy skin, and disorientation are signs of an insulin reaction or insulin shock.

Post-Test Simulation

(300-question, 4-hour post-test)

GENERAL

(Covers medical terminology; anatomy and physiology; medical science and type of medical practice; medical law and ethics; quality assurance and government regulations; and human relations and psychology.)

Directions: Select the ONE best answer for each of the following multiple-choice questions.

1. An additional term added at the end of a medical term that can change the meaning of the word is a

   (A) prefix
   (B) suffix
   (C) word root
   (D) combining vowel
   (E) combining form

2. A hepatic lobectomy is the surgical removal of a lobe of the

   (A) lung
   (B) heart
   (C) stomach
   (D) liver
   (E) gallbladder

3. The lymphatic system includes the

   (A) ureters, urethra, bladder, and kidneys
   (B) uterus, fallopian tubes, ovaries, vagina, and mammary glands
   (C) spleen, lymph vessels, and lymphocytes
   (D) brain, spinal cord, and nerves
   (E) muscles, tendons, bones, and joints

4. The combining vowel or form is

   (A) usually a consonant
   (B) a word root and usually the vowel "o"
   (C) can be found after a prefix
   (D) can be found before a suffix
   (E) B, C, and D only

5. The presence of red blood cells in the urine might indicate

   (A) poorly controlled diabetes and dehydration
   (B) starvation and ingestion of large amounts of aspirin
   (C) arsenic poisoning and trauma
   (D) the use of blood thinners, a reaction to transfusion, and burns
   (E) C and D

6. The Patient's Bill of Rights, which describes the patient-physician relationship, was developed by the

   (A) AAMA
   (B) AMA
   (C) AHA
   (D) CDC
   (E) AMT

7. Nephrosclerosis is a/an

   (A) abnormal renal softening
   (B) abnormal renal hardening
   (C) floating kidney
   (D) bleeding from the kidney
   (E) abnormal softening of nerve tissue

8. The body's constant state of attempting to maintain a balance or equilibrium is called

   (A) histology
   (B) microbiology
   (C) bacteriology
   (D) homeostasis
   (E) homeopathy

9. What plane divides the body into superior and inferior sections?

   (A) transverse
   (B) sagittal
   (C) frontal
   (D) coronal
   (E) midsagittal

10. The study of psychoanalysis was first developed by

    (A) Maslow
    (B) Freud
    (C) Kübler-Ross
    (D) Sabin
    (E) Salk

11. The prefix medi- means

    (A) bad
    (B) one
    (C) middle
    (D) midnight
    (E) one-half

12. What microorganism causes the flu?

    (A) *Escherichia coli (E. coli)*
    (B) human immunodeficiency virus
    (C) hepatitis C
    (D) *Staphylococcus bacterium*
    (E) *Haemophilus influenzae* type B

13. The external genitalia of the female is the

    (A) uterus
    (B) vulva
    (C) cervix
    (D) ovary
    (E) fallopian tube

14. The earliest principles of ethical conduct, established to govern the practice of medicine, were known as the

(A) Patient's Bill of Rights
(B) Code of Ethics of the AAMA
(C) AMA Principles of Medical Ethics
(D) Code of Hammurabi
(E) Hippocratic oath

15. The effacement period of delivery occurs when the

(A) placenta or afterbirth is delivered
(B) buttocks first appear
(C) cervix begins its thinning stage
(D) breast begins secreting milk
(E) cervix is fully dilated

16. The plural form of autopsy is

(A) the same as the singular form
(B) formed by dropping the -y and adding -ies
(C) not necessary since there is never more than one autopsy performed at one time
(D) formed by dropping the -y and adding -es
(E) formed by adding 's

17. A panhysterosalpingo-oophorectomy is

(A) excision of the uterus, including the cervix
(B) surgical removal of the fallopian tubes and ovaries
(C) surgical removal of the uterus, cervix, ovaries, and fallopian tubes
(D) surgical removal of the uterus, cervix, and fallopian tubes, leaving the ovaries for production of estrogen
(E) incision into the uterus for the purpose of viewing the cervix and fallopian tubes

18. A visceral covering refers to

(A) a covering of an organ
(B) the wall of an organ
(C) a direction toward the head
(D) a direction toward the tail or feet
(E) a direction toward the front of the body

19. A tumor of the 8th cranial nerve sheath is called a/an

(A) melanoma
(B) fibroma
(C) lymphoma
(D) acoustic neuroma
(E) sarcoma

20. The combining form enter/o means

(A) liver
(B) blood
(C) uterus
(D) clot
(E) intestines

21. The drug lithium is often prescribed for

(A) manic-depressive disorder
(B) depression
(C) anxiety
(D) schizophrenia
(E) hallucinations

22. The surgical puncture of the chest wall to remove fluids is a

(A) tracheostomy
(B) thoracentesis
(C) tracheotomy
(D) pneumonectomy
(E) thoracostomy

23. An order for persons as well as documents to appear in court is a/an

(A) appellant
(B) defendant
(C) plaintiff
(D) subpoena
(E) felony

24. A pulmonary disease from the dust in the droppings of pigeons and chickens is

(A) *Pneumocystis carinii*
(B) hyaline membrane disease
(C) histoplasmosis
(D) pneumonia
(E) pleurisy

25. A condition in which a person can see things close up but not in the distance is called

(A) presbyopia
(B) astigmatism
(C) esotropia
(D) hyperopia
(E) myopia

26. The combining form carcin/o means

(A) cell
(B) colon
(C) bladder
(D) cancer
(E) gallbladder

27. The absence of oxygen in the blood is

(A) anoxia
(B) hypoxia
(C) anoxemia
(D) stridor
(E) dyspnea

28. Polio vaccine was developed by

(A) Walter Reed
(B) William Morton
(C) Jonas Salk
(D) Albert Sabin
(E) C and D

29. An example of a cognitive disorder is

(A) Alzheimer's disease
(B) delirium
(C) dementia
(D) amnesia
(E) all of the above

30. The color portion of the eye is the

(A) conjunctiva
(B) iris
(C) choroid
(D) retina
(E) sclera

31. A blood count to measure the volume of erythrocytes in a given volume of blood is

(A) hemoglobin
(B) differential
(C) WBCs
(D) hematocrit
(E) platelets

32. A physician who discontinues treatment of a patient without providing sufficient notice of withdrawal or coverage could be charged with

(A) breach of contract
(B) abandonment
(C) a felony
(D) a misdemeanor
(E) rule of discovery

33. Mild emotional disturbances that impair judgment are

(A) hysteria
(B) depression
(C) neuroses
(D) psychoses
(E) hallucinations

34. The disease(s) transmitted by airborne droplets is/are

(A) scabies, impetigo, and wound infections
(B) tuberculosis
(C) measles and chickenpox
(D) meningitis
(E) B and C

35. The suffix -ptosis means

(A) abnormal enlargement
(B) abnormal drooping
(C) abnormal narrowing
(D) abnormal enlargement
(E) abnormal softening

36. Which Canadian physician, along with two other physicians, discovered insulin for the treatment of diabetes mellitus?

(A) Paul Ehrlich
(B) Alexander Fleming
(C) Frederick Banting
(D) William Harvey
(E) Joseph Lister

37. A radiologic procedure to examine a cross-section of the brain after dye has been injected is a/an

(A) MRI
(B) CT scan
(C) PET
(D) TENS
(E) angiogram

38. The reporting of communicable diseases by a physician is a

(A) *respondeat superior*
(B) *res ipsa loquitur*
(C) public duty
(D) misdemeanor
(E) standard of care

39. A chronic disorder of the nervous system with fine tremors, muscular weakness, rigidity, and a shuffling gait is

(A) Huntington's chorea
(B) Reye's syndrome
(C) Bell's palsy
(D) tic douloureaux
(E) Parkinson's disease

40. PPE refers to

(A) clothing
(B) charting
(C) ethical standards
(D) reimbursement
(E) emergency treatment

41. Which nerve carries facial impulses and controls muscles for chewing?

(A) trochlear
(B) oculomotor
(C) trigeminal
(D) olfactory
(E) facial

42. Maslow's hierarchy of needs includes safety and security, which is Level

(A) I
(B) II
(C) III
(D) IV
(E) V

43. An intense feeling of persecution and jealousy is called

(A) narcissism
(B) antisocial reaction
(C) sociopathic behavior
(D) paranoia
(E) hallucination

44. Blood cells that release histamine and heparin to damaged tissue are

(A) neutrophils
(B) basophils
(C) leukocytes
(D) monocytes
(E) erythrocytes

45. The time frame, as set by federal and state governments, during which legal actions can be brought forward is known as

(A) aging of legal actions
(B) standard of care
(C) informed consent
(D) statute of limitations
(E) subpoena *duces tecum*

46. The innominate or hipbone is also called the

(A) epiphysis
(B) diaphysis
(C) periosteum
(D) ileum
(E) os coxae

47. Which agency provides research, prevention, control, and education for the prevention of disease?

(A) OSHA
(B) DEA
(C) BNDD
(D) CDC
(E) FDA

48. Which portion of the brain controls body temperature?

(A) hypothalamus
(B) thalamus
(C) cerebellum
(D) cerebrum
(E) diencephalon

49. Rhinohexis is a nasal

(A) discharge
(B) rupture
(C) suture
(D) surgical repair
(E) bleeding

50. Which protects persons who provide emergency care to injured persons from litigation?

(A) Code of Hammurabi
(B) abandonment
(C) statute of limitations
(D) Good Samaritan Act
(E) public duty

51. A congenital defect present at birth, which is a combination of four symptoms resulting in pulmonary stenosis, septal defect, abnormal blood supply to the aorta, and hypertrophy of the right ventricle, is

(A) mitral stenosis
(B) patent ductus arteriosus
(C) coronary ischemia
(D) tetralogy of Fallot
(E) aortic stenosis

52. Which portion of the brain controls motor function?

(A) temporal lobe
(B) frontal lobe
(C) parietal lobe
(D) occipital lobe
(E) diencephalon

53. Another name for the mitral valve is

(A) tricuspid valve
(B) pulmonary semilunar valve
(C) aortic semilunar valve
(D) intraventricular septum
(E) bicuspid valve

54. Which physician helped conquer yellow fever?

(A) Jenner
(B) Semmelweiss
(C) Ehrlich
(D) Reed
(E) Banting

55. Which hormone, produced by the ovaries, stimulates the development of secondary sex characteristics?

(A) oxytocin
(B) progesterone
(C) estrogen

(D) testosterone
(E) prolactin

56. According to the laws governing the collection of accounts receivable, telephone calls must be made between the hours of

(A) 8 AM and 6 PM
(B) 8 AM and 9 PM
(C) 7 AM and 6 PM

(D) 7 PM and 8 AM
(E) 9 AM and 5 PM

57. The ordinary skill and care that medical practitioners, such as physicians and medical assistants, must use, which is the same skill commonly used by other practitioners, is referred to as

(A) quality of care
(B) standard of care
(C) peer review
(D) a comprehensive performance report (CPR)
(E) A and C

58. A disease resulting from a deficiency in adrenocortical hormone, in which there may be an increased pigmentation of the skin, generalized weakness, and weight loss, is

(A) Addison's disease
(B) Bright's disease
(C) Graves' disease

(D) Hashimoto's disease
(E) myxedema

59. An abnormal increase in the forward curvature of the lumbar spine is also called

(A) scoliosis
(B) humpback of the spine
(C) kyphosis

(D) lordosis
(E) periositis

60. The suffix -lysis means

(A) presence of
(B) disease of
(C) destruction of

(D) inflammation of
(E) removal of

61. A coiled tube that lies on top of the testes within the scrotum is the

(A) seminal vesicles
(B) epididymis
(C) prostate gland

(D) vas deferens
(E) urethra

62. The prefix later/o means

(A) back
(B) front
(C) side

(D) middle
(E) away from

63. Clara Barton is known for her establishment of

  (A) nursing as a profession
  (B) medical assisting as a profession
  (C) the American Red Cross
  (D) the Centers for Disease Control
  (E) the profession of public health

64. Which is caused by a deficiency of vitamin C?

  (A) gout
  (B) scoliosis
  (C) scabies
  (D) scurvy
  (E) rickets

65. Implied consent occurs when

  (A) a person rolls up a sleeve to have blood drawn
  (B) a parent allows a medical assistant to give an immunization to his or her child
  (C) a patient allows a technician to take an EKG
  (D) a patient permits a physician to examine him or her
  (E) all of the above

66. The area between the lungs is called the

  (A) mediastinum
  (B) diaphragm
  (C) abdominopelvic cavity
  (D) dorsal cavity
  (E) ventral cavity

67. A dangerous form of skin cancer is

  (A) Kaposi's sarcoma
  (B) squamous cell carcinoma
  (C) malignant melanoma
  (D) lupus erythematosus
  (E) basal cell carcinoma

68. When the state in which a physician is applying for a license accepts the state licensing requirements from a state in which the physician already holds a license, this is called

  (A) reciprocity
  (B) licensure
  (C) endorsement
  (D) certification
  (E) registration

69. A skin disorder in which the skin becomes taut, thick, and leatherlike is

  (A) eczema
  (B) cellulitis
  (C) scleroderma
  (D) neoplasm
  (E) psoriasis

70. The organization that has developed a continuing education program for the RMA is the

  (A) AAMA
  (B) AMT
  (C) AMTIE
  (D) ACCST
  (E) CAAHEP

71. Myx/o refers to

(A) muscles
(B) mucus
(C) maxilla bone
(D) meninges
(E) spinal cord

72. Professional negligence is also called

(A) criminal action
(B) malpractice
(C) litigation
(D) arraignment
(E) neglect of duty

73. Reports completed by physicians, mandated by Congress, that indicate the types of medical services to Medicare patients are

(A) peer review reports
(B) quality assurance reports
(C) competitive performance reports
(D) preferred provider reports
(E) standard of care reports

74. Which type of practice consists of at least 3 physicians who share the same facility and practice medicine together?

(A) associate practice
(B) solo proprietorship
(C) partnership
(D) group practice
(E) A and C

75. A bone located at the base of the nasal septum is the

(A) sphenoid
(B) parietal
(C) occipital
(D) temporal
(E) vomer

76. A system developed for Medicare to identify reimbursement per condition in a hospital is the

(A) PPO
(B) DRG
(C) EPO
(D) HMO
(E) PCPA

77. A government-controlled insurance for the indigent patient is called

(A) Blue Cross and Blue Shield
(B) Medicare
(C) Medicaid
(D) DRGs
(E) POLs

78. The word root/combining form for the bones of the toes and fingers is

(A) metacarp/o
(B) phalang/o
(C) tibi/o
(D) fibul/o
(E) humer/o

79. A benign neoplasm, which is also referred to as warts, is a/an

(A) furuncle   (D) scabies
(B) ringworm   (E) eczema
(C) verruca

80. A continuous natural sequence of events, without interruption, that produces an injury is known as

(A) precedent   (D) deposition
(B) contributory negligence   (E) breach of duty
(C) proximate cause

81. A medical procedure in which the body and skin are not entered is called a/an

(A) surgical procedure   (D) noninvasive procedure
(B) operative procedure   (E) A and B
(C) invasive procedure

82. A physician specializing in physical medicine and rehabilitation is a

(A) psychiatrist   (D) physician's assistant
(B) physiatrist   (E) physical therapist
(C) psychologist

83. The upper arm bone is the

(A) clavicle   (D) ulna
(B) scapula   (E) humerus
(C) radius

84. A registered nurse who has completed graduate work in a specialty area is called a/an

(A) RN   (D) PA
(B) LPN   (E) CNA
(C) NP

85. A written exception to an insurance contract expanding, decreasing, or modifying coverage of an insurance policy is called

(A) capitation   (D) rider
(B) co-payment   (E) member fee
(C) premium

86. A bone fracture that results in an incomplete break, in which one side of the bone is broken and the other side is bent, is

(A) greenstick   (D) comminuted
(B) transverse   (E) Colles'
(C) compound

87. The basic or general health care a patient receives is

(A) inpatient care

(B) proprietary care

(C) primary care

(D) hospice care

(E) ambulatory care

88. A physician specializing in diagnosing the abnormal changes in tissues that are removed during surgery and postmortem is a/an

(A) oncologist

(B) hematologist

(C) pathologist

(D) radiologist

(E) internist

89. The four D's of negligence include duty, dereliction or neglect of duty, direct cause, and

(A) damages

(B) defamation of character

(C) direct assault

(D) deposition

(E) breach of duty

90. Mortality rate refers to

(A) the incidence of disease in a given population

(B) the incidence of communicable disease in a given population

(C) the incidence of deaths in a given population

(D) the number of handicapped persons in a given population

(E) the number of birth defects in a given population

91. The kneecap is also called the

(A) tibia

(B) femur

(C) popliteal

(D) patella

(E) fibula

92. The initials "OD" stand for

(A) doctor of optometry

(B) doctor of osteopathy

(C) doctor or dental medicine

(D) doctor of chiropractic medicine

(E) doctor of medicine

93. Regulation Z of the Consumer Protection Act requires that a patient

(A) be notified verbally about the interest charges on the outstanding bill

(B) be notified in writing about all interest charges

(C) not be abandoned by the physician

(D) be notified in writing about any interest charges if more than four payments are being made

(E) be notified in writing about any interest charges if more than two payments are being made

94. Surgical removal of a portion of the eardrum is called

(A) myringoscopy
(B) myringectomy
(C) myringotomy
(D) tympanorrhexis
(E) otoscopy

95. A formal written description of an accident that has occurred in a medical setting is a/an

(A) subpoena
(B) stipend
(C) evaluation
(D) incident report
(E) deposition

96. A managed care organization in which there is a fee-for-service on a prepayment or capitation program with the ability to choose one's own physician is a/an

(A) HMO
(B) PPO
(C) EPO
(D) DRG
(E) SNF

97. The clear transparent portion of the eye that is responsible for allowing light to enter the interior of the eye is the

(A) retina
(B) pupil
(C) cornea
(D) sclera
(E) choroid

98. A pouch or saclike area in the first 2 to 3 inches at the beginning of the large intestine is the

(A) appendix
(B) sigmoid colon
(C) jejunum
(D) duodenum
(E) cecum

99. A physician specializing in the care of the elderly is a

(A) gastroenterologist
(B) nephrologist
(C) cardiologist
(D) gerontologist
(E) gynecologist

100. The organs found in the dorsal cavity include

(A) vertebra, spinal cord, and brain
(B) lungs and heart
(C) stomach, spleen, liver, and intestines
(D) uterus, ovaries, and fallopian tubes
(E) A and B

ADMINISTRATIVE

(Covers oral and written communication; appointment scheduling; computers in medicine; fees, billing, collections, and credit; health information technology; insurance and coding; and office management.)

Directions: Select the ONE best answer for each of the following multiple-choice questions.

1. An examination of the financial records of a medical practice for determining the accuracy of the records is called a/an

   (A) account
   (B) reconciliation
   (C) audit
   (D) receipt
   (E) ledger

2. Words that have opposite meanings are

   (A) synonyms
   (B) antonyms
   (C) acronyms
   (D) eponyms
   (E) phonyms

3. The amount of money the insured must pay either monthly or annually for a plan is the

   (A) co-pay
   (B) coinsurance
   (C) premium
   (D) claim
   (E) deductible

4. Newspapers and periodicals are sent via what category of mail?

   (A) first class
   (B) second class
   (C) third class
   (D) fourth class
   (E) any class is acceptable

5. A requirement by some insurance companies for the patient to receive prior approval before having a procedure performed is called

   (A) deductible
   (B) co-pay
   (C) preapproval
   (D) preauthorization
   (E) C and D

6. Money owed by the physician/medical practice to companies and vendors is called

   (A) audit
   (B) double-entry bookkeeping
   (C) accounts receivable
   (D) accounts payable
   (E) aging account

7. The abbreviation a.c. means

   (A) place on account
   (B) take by mouth
   (C) nothing to eat or drink
   (D) take before meals
   (E) none of the above

8. The amount of eligible charges the patient pays each calendar year before the insurance plan begins to pay benefits is called a

   (A) premium
   (B) preapproval
   (C) co-pay
   (D) coinsurance
   (E) deductible

9. Names of diseases based on the physician who first documented the disease are

   (A) acronyms
   (B) antonyms
   (C) synonyms
   (D) phonyms
   (E) eponyms

10. The two-letter abbreviation for Maine is

    (A) MN
    (B) MA
    (C) ME
    (D) MI
    (E) MM

11. A record for each patient of charges, payments, and current balance is a/an

    (A) receipt
    (B) superbill
    (C) ledger
    (D) accounts payable record
    (E) medical record

12. What law affects the hiring of new employees and is an amendment of Title VII of the Civil Rights Act of 1972?

    (A) ERISA
    (B) EEOA
    (C) FUTA
    (D) FICA
    (E) ADA

13. A report completed after the surgeon has performed a procedure is a/an

    (A) consultation report
    (B) autopsy report
    (C) operative note
    (D) pathology report
    (E) history report

14. A small payment given to a physician for a service such as a professional speech is a/an

    (A) royalty
    (B) patent
    (C) draft
    (D) honorarium
    (E) A and D

15. A patient who has moved and left no forwarding address for future billing is a/an

    (A) estate claim
    (B) statute of limitations case
    (C) assignment of benefits case
    (D) skip
    (E) bankruptcy

16. Technology that recognizes the voice of the person dictating the medical record is the

(A) TDD
(B) TActile CONverter
(C) VRT
(D) A and C
(E) A and B

17. Which proofreader's mark means to insert brackets?

(A) [\]
(B) [/]
(C) [
(D)]
(E) ins

18. The International Classification of Diseases is contained in

(A) CPT
(B) DRGs
(C) ICD-9-CM
(D) CPT
(E) HMOs

19. A list of options that is available to the computer user is called

(A) default
(B) sort
(C) error message
(D) menu
(E) batch

20. Current procedural terminology for purposes of categorizing medical procedures in an office is

(A) CPT
(B) CPR
(C) ICD-9-CM
(D) CHAMPUS
(E) CHAMPVA

21. A to-do list should NOT include

(A) nonroutine tasks
(B) complicated tasks
(C) tasks in a random order
(D) dated entries
(E) completed tasks

22. The U.S. Post Office will deliver what type of mail beyond normal working hours?

(A) first-class priority
(B) registered
(C) special handling
(D) special delivery
(E) all of the above

23. ICD-9 coding allows for visits not directly related to illness or injury. This is called

(A) volume codes
(B) V codes
(C) E codes
(D) CPT codes
(E) A and B

24. A patient's written authorization allowing insurance companies to directly pay the physician is called

(A) assignment of plan
(B) assignment of benefits
(C) assignment of action
(D) accounts receivable record
(E) claim against estate

25. Medical insurance that covers retired military personnel and their dependents is

(A) Medicaid
(B) VA insurance
(C) workers' compensation
(D) CHAMPVA
(E) CHAMPUS

26. Which part of speech indicates the relationship between the noun and/or pronoun that follows it and another word in the sentence?

(A) adjective
(B) adverb
(C) interjection
(D) preposition
(E) conjunction

27. What portion of the approved amount for medical service does Medicare pay?

(A) 20 percent
(B) 80 percent
(C) 75 percent
(D) 50 percent
(E) none

28. An assignment of benefits form

(A) must be signed
(B) is good for 1 year
(C) is good indefinitely
(D) A and B
(E) A and C

29. Special handling can be requested for what category of mail?

(A) first class
(B) second class
(C) third class
(D) fourth class
(E) C and D

30. A fifth code number is used in the ICD-9-CM coding system when

(A) there is a V code
(B) there is an E code
(C) certain conditions are present
(D) there is an R/O diagnosis
(E) all of the above

31. Most disability insurance plans have a waiting period of how long before they go into effect?

(A) 1 year
(B) 6 months
(C) 6–8 weeks
(D) 2–4 weeks
(E) 1 week

32. In order to meet postal standards, the last line in an address on an envelope must not exceed

(A) 15 characters
(B) 20 characters
(C) 25 characters
(D) 30 characters
(E) there is no limit

33. What portion of the medical bill does the Medicare patient (or a supplemental insurance carrier) pay?

(A) none
(B) 80 percent
(C) 20 percent
(D) 100 percent
(E) 75 percent

34. The portion of the bill that the patient is responsible for is called a/an

(A) reasonable fee
(B) co-pay
(C) customary fee
(D) usual fee
(E) aging account

35. The maximum weight (in pounds) for priority mail is

(A) 20
(B) 40
(C) 50
(D) 70
(E) 100

36. What type of paperwork can be filed when a Medicare patient wishes to become eligible for Medicaid?

(A) assignment of benefits form
(B) CHAMPUS form
(C) crossover claim
(D) preauthorization form
(E) indemnity schedule

37. A written request for insurance reimbursement is called a/an

(A) claim
(B) premium
(C) deductible
(D) co-pay
(E) indemnity schedule

38. The final determination of what fee is charged for a medical service is made by the

(A) office manager
(B) medical assistant
(C) insurance company
(D) government
(E) physician

39. The length of time that an amount of money is owed to the medical practice is called the

(A) estate claim
(B) assignment of benefits
(C) aging account
(D) accounts receivable
(E) accounts payable

40. A telephone call should be answered on the

(A) first ring
(B) second ring
(C) third ring
(D) fourth ring
(E) fifth ring

41. A brief statement issued to a patient when a payment is made in cash or by check is called a/an

(A) superbill
(B) ledger card
(C) audit
(D) receipt
(E) accounts receivable record

42. A synonym for the word otolaryngology is study of

(A) cancer
(B) the eye
(C) the ear and throat
(D) the ear, nose, and throat
(E) the reproductive system

43. What condition results in the patient being protected by the court from all collection attempts?

(A) statute of limitations
(B) bankruptcy
(C) accounts receivable
(D) aging account
(E) reconciliation

44. A fee that is charged for a procedure by the majority of physicians who have similar training, and who work in the same geographic and socioeconomic area, is a

(A) customary fee
(B) usual fee
(C) reasonable fee
(D) A and B
(E) A and C

45. A telephone caller who has been placed on hold should be checked back with every

(A) 5 minutes
(B) 1 minute
(C) 30 seconds
(D) 20 seconds
(E) 10 seconds

46. A tag appears along with Jean Jones's chart that states "See Mrs. Daniel Jones." This is known as

(A) editing
(B) cross-referencing
(C) cross-tagging
(D) alphabetic filing
(E) unit filing

47. Scheduling two patients during the same time period is called

(A) open office hours
(B) modified wave scheduling
(C) wave scheduling
(D) double booking
(E) specified time scheduling

48. When a patient expires, the bill is sent to

(A) a collection agency
(B) the deceased person's last known address
(C) the estate
(D) the deceased person's insurance company
(E) no one—the bookkeeper will write off the amount

49. Receiving prior approval from an insurance company before a patient can undergo surgery is called a/an

(A) preauthorization
(B) crossover claim
(C) assignment of benefits
(D) rider
(E) fee schedule

50. Canceling a patient's debt is called

(A) bankruptcy
(B) claim of estate
(C) statute of limitations
(D) write-off
(E) skip

51. The amount paid by an insurance company for each procedure or service is called a/an

(A) preauthorization
(B) assignment of benefits
(C) customary fee
(D) usual fee
(E) fee schedule

52. Adopting the feelings of someone else as your own is

(A) disassociation
(B) introjection
(C) rationalization
(D) sublimation
(E) compensation

53. A record for billing and insurance purposes of all services provided to a patient in the medical office is the

(A) ledger
(B) receipt
(C) superbill
(D) audit
(E) medical record

54. Dividing each hour of an office schedule into segments of time, with each patient arriving within 15 to 20 minutes of each other, is called

(A) wave scheduling
(B) modified wave scheduling
(C) open hours
(D) specified time
(E) grouping

55. When an account has been referred to a collection agency, the medical assistant must

(A) work with the agency to collect as much of the bill as possible
(B) immediately send out a letter to the patient with this information
(C) call the patient's employer
(D) not make any attempt to collect
(E) A, B, and C

56. Joseph Kelly has been assigned the ID number 633489. To search for the file, you look under 89, then 63, then 34. What system are you using?

(A) unit numbering
(B) middle digit filing
(C) terminal digit filing
(D) straight numbering
(E) service numbering

57. E codes (as part of the ICD-9 coding system)

   (A) give external causes for an injury or illness
   (B) are required for all diagnoses
   (C) are never used
   (D) are part of the CPT coding system, not the ICD-9 system
   (E) A and B

58. The person who is named as the receiving party of a check is the

   (A) payer
   (B) signee
   (C) payee

   (D) maker
   (E) A and B

59. Justifying thoughts or behavior to avoid the truth is

   (A) denial
   (B) disassociation
   (C) rationalization

   (D) regression
   (E) repression

60. An exception to an insurance contract is called a/an

   (A) modifier
   (B) rider
   (C) exemption

   (D) deductible
   (E) claim

61. The maximum time period set by federal and state governments during which certain legal actions can be brought forward is the

   (A) aging analysis
   (B) claim against estate
   (C) accounts receivable collection

   (D) assignment of benefits period
   (E) statute of limitations

62. Scheduling all school physical exam visits during the same day is an example of

   (A) open office hours
   (B) wave scheduling
   (C) double booking

   (D) grouping
   (E) modified wave scheduling

63. A form of communication in which the conversation is directed back to the patient by repeating the words is called reflecting or

   (A) restating
   (B) mirroring
   (C) clarification

   (D) rationalization
   (E) regression

64. A measure of storage capacity within the computer is the

   (A) gigabyte
   (B) megahertz
   (C) kilobyte

   (D) RAM
   (E) A, C, and D

65. A check endorsement that specifies to whom money should be paid is

(A) blank
(B) restrictive
(C) third-party

(D) postdated
(E) debit

66. The magnetic storage drive within the computer is the

(A) A drive
(B) B drive
(C) C drive

(D) D drive
(E) can be any of the above drives

67. The patient should be greeted within how many minutes after arrival?

(A) 8 minutes
(B) 5 minutes
(C) 3 minutes
(D) 1 minute
(E) the patient does not have to be formally greeted after arrival

68. Telephone calls made outside the caller's area code without the assistance of an operator are

(A) station-to-station calls
(B) direct-distance dialing
(C) conference calls

(D) person-to-person calls
(E) collect calls

69. Which filing system is useful in medical offices with relatively few patients, such as heart surgeons specializing in transplants?

(A) service numbering
(B) straight numbering
(C) alphabetical

(D) middle digit filing
(E) terminal digit filing

70. To start up the computer is referred to as a/an

(A) interface
(B) input
(C) menu

(D) boot
(E) CPU

71. When funds are added to an account, this is a

(A) credit
(B) debit
(C) disbursement

(D) reconciliation
(E) liability

72. Appointments should not be "blocked out" more than how many months in advance?

(A) 1 month
(B) 2 months
(C) 3 months

(D) 6 months
(E) 12 months

73. What is the second indexing unit in the name Trudy Ann Denton-Green (Dr.)?

(A) Trudy
(B) Ann
(C) Green
(D) Dr.
(E) Denton-Green

74. The speed with which the computer can move information from one place to another is

(A) kilobyte
(B) megahertz
(C) RAM
(D) ROM
(E) gigabyte

75. Which prohibits discrimination based on race, color, gender, religion, marital status, national origin, or age when extending credit?

(A) Regulation Z
(B) Equal Credit Opportunity Act
(C) ERISA
(D) Truth in Lending Act
(E) FICA

76. The reason the patient is seeing the physician is the

(A) diagnosis
(B) consultation report
(C) past history
(D) chief complaint
(E) referral

77. Changing unacceptable drives for security, affection, and/or power into socially acceptable channels is called

(A) sublimation
(B) repression
(C) rationalization
(D) introjection
(E) repression

78. The "heart" of the computer is the

(A) RAM
(B) ROM
(C) CPU
(D) DOS
(E) floppy disk

79. A medical condition that has been present for an extended period of time is referred to as a/an

(A) acute condition
(B) chronic condition
(C) emergent condition
(D) critical condition
(E) extended condition

80. Which sets the minimum wage that employers are required to pay their employees?

(A) ERISA
(B) ADA
(C) FLSA
(D) ADEA
(E) Title VII

81. A printed copy of data in a computer file is a

    (A) batch   **(D)** database
    (B) catalog   **(E)** hard copy
    (C) menu

82. A numeric filing system generally uses how many digits?

    (A) 3   **(D)** 6
    (B) 4   **(E)** 7
    (C) 5

83. A small piece of electronic hardware that allows the processing of information in a very small space is a

    (A) boot   **(D)** Chip
    (B) diskette   **(E)** megahertz
    (C) DOS

84. The employer's quarterly federal tax return is the

    (A) W-2   **(D)** ERISA
    (B) W-4   **(E)** FUTA
    (C) Form 941

85. A flashing bar or symbol on a computer screen indicating where the next character is placed is called a

    (A) modem   **(D)** disk
    (B) mouse   **(E)** keyboard
    (C) cursor

86. Which designates that payments must be withheld from the employee's paychecks by the employer?

    (A) Employee Retirement Income Security Act (ERISA)
    (B) Federal Unemployment Tax Act (FUTA)
    (C) Federal Insurance Contributions Act (FICA)
    (D) Old-Age Survivors and Disability Insurance (OASDA)
    (E) Title VII

87. The amount of data on 1,000 floppy disks can be stored on how many CD-ROMs?

    (A) 1   **(D)** 15
    (B) 5   **(E)** 100
    (C) 10

88. Defensive behaviors, which are barriers to effective communication, include

    (A) empathy and sympathy
    (B) compensation and rationalization
    (C) disassociation, introjection, and sublimation
    (D) A and B
    (E) B and C

89. Sheets of microfilm

    (A) comprise a numeric system
    (B) are called microfiche
    (C) are the archives
    (D) are the base of a color-coded filing system
    (E) become obsolete

90. The time during which a computer cannot be used due to maintenance or mechanical failure is

    (A) data debugging   **(D)** interface
    (B) backup   **(E)** format
    (C) downtime

91. Which prohibits the unfair employment practices against handicapped persons and those with AIDS?

    (A) ADEA   **(D)** FLSA
    (B) ADA   **(E)** ERISA
    (C) DEA

92. A computer light wand is also called a

    (A) joystick   **(D)** pen
    (B) mouse   **(E)** peripheral
    (C) pad

93. A computer that processes binary or discrete numerical data is the

    (A) ASCII   **(D)** plotter
    (B) disk drive   **(E)** floppy
    (C) digital

94. Medical files relating to patients who have not been seen for period of time, usually 5 years, are

    (A) still active   **(D)** archives
    (B) inactive   **(E)** numeric
    (C) closed

95. Which key on the computer keyboard causes computer operations to become suspended?

    (A) delete   **(D)** backspace
    (B) escape   **(E)** break
    (C) insert

96. A form that is a record of earnings and taxes withheld is the

    (A) W-4   **(D)** ERISA
    (B) W-2   **(E)** Title VII
    (C) Form 941

97. Which stores computer data to process at periodic intervals?

   (A) hard copy
   (B) modem
   (C) database
   (D) batch
   (E) catalog

98. An insurance form that is generally accepted by most insurance companies is

   (A) HCFA-1500
   (B) HCFA-1400
   (C) Medicaid
   (D) there is no one widely accepted form
   (E) insurance companies will accept any standard form

99. A long waiting period may result from which appointment scheduling system?

   (A) double booking
   (B) grouping
   (C) wave
   (D) modified wave
   (E) open booking

100. Medical records that are no longer needed, but that must still be kept, are

   (A) kept for a period of 5 years
   (B) archives
   (C) closed files
   (D) active files
   (E) numeric files

CLINICAL

(Covers infection control; vital signs and measurements; assisting with physical examinations; assisting with medical specialties; assisting with minor surgery; assisting patients with special physical needs; urinalysis; microbiology; hematology; pharmacology and medication administration; patient education and nutrition; electrocardiology, radiology, and physical therapy; and emergency services.)

Directions: Select the ONE best answer for each of the following multiple-choice questions.

1. During the inflammatory response, white blood cells overpower and consume the pathogenic microorganisms in a process called

   (A) suppuration
   (B) phagocytosis
   (C) septicemia
   (D) specific defense
   (E) nonspecific defense

2. The gradual drop of a fever is

   (A) lysis
   (B) crisis
   (C) intermittent
   (D) remittent
   (E) continuous

3. The section of the patient history that is the reason for the office visit is

   (A) past medical history
   (B) personal history
   (C) family medical history
   (D) chief complaint
   (E) assessment by the physician of body systems

4. Which wave on an EKG represents the electrical impulse as it passes through the ventricles?

   (A) T wave
   (B) QRS
   (C) P wave
   (D) U wave
   (E) QRSTU

5. The local anesthetic Xylocaine is

   (A) benzocaine
   (B) procaine
   (C) lidocaine
   (D) chloroprocaine
   (E) mepivacaine

6. Normal specific gravity ranges from

   (A) 1.010 to 1.030
   (B) 1.010 to 1.014
   (C) 1.010 to 1.020
   (D) 1.005 to 1.010
   (E) 1.000 to 1.005

7. The abbreviation ss means

   (A) after meals
   (B) before meals
   (C) hour of sleep
   (D) one-half
   (E) without

8. What color top tube for blood collecting contains heparin?

   (A) red top
   (B) purple top
   (C) purple/lavender top
   (D) marbled top
   (E) green top

9. An accurate axillary temperature registers approximately how many degrees lower than a rectal temperature?

   (A) four
   (B) three
   (C) two
   (D) one
   (E) it registers the same as a rectal temperature

10. The entrance of a disease-producing organism into a cell or organism is referred to as a/an

   (A) disease
   (B) infection
   (C) pathogen
   (D) microorganism
   (E) infestation

11. The smallest-gauge suture material is

    (A) 00
    (B) 000
    (C) 0000
    (D) 00000
    (E) 000000

12. Surgical scrub clothes should

    (A) be white only
    (B) be changed between each patient
    (C) never be worn home
    (D) be washed separately from other surgical scrub clothes
    (E) be sterile

13. A deflection in an EKG caused by electrical activity other than from the heart is a/an

    (A) sensor
    (B) artifact
    (C) tracing
    (D) lead
    (E) channel

14. Signs that are perceptible to others, such as those found by the physician upon examination of the patient, are found in the POMR under

    (A) database
    (B) initial plan
    (C) progress notes
    (D) objective findings
    (E) problem list

15. When taking an aural temperature on a child, the medical assistant should

    (A) gently pull the outer ear downward
    (B) gently pull the outer ear upward
    (C) place the child in a prone position
    (D) use a mercury thermometer
    (E) none of the above

16. A refractometer is used to measure

    (A) pH
    (B) RBCs and WBCs
    (C) glucose
    (D) hemoglobin
    (E) specific gravity

17. A surgical instrument used to grasp is the

    (A) curette
    (B) scalpel
    (C) forceps
    (D) trocar
    (E) sound

18. A procedure in which the body and/or skin is entered is a/an

    (A) elective procedure
    (B) optional procedure
    (C) noninvasive procedure
    (D) invasive procedure
    (E) assessment procedure

19. OS is an abbreviation for

    (A) right eye
    (B) left eye
    (C) right ear
    (D) left ear
    (E) after meals

20. Which aids in the blood-clotting process?

    (A) leukocyte
    (B) reticulocyte
    (C) platelet
    (D) phagocyte
    (E) plasma

21. A form resistant to heat, drying, and chemicals but that can be killed by steam under pressure is

    (A) virus
    (B) TB
    (C) ARC
    (D) spore
    (E) HIV

22. What is used to determine the number of red and white blood cells in a specimen?

    (A) urinometer
    (B) hemacytometer
    (C) specific gravity
    (D) GTT
    (E) hemoglobinometer

23. The "startle" infant reflex test is called the

    (A) China doll reflex
    (B) palmar grasp reflex
    (C) Moro reflex
    (D) rooting reflex
    (E) Apgar scale

24. The small squares on EKG paper are

    (A) 2-mm square and represent 0.1 mv of voltage
    (B) 1-mm square and represent 0.0 mv of voltage
    (C) 1-mm square and represent 0.1 mv of voltage
    (D) 5-mm square and represent 0.1 mv of voltage
    (E) 5-mm square and represent 0.2 mv of voltage

25. A position used for rectal examinations is

    (A) supine
    (B) Fowler's
    (C) Sims'
    (D) knee-chest
    (E) C and D

26. Rx is Latin for

    (A) prescription
    (B) take thou
    (C) mark
    (D) name
    (E) taken by mouth

27. As age increases

(A) respirations increase
(B) pulse rate increases
(C) pulse rate decreases
(D) pulse rate remains the same throughout life
(E) blood pressure decreases dramatically

28. Which instrument fits inside a speculum or scope and assists in guiding the instrument?

(A) probe
(B) obturator
(C) sound
(D) trocar
(E) anoscope

29. Which form of bacteria forms grape-like clusters of pus-producing organisms that stain gram-positive?

(A) diplococci
(B) streptococci
(C) staphylococci
(D) bacilli
(E) spirilla

30. A landmark used for chest leads when taking an EKG is the

(A) 4th intercostal space
(B) 3rd intercostal space
(C) 2nd intercostal space
(D) right axilla
(E) supracostal space

31. A lighted instrument used to examine the superficial rectum is the

(A) anoscope
(B) sigmoidoscope
(C) proctoscope
(D) otoscope
(E) cystoscope

32. A visual examination of the cervix and vagina using a lighted instrument is called

(A) cystoscopy
(B) cystocele
(C) colposcopy
(D) eclampsia
(E) endoscopy

33. Micronase is classified as a/an

(A) antibiotic
(B) antacid
(C) antihypertensive
(D) oral hyperglycemic agent
(E) decongestant

34. The area that is considered sterile on a draped Mayo stand is

(A) inside a 2-inch border
(B) inside a 1-inch border
(C) outside a 2-inch border
(D) outside a 3-inch border
(E) the entire drape is sterile

35. The duration of the PR interval is normally how many blocks wide?

(A) 2.5
(B) 3
(C) 3–5
(D) 5
(E) can be all of the above

36. A glass/mercury thermometer should remain in the anal opening for

(A) 3 minutes
(B) 5 minutes
(C) 10 minutes
(D) 15 minutes
(E) as long as it takes to register

37. Inner ear infection is also called

(A) anacusis
(B) otosclerosis
(C) presbycusis
(D) otitis media
(E) Meniere's disease

38. A position used to treat shock is

(A) Fowler's
(B) Sims'
(C) Trendelenburg
(D) knee-chest
(E) none of the above

39. Diseases caused by fungi are

(A) amebic dysentery, malaria, trichomonas, and giardiasis
(B) Rocky Mountain spotted fever, typhus, rickettsial pox, and trench fever
(C) herpes I and II, HIV, common cold, influenza, hepatitis A and B, polio, and warts
(D) thrush, diphtheria, whooping cough, syphilis, boils, and meningitis
(E) tetanus, athlete's foot, jock itch, ringworm, and candidiasis

40. Acetaminophen is the generic name for

(A) Valium
(B) Demerol
(C) Advil
(D) aspirin
(E) Tylenol

41. Which instrument is used to perform surgery using freezing temperatures?

(A) laser
(B) cryosurgical unit
(C) hyfrecator
(D) trocar
(E) none of the above

42. An increase in intraocular pressure is found in

(A) Cushing's syndrome
(B) lazy eye
(C) cataracts
(D) glaucoma
(E) farsightedness

43. Leads 1, 2, 3 (I, II, III) of an electrocardiogram are called

(A) standard limb or bipolar leads
(B) augmented leads
(C) chest leads
(D) precordial leads
(E) Welch sensors

44. A tetanus booster should be given every

(A) year
(B) 2 years
(C) 5 years
(D) 7 years
(E) 10 years

45. The need to urinate during the night is called

(A) nocturia
(B) dysuria
(C) oliguria
(D) anuria
(E) albuminuria

46. Which instrument is used to test hearing ability?

(A) ophthalmoscope
(B) otoscope
(C) tuning fork
(D) stethoscope
(E) percussion hammer

47. A drug classification that controls bleeding is

(A) hypoglycemic
(B) antihypertensive
(C) antihistaminic
(D) hemostatic
(E) hyperglycemic

48. The normal adult male hemoglobin is

(A) 14 to 18 g/dl
(B) 12 to 16 g/dl
(C) 8 to 12 g/dl
(D) 6 to 8 g/dl
(E) 20 to 30 g/dl

49. Three dashes (---) on EKG paper indicate

(A) lead I
(B) AVF lead
(C) V1 lead
(D) lead II
(E) lead III

50. Which can be caused by either bacteria or a virus?

(A) tetanus
(B) pneumonia
(C) meningitis
(D) malaria
(E) B and C

51. Amyotropic lateral sclerosis is also known as

(A) Bell's palsy
(B) Lou Gehrig's disease
(C) Addison's disease
(D) Bright's disease
(E) Cushing's syndrome

52. The portion of the microscope that regulates the intensity of light is the

(A) substage
(B) diaphragm
(C) rheostat
(D) stage
(E) revolving nosepiece

53. The force or strength of a pulse is referred to as

(A) rhythm
(B) rate
(C) pulse pressure
(D) volume
(E) tone

54. Fainting is also called

(A) syndrome
(B) syncope
(C) myxedema
(D) prognosis
(E) aneurysm

55. Movement that bends a body part backward is

(A) supination
(B) pronation
(C) dorsiflexion
(D) rotation
(E) inversion

56. The position in which the patient is lying face down on the exam table is

(A) Fowler's
(B) Sims'
(C) supine
(D) prone
(E) lithotomy

57. A permanent form of birth control for the male, which consists of cutting the vas deferens, is called

(A) epididymectomy
(B) TUR
(C) orchiectomy
(D) orchidopexy
(E) vasectomy

58. Which schedule of drugs has a moderate to low potential for addiction?

(A) Schedule I
(B) Schedule II
(C) Schedule III
(D) Schedule IV
(E) Schedule V

59. Gram-positive bacteria, when stained, retain the

(A) pink color
(B) violet color
(C) green/blue color
(D) blue color
(E) lavender color

60. The most common site for taking a pulse on an infant or young child is

(A) brachial
(B) pedis
(C) radial
(D) apical
(E) carotid

61. A blood clot causing a heart attack is a/an

(A) aneurysm
(B) infarction
(C) syncope
(D) TIA
(E) CVA

62. Which of the following conditions is NOT favorable for the growth of bacteria?

(A) moisture

(B) temperature of 98.6°F

(C) direct sunlight

(D) oxygen

(E) dampness

63. A crutch gait in which the crutches are moved forward and the weaker leg is brought through the crutches is

(A) swing-through

(B) one-point

(C) two-point

(D) three-point

(E) four-point

64. The branch of medicine that deals with disorders and diseases of the kidney is

(A) neurology

(B) nephritis

(C) urology

(D) nephrology

(E) gynecology

65. The drug classification that produces a lack of feeling, which may be of local or general effect, is

(A) adrenergic

(B) anesthetic

(C) antibiotic

(D) antiseptic

(E) antidote

66. Tests ordered for a CPX include all of the following EXCEPT

(A) CBC

(B) blood chemistry profile

(C) EKG

(D) EEG

(E) visual acuity

67. Burns are classified according to

(A) depth and surface area

(B) pain

(C) length

(D) breadth

(E) age of patient

68. A resuscitation procedure that involves both respiratory and cardiac maneuvers is

(A) CBC

(B) DNR

(C) CVA

(D) CAN

(E) CPR

69. Ringing in the ears is

(A) urticaria

(B) tinnitus

(C) cyanosis

(D) hemoptysis

(E) laryngitis

70. A pulse rate above 100 is called

(A) bradycardia

(B) tachycardia

(C) tachypenia

(D) pulse deficit

(E) pulse pressure

71. When performing two-person CPR, the compression:breath ratio is

(A) 1:10
(B) 10:1
(C) 5:1
(D) 1:5
(E) 15:2

72. The round, raised skin lesions with itching that are a positive sign of reaction to allergy testing are called

(A) nodules
(B) papules
(C) vesicles
(D) macules
(E) wheals

73. To change grams to milligrams, the decimal point is moved how many spaces?

(A) 3 spaces to the left
(B) 3 spaces to the right
(C) 2 spaces to the left
(D) 2 spaces to the right
(E) 1 space to the right

74. A blood test for HIV, used as a backup for ELISA, is

(A) ARC
(B) TIA
(C) Western blot
(D) Eastern blot
(E) RAIU

75. The equivalent metric measurement of the apothecary measurement of 1 oz. is

(A) 5 cc
(B) 10 cc
(C) 15 cc
(D) 30 cc
(E) 50 cc

76. Which measures the intraocular pressure of the eye?

(A) ophthalmoscope
(B) otoscope
(C) penlight
(D) tonometer
(E) litmus paper

77. All of the following may cause the pulse to increase EXCEPT

(A) brain injuries and depression
(B) fever
(C) shock
(D) fear, anxiety, and anger
(E) all of the above cause the pulse rate to increase

78. A surgical opening created in the large intestine for the purpose of allowing waste material to drain is a/an

(A) iliostomy
(B) ileostomy
(C) colostomy
(D) stoma
(E) I & D

79. A recessive hereditary disease caused by lack of an enzyme, which can result in severe mental retardation if not detected soon after birth, is

(A) Down syndrome
(B) PKU
(C) CPU
(D) anaphylactic shock
(E) cystic fibrosis

80. The crushing of gallstones in the common bile duct is called

(A) choledochal
(B) cholelithiasis
(C) cholecystitis
(D) cholelithotripsy
(E) cystolithotripsy

81. A contagious skin disease caused by an egg-laying mite that causes intense itching is

(A) scabies
(B) tinea
(C) verruca
(D) herpes simplex
(E) herpes zoster

82. Which is used to calculate a pediatric dosage based on a child's weight?

(A) Fried's law
(B) Young's rule
(C) West's nomogram
(D) Clark's rule
(E) Westergren test

83. The minute air sacs in the lungs are called

(A) capillaries
(B) bronchioles
(C) alveoli
(D) bronchi
(E) B and C

84. Taking medicine by placing it under the tongue is called

(A) topical
(B) buccal
(C) sublingual
(D) parenteral
(E) inhalation

85. A condition in which acid from the stomach backs up into the esophagus, causing inflammation and pain, is called

(A) ileitis
(B) reflux esophagitis
(C) diverticulosis
(D) intussusception
(E) inguinal hernia

86. An intradermal injection is given for

(A) insulin therapy
(B) iron-replacement therapy
(C) pain management
(D) antibiotic therapy
(E) tuberculin skin testing

87. An overgrowth and thickening of cells in the epithelium is called

(A) lipoma
(B) hemangioma
(C) leukoplakia
(D) keratosis
(E) Kaposi's sarcoma

88. The agency that issues universal precautions pertaining to the handling of body fluids is

(A) FDA
(B) AMA
(C) OSHA
(D) DEA
(E) AAMA

89. A test used to measure the levels of hormones in blood plasma is the

(A) RAIU
(B) RIA
(C) PBI
(D) GTT
(E) T4

90. An unusual or abnormal response to a drug or food is called a/an

(A) toxicity
(B) contraindication
(C) habituation
(D) prophylaxis
(E) idiosyncrasy

91. When a patient needs to collect a routine urine specimen, the patient should be told to fill the container

(A) ½ full
(B) ¾ full
(C) ⅔ full
(D) ⅝ full
(E) completely full

92. A condition resulting in severe pain and constriction around the heart is called

(A) thrombophlebitis
(B) Reynaud's phenomenon
(C) arteriosclerosis
(D) angina pectoris
(E) aortic insufficiency

93. The official federal agency with responsibility for the regulation of food, drugs, cosmetics, and medical devices is the

(A) PDR
(B) DEA
(C) USP-NF
(D) BNDD
(E) FDA

94. Difficulty breathing while lying down is

(A) tachypnea
(B) orthopnea
(C) dyspnea
(D) apnea
(E) bradycardia

95. Cyanosis is due to

(A) an increase in carbon dioxide
(B) a decrease in carbon dioxide
(C) an increase in oxygen
(D) rich oxygen levels
(E) poor carbon dioxide levels

96. A disorder resulting from overactivity of the thyroid, which can result in a crisis situation, is

(A) Cushing's syndrome
(B) myasthenia gravis
(C) Graves' disease
(D) Addison's disease
(E) Bright's disease

97. A shrill, harsh sound heard more clearly during inspiration is called

(A) rales
(B) stertorous sound
(C) rhonchi
(D) stridor
(E) wheeze

98. The result of an excess of ketone bodies in the blood, which can result in death for the diabetic patient if not reversed, is called

(A) thyrotoxicosis
(B) alkalosis
(C) ketoacidosis
(D) myxedema
(E) Cushing's syndrome

99. The average blood pressure reading for adults is

(A) 138/86
(B) 100/65
(C) 118/76
(D) 120/80
(E) 95/65

100. Which of the following will cause a decreased respiratory rate?

(A) allergic reactions
(B) epinephrine
(C) morphine
(D) asthma
(E) fever

POST-TEST ANSWERS

GENERAL
1. B
2. D
3. C
4. E
5. E
6. C
7. B
8. D
9. A
10. B
11. C
12. E
13. B
14. D
15. C
16. B
17. C
18. A
19. D
20. E
21. A
22. B
23. D
24. C
25. E
26. D
27. C
28. E
29. E
30. B
31. D
32. B
33. C
34. E
35. B
36. C
37. B
38. C
39. E
40. A
41. C
42. B
43. D
44. B
45. D
46. E
47. D
48. A
49. B
50. D
51. D
52. B
53. E
54. D
55. C
56. B
57. B
58. A
59. D
60. C
61. B
62. C
63. C
64. D
65. E
66. A
67. C
68. A
69. C
70. C
71. B
72. B
73. C
74. D
75. E
76. B
77. C
78. B
79. C
80. C
81. D
82. B
83. E
84. C
85. D
86. A
87. C
88. C
89. A
90. C
91. D
92. A
93. D
94. B
95. D
96. B
97. C
98. E
99. D
100. A

ADMINISTRATIVE
1. C
2. B
3. C
4. B
5. E
6. D
7. D
8. E
9. E
10. C
11. C
12. B
13. C
14. D
15. D
16. C
17. B
18. C
19. D
20. A
21. E
22. D
23. B
24. B
25. E
26. D
27. B
28. D
29. E
30. C
31. D
32. B
33. C
34. B
35. D
36. C
37. A
38. E
39. C
40. B
41. D
42. C
43. B
44. A
45. C
46. B
47. D
48. C
49. A
50. D
51. E
52. B
53. C
54. B
55. D
56. C
57. A
58. C
59. C
60. B
61. E
62. D
63. B
64. E
65. B
66. C
67. D
68. B
69. C
70. D
71. A
72. D
73. A
74. B
75. B
76. D
77. A
78. C
79. B
80. C
81. E
82. D
83. D
84. C
85. C
86. C
87. A
88. E
89. B
90. C
91. B
92. D
93. C

94. B	20. C	48. A	76. D
95. E	21. D	49. B	77. A
96. B	22. B	50. E	78. C
97. D	23. D	51. B	79. B
98. A	24. C	52. C	80. D
99. C	25. E	53. D	81. A
100. B	26. B	54. B	82. D
	27. C	55. C	83. C
CLINICAL	28. B	56. D	84. C
1. B	29. C	57. E	85. B
2. A	30. A	58. C	86. E
3. D	31. A	59. B	87. D
4. B	32. C	60. D	88. C
5. C	33. D	61. B	89. B
6. A	34. B	62. C	90. E
7. D	35. C	63. D	91. C
8. E	36. B	64. D	92. D
9. C	37. D	65. B	93. E
10. B	38. C	66. D	94. B
11. E	39. D	67. A	95. A
12. C	40. E	68. E	96. C
13. B	41. B	69. B	97. D
14. D	42. D	70. B	98. C
15. A	43. A	71. C	99. D
16. E	44. E	72. E	100. C
17. C	45. A	73. B	
18. D	46. C	74. C	
19. B	47. D	75. D	

Pre-Test Simulation
(150-question, 2-hour test)

DIRECTIONS:
1. Fill in only one circle, using a number 2 pencil.
2. Keep all marks inside the circle.
3. Blacken the circle completely.
4. Completely erase any answer you wish to change, and make no stray marks.

Correct: Ⓐ Ⓑ ● Ⓓ Ⓔ   Wrong: Ⓐ Ⓑ Ⓒ Ⓓ Ⓔ

GENERAL

1. Ⓐ Ⓑ Ⓒ Ⓓ Ⓔ
2. Ⓐ Ⓑ Ⓒ Ⓓ Ⓔ
3. Ⓐ Ⓑ Ⓒ Ⓓ Ⓔ
4. Ⓐ Ⓑ Ⓒ Ⓓ Ⓔ
5. Ⓐ Ⓑ Ⓒ Ⓓ Ⓔ
6. Ⓐ Ⓑ Ⓒ Ⓓ Ⓔ
7. Ⓐ Ⓑ Ⓒ Ⓓ Ⓔ
8. Ⓐ Ⓑ Ⓒ Ⓓ Ⓔ
9. Ⓐ Ⓑ Ⓒ Ⓓ Ⓔ
10. Ⓐ Ⓑ Ⓒ Ⓓ Ⓔ
11. Ⓐ Ⓑ Ⓒ Ⓓ Ⓔ
12. Ⓐ Ⓑ Ⓒ Ⓓ Ⓔ
13. Ⓐ Ⓑ Ⓒ Ⓓ Ⓔ
14. Ⓐ Ⓑ Ⓒ Ⓓ Ⓔ
15. Ⓐ Ⓑ Ⓒ Ⓓ Ⓔ
16. Ⓐ Ⓑ Ⓒ Ⓓ Ⓔ
17. Ⓐ Ⓑ Ⓒ Ⓓ Ⓔ
18. Ⓐ Ⓑ Ⓒ Ⓓ Ⓔ
19. Ⓐ Ⓑ Ⓒ Ⓓ Ⓔ
20. Ⓐ Ⓑ Ⓒ Ⓓ Ⓔ
21. Ⓐ Ⓑ Ⓒ Ⓓ Ⓔ
22. Ⓐ Ⓑ Ⓒ Ⓓ Ⓔ
23. Ⓐ Ⓑ Ⓒ Ⓓ Ⓔ
24. Ⓐ Ⓑ Ⓒ Ⓓ Ⓔ
25. Ⓐ Ⓑ Ⓒ Ⓓ Ⓔ
26. Ⓐ Ⓑ Ⓒ Ⓓ Ⓔ
27. Ⓐ Ⓑ Ⓒ Ⓓ Ⓔ
28. Ⓐ Ⓑ Ⓒ Ⓓ Ⓔ
29. Ⓐ Ⓑ Ⓒ Ⓓ Ⓔ
30. Ⓐ Ⓑ Ⓒ Ⓓ Ⓔ
31. Ⓐ Ⓑ Ⓒ Ⓓ Ⓔ
32. Ⓐ Ⓑ Ⓒ Ⓓ Ⓔ
33. Ⓐ Ⓑ Ⓒ Ⓓ Ⓔ
34. Ⓐ Ⓑ Ⓒ Ⓓ Ⓔ
35. Ⓐ Ⓑ Ⓒ Ⓓ Ⓔ
36. Ⓐ Ⓑ Ⓒ Ⓓ Ⓔ
37. Ⓐ Ⓑ Ⓒ Ⓓ Ⓔ
38. Ⓐ Ⓑ Ⓒ Ⓓ Ⓔ
39. Ⓐ Ⓑ Ⓒ Ⓓ Ⓔ
40. Ⓐ Ⓑ Ⓒ Ⓓ Ⓔ
41. Ⓐ Ⓑ Ⓒ Ⓓ Ⓔ
42. Ⓐ Ⓑ Ⓒ Ⓓ Ⓔ
43. Ⓐ Ⓑ Ⓒ Ⓓ Ⓔ
44. Ⓐ Ⓑ Ⓒ Ⓓ Ⓔ
45. Ⓐ Ⓑ Ⓒ Ⓓ Ⓔ
46. Ⓐ Ⓑ Ⓒ Ⓓ Ⓔ
47. Ⓐ Ⓑ Ⓒ Ⓓ Ⓔ
48. Ⓐ Ⓑ Ⓒ Ⓓ Ⓔ
49. Ⓐ Ⓑ Ⓒ Ⓓ Ⓔ
50. Ⓐ Ⓑ Ⓒ Ⓓ Ⓔ

ADMINISTRATIVE

1. Ⓐ Ⓑ Ⓒ Ⓓ Ⓔ
2. Ⓐ Ⓑ Ⓒ Ⓓ Ⓔ
3. Ⓐ Ⓑ Ⓒ Ⓓ Ⓔ
4. Ⓐ Ⓑ Ⓒ Ⓓ Ⓔ
5. Ⓐ Ⓑ Ⓒ Ⓓ Ⓔ
6. Ⓐ Ⓑ Ⓒ Ⓓ Ⓔ
7. Ⓐ Ⓑ Ⓒ Ⓓ Ⓔ
8. Ⓐ Ⓑ Ⓒ Ⓓ Ⓔ
9. Ⓐ Ⓑ Ⓒ Ⓓ Ⓔ
10. Ⓐ Ⓑ Ⓒ Ⓓ Ⓔ
11. Ⓐ Ⓑ Ⓒ Ⓓ Ⓔ
12. Ⓐ Ⓑ Ⓒ Ⓓ Ⓔ
13. Ⓐ Ⓑ Ⓒ Ⓓ Ⓔ
14. Ⓐ Ⓑ Ⓒ Ⓓ Ⓔ
15. Ⓐ Ⓑ Ⓒ Ⓓ Ⓔ
16. Ⓐ Ⓑ Ⓒ Ⓓ Ⓔ
17. Ⓐ Ⓑ Ⓒ Ⓓ Ⓔ
18. Ⓐ Ⓑ Ⓒ Ⓓ Ⓔ
19. Ⓐ Ⓑ Ⓒ Ⓓ Ⓔ
20. Ⓐ Ⓑ Ⓒ Ⓓ Ⓔ
21. Ⓐ Ⓑ Ⓒ Ⓓ Ⓔ
22. Ⓐ Ⓑ Ⓒ Ⓓ Ⓔ
23. Ⓐ Ⓑ Ⓒ Ⓓ Ⓔ
24. Ⓐ Ⓑ Ⓒ Ⓓ Ⓔ
25. Ⓐ Ⓑ Ⓒ Ⓓ Ⓔ

CLINICAL

1. Ⓐ Ⓑ Ⓒ Ⓓ Ⓔ
2. Ⓐ Ⓑ Ⓒ Ⓓ Ⓔ
3. Ⓐ Ⓑ Ⓒ Ⓓ Ⓔ
4. Ⓐ Ⓑ Ⓒ Ⓓ Ⓔ
5. Ⓐ Ⓑ Ⓒ Ⓓ Ⓔ
6. Ⓐ Ⓑ Ⓒ Ⓓ Ⓔ
7. Ⓐ Ⓑ Ⓒ Ⓓ Ⓔ
8. Ⓐ Ⓑ Ⓒ Ⓓ Ⓔ
9. Ⓐ Ⓑ Ⓒ Ⓓ Ⓔ
10. Ⓐ Ⓑ Ⓒ Ⓓ Ⓔ
11. Ⓐ Ⓑ Ⓒ Ⓓ Ⓔ
12. Ⓐ Ⓑ Ⓒ Ⓓ Ⓔ
13. Ⓐ Ⓑ Ⓒ Ⓓ Ⓔ
14. Ⓐ Ⓑ Ⓒ Ⓓ Ⓔ
15. Ⓐ Ⓑ Ⓒ Ⓓ Ⓔ
16. Ⓐ Ⓑ Ⓒ Ⓓ Ⓔ
17. Ⓐ Ⓑ Ⓒ Ⓓ Ⓔ
18. Ⓐ Ⓑ Ⓒ Ⓓ Ⓔ
19. Ⓐ Ⓑ Ⓒ Ⓓ Ⓔ
20. Ⓐ Ⓑ Ⓒ Ⓓ Ⓔ
21. Ⓐ Ⓑ Ⓒ Ⓓ Ⓔ
22. Ⓐ Ⓑ Ⓒ Ⓓ Ⓔ
23. Ⓐ Ⓑ Ⓒ Ⓓ Ⓔ
24. Ⓐ Ⓑ Ⓒ Ⓓ Ⓔ
25. Ⓐ Ⓑ Ⓒ Ⓓ Ⓔ
26. Ⓐ Ⓑ Ⓒ Ⓓ Ⓔ
27. Ⓐ Ⓑ Ⓒ Ⓓ Ⓔ
28. Ⓐ Ⓑ Ⓒ Ⓓ Ⓔ
29. Ⓐ Ⓑ Ⓒ Ⓓ Ⓔ
30. Ⓐ Ⓑ Ⓒ Ⓓ Ⓔ
31. Ⓐ Ⓑ Ⓒ Ⓓ Ⓔ
32. Ⓐ Ⓑ Ⓒ Ⓓ Ⓔ
33. Ⓐ Ⓑ Ⓒ Ⓓ Ⓔ
34. Ⓐ Ⓑ Ⓒ Ⓓ Ⓔ
35. Ⓐ Ⓑ Ⓒ Ⓓ Ⓔ
36. Ⓐ Ⓑ Ⓒ Ⓓ Ⓔ
37. Ⓐ Ⓑ Ⓒ Ⓓ Ⓔ
38. Ⓐ Ⓑ Ⓒ Ⓓ Ⓔ
39. Ⓐ Ⓑ Ⓒ Ⓓ Ⓔ
40. Ⓐ Ⓑ Ⓒ Ⓓ Ⓔ
41. Ⓐ Ⓑ Ⓒ Ⓓ Ⓔ
42. Ⓐ Ⓑ Ⓒ Ⓓ Ⓔ
43. Ⓐ Ⓑ Ⓒ Ⓓ Ⓔ
44. Ⓐ Ⓑ Ⓒ Ⓓ Ⓔ
45. Ⓐ Ⓑ Ⓒ Ⓓ Ⓔ
46. Ⓐ Ⓑ Ⓒ Ⓓ Ⓔ
47. Ⓐ Ⓑ Ⓒ Ⓓ Ⓔ
48. Ⓐ Ⓑ Ⓒ Ⓓ Ⓔ
49. Ⓐ Ⓑ Ⓒ Ⓓ Ⓔ
50. Ⓐ Ⓑ Ⓒ Ⓓ Ⓔ

(Additional columns of answer bubbles numbered 13–50 continue across the sheet.)

Post-Test Simulation
(300-question, 4-hour test)

DIRECTIONS:
1. Fill in only one circle, using a number 2 pencil.
2. Keep all marks inside the circle.
3. Blacken the circle completely.
4. Completely erase any answer you wish to change, and make no stray marks.

Correct: (A) (B) ● (D) (E)   Wrong: (Ⓐ) (Ⓑ) (Ⓧ) (Ⓓ) (Ⓔ)

GENERAL

1. (A) (B) (C) (D) (E)
2. (A) (B) (C) (D) (E)
3. (A) (B) (C) (D) (E)
4. (A) (B) (C) (D) (E)
5. (A) (B) (C) (D) (E)
6. (A) (B) (C) (D) (E)
7. (A) (B) (C) (D) (E)
8. (A) (B) (C) (D) (E)
9. (A) (B) (C) (D) (E)
10. (A) (B) (C) (D) (E)
11. (A) (B) (C) (D) (E)
12. (A) (B) (C) (D) (E)
13. (A) (B) (C) (D) (E)
14. (A) (B) (C) (D) (E)
15. (A) (B) (C) (D) (E)
16. (A) (B) (C) (D) (E)
17. (A) (B) (C) (D) (E)
18. (A) (B) (C) (D) (E)
19. (A) (B) (C) (D) (E)
20. (A) (B) (C) (D) (E)
21. (A) (B) (C) (D) (E)
22. (A) (B) (C) (D) (E)
23. (A) (B) (C) (D) (E)
24. (A) (B) (C) (D) (E)
25. (A) (B) (C) (D) (E)
26. (A) (B) (C) (D) (E)
27. (A) (B) (C) (D) (E)
28. (A) (B) (C) (D) (E)
29. (A) (B) (C) (D) (E)
30. (A) (B) (C) (D) (E)
31. (A) (B) (C) (D) (E)
32. (A) (B) (C) (D) (E)
33. (A) (B) (C) (D) (E)
34. (A) (B) (C) (D) (E)
35. (A) (B) (C) (D) (E)
36. (A) (B) (C) (D) (E)
37. (A) (B) (C) (D) (E)
38. (A) (B) (C) (D) (E)

39. (A) (B) (C) (D) (E)
40. (A) (B) (C) (D) (E)
41. (A) (B) (C) (D) (E)
42. (A) (B) (C) (D) (E)
43. (A) (B) (C) (D) (E)
44. (A) (B) (C) (D) (E)
45. (A) (B) (C) (D) (E)
46. (A) (B) (C) (D) (E)
47. (A) (B) (C) (D) (E)
48. (A) (B) (C) (D) (E)
49. (A) (B) (C) (D) (E)
50. (A) (B) (C) (D) (E)
51. (A) (B) (C) (D) (E)
52. (A) (B) (C) (D) (E)
53. (A) (B) (C) (D) (E)
54. (A) (B) (C) (D) (E)
55. (A) (B) (C) (D) (E)
56. (A) (B) (C) (D) (E)
57. (A) (B) (C) (D) (E)
58. (A) (B) (C) (D) (E)
59. (A) (B) (C) (D) (E)
60. (A) (B) (C) (D) (E)
61. (A) (B) (C) (D) (E)
62. (A) (B) (C) (D) (E)
63. (A) (B) (C) (D) (E)
64. (A) (B) (C) (D) (E)
65. (A) (B) (C) (D) (E)
66. (A) (B) (C) (D) (E)
67. (A) (B) (C) (D) (E)
68. (A) (B) (C) (D) (E)
69. (A) (B) (C) (D) (E)
70. (A) (B) (C) (D) (E)
71. (A) (B) (C) (D) (E)
72. (A) (B) (C) (D) (E)
73. (A) (B) (C) (D) (E)
74. (A) (B) (C) (D) (E)
75. (A) (B) (C) (D) (E)
76. (A) (B) (C) (D) (E)
77. (A) (B) (C) (D) (E)

78. (A) (B) (C) (D) (E)
79. (A) (B) (C) (D) (E)
80. (A) (B) (C) (D) (E)
81. (A) (B) (C) (D) (E)
82. (A) (B) (C) (D) (E)
83. (A) (B) (C) (D) (E)
84. (A) (B) (C) (D) (E)
85. (A) (B) (C) (D) (E)
86. (A) (B) (C) (D) (E)
87. (A) (B) (C) (D) (E)
88. (A) (B) (C) (D) (E)
89. (A) (B) (C) (D) (E)
90. (A) (B) (C) (D) (E)
91. (A) (B) (C) (D) (E)
92. (A) (B) (C) (D) (E)
93. (A) (B) (C) (D) (E)
94. (A) (B) (C) (D) (E)
95. (A) (B) (C) (D) (E)
96. (A) (B) (C) (D) (E)
97. (A) (B) (C) (D) (E)
98. (A) (B) (C) (D) (E)
99. (A) (B) (C) (D) (E)
100. (A) (B) (C) (D) (E)

ADMINISTRATIVE

1. (A) (B) (C) (D) (E)
2. (A) (B) (C) (D) (E)
3. (A) (B) (C) (D) (E)
4. (A) (B) (C) (D) (E)
5. (A) (B) (C) (D) (E)
6. (A) (B) (C) (D) (E)
7. (A) (B) (C) (D) (E)
8. (A) (B) (C) (D) (E)
9. (A) (B) (C) (D) (E)
10. (A) (B) (C) (D) (E)
11. (A) (B) (C) (D) (E)
12. (A) (B) (C) (D) (E)
13. (A) (B) (C) (D) (E)
14. (A) (B) (C) (D) (E)

15. (A) (B) (C) (D) (E)
16. (A) (B) (C) (D) (E)
17. (A) (B) (C) (D) (E)
18. (A) (B) (C) (D) (E)
19. (A) (B) (C) (D) (E)
20. (A) (B) (C) (D) (E)
21. (A) (B) (C) (D) (E)
22. (A) (B) (C) (D) (E)
23. (A) (B) (C) (D) (E)
24. (A) (B) (C) (D) (E)
25. (A) (B) (C) (D) (E)
26. (A) (B) (C) (D) (E)
27. (A) (B) (C) (D) (E)
28. (A) (B) (C) (D) (E)
29. (A) (B) (C) (D) (E)
30. (A) (B) (C) (D) (E)
31. (A) (B) (C) (D) (E)
32. (A) (B) (C) (D) (E)
33. (A) (B) (C) (D) (E)
34. (A) (B) (C) (D) (E)
35. (A) (B) (C) (D) (E)
36. (A) (B) (C) (D) (E)
37. (A) (B) (C) (D) (E)
38. (A) (B) (C) (D) (E)
39. (A) (B) (C) (D) (E)
40. (A) (B) (C) (D) (E)
41. (A) (B) (C) (D) (E)
42. (A) (B) (C) (D) (E)
43. (A) (B) (C) (D) (E)
44. (A) (B) (C) (D) (E)
45. (A) (B) (C) (D) (E)
46. (A) (B) (C) (D) (E)
47. (A) (B) (C) (D) (E)
48. (A) (B) (C) (D) (E)
49. (A) (B) (C) (D) (E)
50. (A) (B) (C) (D) (E)
51. (A) (B) (C) (D) (E)
52. (A) (B) (C) (D) (E)
53. (A) (B) (C) (D) (E)

54	(A) (B) (C) (D) (E)	92	(A) (B) (C) (D) (E)	27	(A) (B) (C) (D) (E)	65	(A) (B) (C) (D) (E)
55	(A) (B) (C) (D) (E)	93	(A) (B) (C) (D) (E)	28	(A) (B) (C) (D) (E)	66	(A) (B) (C) (D) (E)
56	(A) (B) (C) (D) (E)	94	(A) (B) (C) (D) (E)	29	(A) (B) (C) (D) (E)	67	(A) (B) (C) (D) (E)
57	(A) (B) (C) (D) (E)	95	(A) (B) (C) (D) (E)	30	(A) (B) (C) (D) (E)	68	(A) (B) (C) (D) (E)
58	(A) (B) (C) (D) (E)	96	(A) (B) (C) (D) (E)	31	(A) (B) (C) (D) (E)	69	(A) (B) (C) (D) (E)
59	(A) (B) (C) (D) (E)	97	(A) (B) (C) (D) (E)	32	(A) (B) (C) (D) (E)	70	(A) (B) (C) (D) (E)
60	(A) (B) (C) (D) (E)	98	(A) (B) (C) (D) (E)	33	(A) (B) (C) (D) (E)	71	(A) (B) (C) (D) (E)
61	(A) (B) (C) (D) (E)	99	(A) (B) (C) (D) (E)	34	(A) (B) (C) (D) (E)	72	(A) (B) (C) (D) (E)
62	(A) (B) (C) (D) (E)	100	(A) (B) (C) (D) (E)	35	(A) (B) (C) (D) (E)	73	(A) (B) (C) (D) (E)
63	(A) (B) (C) (D) (E)			36	(A) (B) (C) (D) (E)	74	(A) (B) (C) (D) (E)
64	(A) (B) (C) (D) (E)	**CLINICAL**		37	(A) (B) (C) (D) (E)	75	(A) (B) (C) (D) (E)
65	(A) (B) (C) (D) (E)	1	(A) (B) (C) (D) (E)	38	(A) (B) (C) (D) (E)	76	(A) (B) (C) (D) (E)
66	(A) (B) (C) (D) (E)	2	(A) (B) (C) (D) (E)	39	(A) (B) (C) (D) (E)	77	(A) (B) (C) (D) (E)
67	(A) (B) (C) (D) (E)	3	(A) (B) (C) (D) (E)	40	(A) (B) (C) (D) (E)	78	(A) (B) (C) (D) (E)
68	(A) (B) (C) (D) (E)	4	(A) (B) (C) (D) (E)	41	(A) (B) (C) (D) (E)	79	(A) (B) (C) (D) (E)
69	(A) (B) (C) (D) (E)	5	(A) (B) (C) (D) (E)	42	(A) (B) (C) (D) (E)	80	(A) (B) (C) (D) (E)
70	(A) (B) (C) (D) (E)	6	(A) (B) (C) (D) (E)	43	(A) (B) (C) (D) (E)	81	(A) (B) (C) (D) (E)
71	(A) (B) (C) (D) (E)	7	(A) (B) (C) (D) (E)	44	(A) (B) (C) (D) (E)	82	(A) (B) (C) (D) (E)
72	(A) (B) (C) (D) (E)	8	(A) (B) (C) (D) (E)	45	(A) (B) (C) (D) (E)	83	(A) (B) (C) (D) (E)
73	(A) (B) (C) (D) (E)	9	(A) (B) (C) (D) (E)	46	(A) (B) (C) (D) (E)	84	(A) (B) (C) (D) (E)
74	(A) (B) (C) (D) (E)	10	(A) (B) (C) (D) (E)	47	(A) (B) (C) (D) (E)	85	(A) (B) (C) (D) (E)
75	(A) (B) (C) (D) (E)	11	(A) (B) (C) (D) (E)	48	(A) (B) (C) (D) (E)	86	(A) (B) (C) (D) (E)
76	(A) (B) (C) (D) (E)	12	(A) (B) (C) (D) (E)	49	(A) (B) (C) (D) (E)	87	(A) (B) (C) (D) (E)
77	(A) (B) (C) (D) (E)	13	(A) (B) (C) (D) (E)	50	(A) (B) (C) (D) (E)	88	(A) (B) (C) (D) (E)
78	(A) (B) (C) (D) (E)	14	(A) (B) (C) (D) (E)	51	(A) (B) (C) (D) (E)	89	(A) (B) (C) (D) (E)
79	(A) (B) (C) (D) (E)	15	(A) (B) (C) (D) (E)	52	(A) (B) (C) (D) (E)	90	(A) (B) (C) (D) (E)
80	(A) (B) (C) (D) (E)	16	(A) (B) (C) (D) (E)	53	(A) (B) (C) (D) (E)	91	(A) (B) (C) (D) (E)
81	(A) (B) (C) (D) (E)	17	(A) (B) (C) (D) (E)	54	(A) (B) (C) (D) (E)	92	(A) (B) (C) (D) (E)
82	(A) (B) (C) (D) (E)	18	(A) (B) (C) (D) (E)	55	(A) (B) (C) (D) (E)	93	(A) (B) (C) (D) (E)
83	(A) (B) (C) (D) (E)	19	(A) (B) (C) (D) (E)	56	(A) (B) (C) (D) (E)	94	(A) (B) (C) (D) (E)
84	(A) (B) (C) (D) (E)	20	(A) (B) (C) (D) (E)	57	(A) (B) (C) (D) (E)	95	(A) (B) (C) (D) (E)
85	(A) (B) (C) (D) (E)	21	(A) (B) (C) (D) (E)	58	(A) (B) (C) (D) (E)	96	(A) (B) (C) (D) (E)
86	(A) (B) (C) (D) (E)	22	(A) (B) (C) (D) (E)	59	(A) (B) (C) (D) (E)	97	(A) (B) (C) (D) (E)
87	(A) (B) (C) (D) (E)	23	(A) (B) (C) (D) (E)	60	(A) (B) (C) (D) (E)	98	(A) (B) (C) (D) (E)
88	(A) (B) (C) (D) (E)	24	(A) (B) (C) (D) (E)	61	(A) (B) (C) (D) (E)	99	(A) (B) (C) (D) (E)
89	(A) (B) (C) (D) (E)	25	(A) (B) (C) (D) (E)	62	(A) (B) (C) (D) (E)	100	(A) (B) (C) (D) (E)
90	(A) (B) (C) (D) (E)	26	(A) (B) (C) (D) (E)	63	(A) (B) (C) (D) (E)		
91	(A) (B) (C) (D) (E)			64	(A) (B) (C) (D) (E)		

SOFTWARE INSTRUCTIONS

Instructions for Installing Software to Accompany *Medical Assistant Exam Review Programmed Learner* by Fremgen, Wallington, and King

Introduction

This software consists of a quiz player and quiz files. The quiz player file is the executable file that is used to read and take the quizzes. The quiz files contain the review questions. The quizzes correspond to chapters in *Essentials of Medical Assisting*, by Bonnie Fremgen. The table at the end of this document lists each file by name and the chapter each file represents. There is also a cumulative review consisting of 100 questions taken from all chapters.

    This software is distributed on three 3.5" diskettes. Two diskettes contain the player software and one diskette contains the quiz files. It is designed to be installed on a hard disk. For ease of use we recommend installing the quiz player and the quiz files in the same subdirectory.

System Requirements

- 486 processor or better
- Windows 3.1 or later
- 8 megabytes of RAM
- 4 megabytes hard disk space
- Color monitor and video card set to display 256 colors

Installing Quiz Player and Quiz Files

1. Start your PC and launch Windows.
2. Insert the diskette labeled "Windows 3.1 Quiz Player" and "Disk 1 of 2" into your computer's diskette drive.
3. In Windows 3.1, launch Program Manager and choose "Run" from the File menu. In Windows 95, click on the Start menu and choose "Run."
4. In the Command Line box, type "a:setup" or "b:setup" depending on whether your diskette drive is designated as drive "A" or drive "B."
5. Click "OK."
6. Follow the instructions displayed on your screen.
7. When the installation is complete, remove the quiz player diskettes and store them in a safe place.
8. Insert the diskette labeled "Quiz Files" into your computer's diskette drive.

9. Using File Manager (Windows 3.1) or Windows Explorer (Windows 95) copy the quiz files into the directory where the quiz player has been installed. The quiz files have a ".QFT" extension.

Launching Quiz Player and Playing the Sample Quiz

1. Using File Manager (Windows 3.1) or Windows Explorer (Windows 95) locate the icon for the quiz player. It will be called "Quiz Factory Player." Double-click on the icon to launch the player.
2. Click "Open File."
3. Select "SAMPLE.QFT" from the dialog box and press "OK."
4. Click "NEW" for a new player.
5. Type in your name and other information.
6. Click on messages to read them.
7. Click "Test" to begin sample test.
8. Click "Quit" to exit the quiz player.

Launching Quiz Player and Taking a Quiz

1. Using File Manager (Windows 3.1) or Windows Explorer (Windows 95) locate the icon for the quiz player. It will be called "Quiz Factory Player." Double-click on the icon to launch the player.
2. Click "Open File."
3. Select "CHAP01.QFT" from the dialog box and press "OK."
4. Click "NEW" for a new player.
5. Type in your name.
6. Click "Test" to begin quiz.
7. When you finish the quiz you can check your results, review the questions you answered correctly, and review the questions you answered incorrectly. As you review the questions you answered incorrectly Quiz Factory Player can show you the correct answer. Click on the "Show Correct" button to see which answer is correct.
8. The quizzes in this package have been set up to allow you to quit in mid-quiz and resume later. You also can take the same quiz again at a later time. The program erases your previous score for that quiz if you take the quiz again.
9. Click "Quit" to exit the quiz player.

Technical Support

If you are having problems with the software, call (201)236-3477 between 9:00 a.m. and 4:30 p.m. EST, Monday through Friday. You can also send a message to tech_support@prenhall.com.

Our technical support staff will need to know certain things about your system in order to help us solve your problems more quickly and efficiently. If possible, please be at your computer when you call for support. You should have the following information ready:

- product title and product ISBN
- computer make and model
- CD-ROM drive make and model
- RAM available
- hard disk space available
- graphics card type
- sound card type
- printer make and model
- network connection
- detailed description of the problem, including the exact wording of any error messages.

About The Software

The quizzes in this package have been developed using Quiz Factory. Quiz Factory is a trademark of LearningWare, Inc.

Windows is a registered trademark of Microsoft Corporation.

Known Errors

Occasionally the first multiple-choice question in a quiz will have one answer choice that appears to be highlighted, as if the correct answer were preselected. However, the check box will not be checked, indicating that an answer still must be selected. You still must select the correct answer by clicking in the answer area. There is nothing wrong with your system and this error does not affect the operation of the software in any other way.

List of Files

The following table lists the files on the Question Files diskette and identifies the corresponding chapter in *Essentials of Medical Assisting*.

File name	Chapter	Chapter title
chap01.qft	Chapter 1	Medical Assisting: The Profession
chap02.qft	Chapter 2	Medical Science: History and Practice
chap03.qft	Chapter 3	Health Care Environment
chap04.qft	Chapter 4	Medical Ethics
chap05.qft	Chapter 5	Medicine and the Law
chap06.qft	Chapter 6	Quality Assurance and the Medical Assistant
chap07.qft	Chapter 7	Communication: Verbal and Nonverbal
chap08.qft	Chapter 8	Patient Reception
chap09.qft	Chapter 9	Appointment Scheduling
chap10.qft	Chapter 10	Office Safety, Facilities, and Equipment
chap11.qft	Chapter 11	Written Communication
chap12.qft	Chapter 12	Computers in Medicine

File name	Chapter	Chapter title
chap13.qft	Chapter 13	Medical Records and Transcription
chap14.qft	Chapter 14	Fees, Billing, Collections, and Credit
chap15.qft	Chapter 15	Financial Management
chap16.qft	Chapter 16	Banking Procedures
chap17.qft	Chapter 17	Insurance
chap18.qft	Chapter 18	Office Management
chap19.qft	Chapter 19	Infection Control: Asepsis
chap20.qft	Chapter 20	Vital Signs and Measurements
chap21.qft	Chapter 21	Assisting with Physical Examinations
chap22.qft	Chapter 22	Assisting with Medical Specialties
chap23.qft	Chapter 23	Assisting with Minor Surgery
chap24.qft	Chapter 24	Patients with Special Physical and Emotional Needs
chap25.qft	Chapter 25	Microbiology
chap26.qft	Chapter 26	Urinalysis
chap27.qft	Chapter 27	Hematology
chap28.qft	Chapter 28	Radiology
chap29.qft	Chapter 29	Electrocardiography and Pulmonary Function
chap30.qft	Chapter 30	Physical Therapy and Rehabilitation
chap31.qft	Chapter 31	Pharmacology
chap32.qft	Chapter 32	Administering Medications
chap33.qft	Chapter 33	Patient Education and Nutrition
chap34.qft	Chapter 34	Emergency First Aid
chap35.qft	Chapter 35	Externship and Career Opportunities
chap36.qft		Anatomy, Physiology, and Medical Terminology*
review.qft		Cumulative review
readme.txt		This document

*Note: This is not a numbered chapter in the textbook, *Essentials of Medical Assisting*. Anatomy and physiology are covered in an appendix in the textbook.

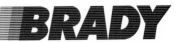

Medical Assistant
Test Review
Programmed
Learner

–

Bonnie Fremgen, PhD
Kathleen Wallington, CMA
Mary King-Lesniewski, CMA

Thank you for purchasing this book. We at Brady/Prentice Hall wish you well in your career as a Medical Assistant.

This bookmark can be used to cover the correct answers and explanations as you answer the review questions.

BRADY
Prentice Hall
Upper Saddle River, New Jersey 07458